CRACKING THE
OBESITY CRISIS

Veronica M. McNally

authorHOUSE®

AuthorHouse™ UK
1663 Liberty Drive
Bloomington, IN 47403 USA
www.authorhouse.co.uk
Phone: 0800.197.4150

Published by AuthorHouse 03/16/2017

ISBN: 978-1-5246-3717-0 (sc)
ISBN: 978-1-5246-6200-4 (hc)
ISBN: 978-1-5246-6199-1 (e)

Print information available on the last page.

Any people depicted in stock imagery provided by Thinkstock are models,
and such images are being used for illustrative purposes only.
Certain stock imagery © Thinkstock.

This book is printed on acid-free paper.

I wish to thank my daughter Maeve for drawing the art on the front cover of the book and also the hard work of Aiden and Richard in the creation of this book.

INTRODUCTION

Very few people would think that defending our borders, in short out national security has anything to do with the food we eat, but a logical link can be made. The British Government said that you are allowed to use the word "fat" since 2012.

Fat people are basically insecure, unhappy people trapped inside very unattractive bodies and discrimination is emerging, in Britain including in some chain stores where unless you are over a size 12, clothing is not available for purchase.

The disadvantage associated with fat people is if we ever had to defend our borders, for example from the Islamic State, that because of their body mass, a fat person male or female could not hold a machine gun effectively as the fat on their bodies would put them in an awkward position holding a machine gun, although some fat people may qualify to hold a revolver, if necessary, if we need to defend these it would be very difficult to find enough ground forces.

The psychology of fat people is even if they are five stone overweight they will say "I'm not the worst, there is worse out there than me." They are trying to lead fashion to make slim people feel "Out of fashion", no longer in vogue.

The Islamic people however are at an advantage as they do Ramadan and they are not overweight. A leader has not yet emerged to organise an attack on their isles amongst the Islamic State, but that does not mean it is not possible.

Slim men and women in the UK and Ireland need to remain on "High alert" in case we need to defend ourselves and our country. Most fat people would say "Let's eat, drink and be merry for tomorrow we may die", or as people sang during the Black Death in Europe in the 1400's when they were dying:

"Ring a ring a rosies,
A pocket full of posies,
A tischo, a tischo,
We all fall down."

As a nutritional consultant, with my highest qualification being a Bachelor of Science, I wish to present my research, as a user of medication to treat bi-polar disorder, gained three stone because prescribed medication, but losing the weight be stopping a tablet called "Depakote", and suffered the pain of allowing my stomach to shrink naturally. I have been a stable 9 stone for several years as I was before I took this tablet.

I think there is hope for overweight and obese people, but I don't see a way back for the clinically aid morbidly obese.

I wish to share my research and findings with others.

"But you must suffer the pain of letting your stomach shrink naturally by fasting – no gain without pain, if you are truly patriotic."

Smoking a cigarette is not as dangerous as letting our islands being overrun by the Islamic State because some of us are overweight and unfit.

It's too risky to wait for the obesity crisis to resolve itself naturally. If we wish to defend our borders against an invasion from the Islamic state while the British are sitting up overeating. But at least we can depend on a few fit and slim women to be successful in the British

Army and the Royal Navy as there is currently a shortage of men as many are too fat to fight.

If there is a war at any time in the future, women may not be suited to actually be on the front line, but as women's hands are smooth and soft in many cases, females would be useful behind soldiers to be there as assistants to men quickly reloading magazines of bullets speedily, making it easier to allow male soldiers to keep shooting the enemy, if and when that day comes. But in the meantime, those with a conscience and who are patriotic need to keep ourselves slim and fit in Britain and Ireland instead of being too fat to fight.

The research which I wish to present to the general public is hopefully of interest to others so that they can take responsibility for their own health in some situations. Nutrition does not have the answer to all ailments but it does help with certain conditions and give us strength to live to see another day.

Overweight and obese people certainly are a threat to National Security. The reason is, who is going to know the difference in a fat terrorist or a slim terrorist, strapped with explosives around their body covered by a jacket? Is it a very difficult dilemma for security in the UK and Ireland as they have not yet hit us. It would be easier for Ireland, North and South, to detect possible suicide bombers, as there are not many Muslim men in this country, and they could be frisked at airports and coming off boats entering Northern Ireland, The Republic of Ireland and Scotland. It is much more of a nightmare in England as there are so many Muslim men in the country already which makes it much more difficult to identify possible suicide bombers.

This research does have an underlying religious theme as it is educational, not just about diet, but most especially about those who are eating too much, as gluttony is one of the seven deadly sins. For some people, food is simply an addiction but otherwise they are good people.

Religion is important as a means of moral guidance, but in the past and in the present religious differences can cause wars or potential wars, certainly a lot of conflict between people down through the ages.

In the spiritual world it is Jesus Christ up against Mohammad. But Christians need to be confident and not have too much anxiety as good always wins over evil. Christians just need to keep vigilant, try to keep slim and fit in order to defend our borders.

On Tuesday 15th March 2016 The Chancellor of the Exchequer made a very clever move by increasing tax on the cheapest but most dangerous substance available in Britain, commonly known as cane sugar or sucrose to try and save the Health of the Nation.

Nutrition scientifically is defined as:

"The science of the substances to sustain health, promote energy for living. It also refers to eating the right foods in the proper amounts and excluding edible substances not needed".

(1982 Fundamentals of General, Organic and Biological Chemistry. Holum John. R.)

A POTENTIAL CATASTROPHE

Until 14th July 2016 with the atrocious attack on hundreds of innocent people in Nice, France – a potential war seemed maybe unrealistic to some people. But, with our new Prime Minister Theresa May, the English politicians are feeling very defensive and are admitting to the House of Commons that the terrorists have weapons of mass destruction, capable of killing more people than the nuclear bomb dropped on Hiroshima in 1945 which killed 140,000 people, but yet there is a feeling of compassion for innocent Muslims who do not agree with the behaviour of ISIS as they are saying it is not a true representation of the Islamic religion.

There could be hard times ahead for a lot of people. The issue about the health of the nation is not being addressed to the House of Commons at all these days. It is very low on the agenda of our new Prime Minister Theresa May. This could possibly be because she knows that there are many people beyond help as they are so obese, and the trend is set to continue of thousands dying in hospitals today in Britain. It would be scary going into hospital in Britain today as there is a good chance you could be leaving the hospital in a 'Wooden Coat".

If we are facing hard times in the context of another war, it is important for people in Britain to keep themselves in a fit and healthy condition. The reason is illustrated in the 19th Century by Sir Charles Darwin with his theory of Natural Selection, and survival of the fittest. In other words, if you have obesity and complications never mind any other sort of illness, the chances of surviving this potential catastrophe are better if you are healthy and fit in order to survive hard times ahead.

It is difficult for the British Health Secretary, Mr Jeremy Hunt because of the fact that the Health of the Nation is so impossible to cure with 52% of the nation on monthly prescriptions and an eight hour queue to speak to an out of hours doctor. Patients going home Accident & Emergency wards because they were too ill to wait to see a doctor, and no apparent breakthrough with one of the Western World's greatest enemies – cancer. Should scientists turn to investigate food science? Until the 20th Century, there was no tinned, packet or processed foods produced and cancer was not a big issue.

Brilliant discoveries are currently being made in laboratories, probably around Oxford and Cambridge Universities that "Yes" there is links to be made between diet and conquering cancer, which is wonderful news. It is best to know as much as you can about food in order to avoid this plague which we are suffering in the 21st century and become slim and healthy as well. Its typical of the English to make great scientific breakthroughs.

A CASE STUDY

My son Joseph aged 22 is a graduate in History from Queen's University, Belfast and is not entering his final year in an M.A. in Law in University College, Dublin. He has always been fit and well and he is his ideal weight for his height. He is an athlete and plays Gaelic football and hurling (An Irish version of ice hockey). He will not eat anything from a tin, not even a tin of baked beans. He has never had any medical complications only for glandular fever when he was a teenager which he recovered from.

This is partly my influence as I gave him fresh food from babyhood. His older sister Maeve doesn't follow such a strict dietary regime, but she is a keen cook and eats mostly healthy foods as she was educated to eat from a baby too – by me. Thank God both of my children are physically healthy and well. So far – so good.

Why Diet?

There are many slimming weight loss programmes on the market but very few come down to good honest home cooking.

The recipe portfolio includes many meals which can be cooked at home ranging from a simple family lunch to a three course à la carte menu. One missing utensil used in most kitchens is absent, the deep fat fryer.

Diet isn't just about diet foods; it is about developing a whole new relationship with food. It is not just that we eat but about what we eat. A portion means a portion. If it says serve 4, then you should eat quarter portions at a time. It would be impossible to lose weight even without using the deep fat fryer and substituting it with extra-virgin olive oil, unless we eat small average portions, not easy to be done with these delicious recipes. Extra portions for a single person can be refrigerated in small containers or put into the freezer.

Clients will be advised by their GP about their ideal weight range for their height which should fall within their Body Mass Index.

Before commencing a weight reduction diet, clients should consult their GP about their target weight. Clients should consult their GP if they have insulin or non-insulin dependent diabetes, crohn's disease or any other type of bowel disorder, diverticular disease, ulcerative colitis, coeliac disease or bowel cancer.

Free foods are listed which can help not only to provide valuable vitamins and minerals but also to help ease the feeling of hunger in the form of fruit and vegetables.

The calories used in various exercise is listed indicating how much exercise is needed to lose weight and stay healthy.

According to the profession of Human Nutrition and Dietetics, I as a Nutritional Consultant, a healthy diet is low in saturated fat, low in sugar, low in salt and high in fibre in accordance with the NACNE Report 1983, National Advisory Council for Nutritional Education.

Unfortunately this portfolio of recipes does nothing to help the obese and clinically obese. Unless they are prepared to turn around, give up junk food, tolerate hunger pains, eat lots of fresh fruits and vegetables and start eating healthy options, they are literally past the point of rescue and are eating themselves into an early grave.

With the Government and the whole of the British Isles under severe economic crisis, the money to is just not available to do major surgery on obese and clinically obese people, putting a gastric band around their stomach and removing large quantities of fat surgically from the human body. It can be done but it is such a huge burden on a Government trying to deal with rising unemployment this strategy is not commercially viable.

While trying to lose weight, sugary desserts are best avoided except for a special dinner party. Alcohol used in cooking is not counted as being of calorific value as during cooking alcohol evaporates at 78 degrees centigrade and all that is left is the taste of alcohol.

The achieve the optimum health The Royal College of Physicians again recommend a diet low in fat, sugar, salt and high in fibre. No more than 10 cigarettes a day, no more than 14 units of alcohol per week for women, i.e. 10 glasses of wine, spirits or glasses of beer and 21 units of alcohol per week for a man, i.e. 10.5 units or 21 units of spirits.

Recipes which are considered a healthy option can be incorporated into a client's daily calorie intake making healthy eating actually pleasant and fun for all the family and presentation can be left to the cook's imagination as often seen on television programmes.

The unfortunate thing about health and disease is that in health and social care, there are plenty of social workers "on the ground" but a severe lack of dieticians in the community and health promoters "on the ground", and the real honest true information about what is a healthy diet and a healthy lifestyle is withheld from the general public.

In most cases nobody sees a dietician until they are practically on their death bed.

It is often too late when are in the cardiovascular ward, having survived a myocardial infarction (heart attack), knowing a more severe heart attack or stroke is likely to come along.

It is often too late when you have become clinically obese to reverse the situation especially by yourself without professional help.

With three years training as a dietician behind me a diploma in Nutrition, a certificate in Health Promotion and a certificate in Health & Social Care as well as an overall Bachelor of Science, I am trying to help people gain knowledge they may not be able to get from health professionals.

In the field of Health Promotion they talk about Health Education, Health Protection, Health Promotion but very little of this filters through to the general public, only for an occasional poster on a bus or in a doctor's surgery.

In the field of Health Promotion they see health as an iconic state rarely achieved in real life.

According to The World Health Organisation 1945

"Health is a state of physical, mental and social wellbeing with the absence of disease and infirmity."

This is the idealistic dream health professionals have had since the end of World War II, but mainly because of what people are taking into their bodies, this iconic dream seems further and further away from becoming true.

A buzz word in the Health Promotion profession is "empowerment". In an indirect way I am hoping to empower the community into turning to healthier eating habits.

The information about vitamins and minerals is not widely known by the general public. It is known to doctors, pharmacists, dieticians and perhaps home economics teachers but the rest of it is kept to the archives of Universities, and little true facts filter through to the general public.

If people really want to achieve optimum health it is time to forget fad-diets and take a brave step. Recycle the deep fat fryer and buy a food blender. I did it ten years ago and I have no regrets. We don't just need to consider ourselves, we need to consider our children's health and weight as they are the next generation. I don't just advertise these recipes I cook them all the time. Some of them may look expensive but it is cheaper to cook at home than to buy out of a chip shop.

It is not a cardinal sin to eat chips occasionally in a restaurant or café. Neither is it unhealthy to eat a Chinese or Indian meal in a restaurant or take away occasionally. It is just best to avoid fast food takeaways in general as much as possible, moderation being the operative word in food consumption.

This diet plan consists of a weight loss programme combined with exercise to help people become within their ideal weight range. It is a calorie controlled diet to try and achieve and maintain correct weight for height and age group. As you get older you are expected to gain a bit of weight, so you cannot expect to be the same weight as you were at the age of 18.

This diet obviously contains a lot of fruits and vegetables. This is designed to create bulk in the diet and fight the hunger pains.

This diet does not have to be adhered to religiously. There is room for manoeuvre. Meal times can be switched about. Meals can be omitted or changed around to suit oneself. It is just a blueprint of what is achievable on a calorie controlled diet. But meals cannot be increased or weight loss will never be achieved.

Alcohol cannot be taken on this diet unless a lot of meals are omitted, not advisable as in most cases, alcohol contains empty calories.

When target weight is achieved, a range of recipes are included which are low enough in saturated fat, sugar, etc. which will help maintain a healthy diet. But do not disregard the calorie controlled diet once weight loss begins.

Nobody can take it away from the British. They are good cooks. A lot of these recipes are historically British. They are not my recipes. I am not a chef, although I have a keen interest in cooking. But a lot of these recipes what were served amongst Royalty and The Aristocrats in the past. A lot of them would have been brought to Britain by William the Conqueror in 1066 and have gradually filtered into society.

Today's middle class society in this recession would probably not be able to afford to eat such exquisite cuisine in Restaurants and Hotels but they could afford to cook it at home.

With a mixture of international cuisine, hopefully a lot of people will find these recipes healthy, affordable, and interesting to cook and eat at home.

With a more holistic approach to the obesity crisis, involving not only losing weight to become within acceptable limits i.e. a size 8-16; we need to at the wider picture. This includes investigating the reasons why we become overweight such as depression, mood swings and the complications medication cause, for example, slowing down the metabolism and how we can lose weight under these circumstances.

The complication of medical conditions such as coronary heart disease and bowel disorders need to be addressed, as well as the importance regular exercise as part of a strict weight reduction regime.

What is a balanced diet?

A balanced diet is a diet low in saturated fat, sugar, and salt and high in fibre including plenty of fresh fruit and vegetables. It is better to eat fat which comes from plant sources rather than animal sources as it is lower in cholesterol.

When does the body need to be well nourished?

Proteins

Proteins provide amino acids necessary to produce enzymes, antibodies, for cell growth and maintenance and repair of tissues. Enzymes are needed to regulate body processes. Antibodies fight infection and disease.

Proteins are found in the diet in fish, meat, milk, poultry, eggs and cheese.

Carbohydrates

Carbohydrates are primarily an energy source. Complex carbohydrates, such as fruits, vegetables, beans, lentils and whole grains also provide fibre in the diets. Simple carbohydrates are found in sugars and starches.

Fats

Fats provide a concentrated source of energy. Fat protects vital organs and provides body insulation. Fat is especially helpful in making food palatable but consumption of fats in excess is sure to result in weight gain. Apart from the obvious sources of fats, cooking oils fats are found in meat, eggs, cheese, milk, poultry and nuts.

DIET THERAPY

Dieting can literally be therapeutic for those of us who are wishing and hoping to achieve a weight which is within our ideal weight range. It is not only good for our health but also our self esteem, how we look at ourselves and hw others look at us.

Becoming inside our ideal weight range is integral at how we look at ourselves regarding not only our own self image, but also how we feel about fashion, make-up and beauty. Achieving our ideal weight can actually make us look younger, fitter and more confident within ourselves.

We need to break the cycle of over indulgence in food and alcohol, and develop a whole new relationship with food, and to also develop positive mental attitude about ourselves.

We don't need to always be slaving over a hot cooker. Instead it is necessary to be aware of the calorific content of various foods and beverages and have the autonomy or independence to create our own menus.

We need to limit the quantities of food we are eating and suffer the pain of our stomach's shrinking, as we decrease the amount of food we eat. Overweight people are literally just eating too much, more than we need. The key is to learn to eat only as much as the body needs, and no more, which means eating healthy options in small quantities. A portion means a portion. If it says 'serves 4', then you should only eat a quarter portion, and refrigerate or freeze the extra portions.

If you are serious about losing weight, throw out the deep fat fryer and buy a steamer. A steamer cooks the food without adding any extra calories. You can cook potatoes, vegetables, chicken, or fish in the steamer and it can be left unattended for up for half an hour, as long as you don't allow the water in the base of the steamer to evaporate. If you boil potatoes or vegetables in water, the vitamins are leeched out into the water and destroyed. But in a steamer, the vitamins are preserved, which is much healthier.

If you are frying it is healthiest to adopt the Mediterranean lifestyle, and cook in a little olive oil, extra virgin olive oil, or rapeseed oil made in Ireland, which are a natural source of omega 9. People in Mediterranean countries whose diet includes cooking with olive oil, plenty of fruit and vegetables, and a high intake of fish, have a lower incidence of coronary heart disease than in Britain and Ireland.

There is a portfolio of recipies in this book, but not everybody has the time to cook a meal for themselves and their family all the time. In today's busy world, we often 'Eat on the go'.

It is however very necessary to be aware of the number of calories we can consume and still lose weight. In table 1.1, there is a list of the calorific content of foods generally available in British supermarkets.

Dieters can therefore have the autonomy or freedom to create their own menus as well as knowing the calorific content of snack foods.

The major difference between slim people and overweight or obese people is that slim people are only eating as much food as they need to stay a healthy weight. Whereas obese people are basically taking in more food than they need and the excess energy is being converted to fat and stored in the adipose tissue in the body.

There is a strong association between high intakes of saturated fats, mostly from meat and dairy products and cardiovascular disease, and the reverse is true in countries such as Italy whose diet includes large quantities of olive oil.

There are two basic kinds of fat, saturated (hard fat) and unsaturated fat. Saturated fat is found in meat, lard and dairy products. It is healthiest not to eat saturated fat.

There are two kinds of unsaturated fats, monounsaturated fat which olive oil is a rich source and polyunsaturated fats found in nuts, seed oils and fish.

In 1983, the N.A.C.N.E. report was published National Advisory Council for Nutritional Education. It stated that we need to lower our intake of saturated fat, sugar, salt and increase our fibre intake.

To achieve optimum health, the Royal College of Physicians published a similar report recommending a diet low in fat, sugar, salt and high in fibre, limiting or stopping smoking and limiting alcohol to no more than 14 small glasses of wine per week for women, or 21 glasses of beer for men in the week.

Alcohol used in cookery is not counted as being of calorific value as during cooking, alcohol evaporates at 78 degrees centigrade and the calories are lost. All that remains is the taste of alcohol.

The unfortunate thing about health professionals is that there is a severe lack of dieticians in the community, or health promotions in the community. The real honest, true information about what is a healthy diet and a healthy lifestyle is withheld from the general public.

Losing or gaining weight is an exact science. In order to lose a pound in fat, it is necessary to expend 3,500 kilo calories in energy. This can be achieved by going on a weight reduction diet of 1,200 calories per day for a woman, and 1,500 calories per day for a man, and the body will start to use the excess fat on the body as energy, and this will result in weight loss.

It is advisable to exercise as well as diet to lose weight, having a treadmill in your house or garage is beneficial as a means of using calories, to lose weight, even running up the stairs briskly will use up calories, or going for a long brisk walk. Swimming is also an effective way of using up calories. Most public swimming pools have hoists and lifts to help obese people get in and out of swimming pools.

There is a wide variety of slimming clubs in Britain and they are generally successful and work of the same principle of losing weight by reducing calorific intake.

It is unfortunate for men however that this wide variety of slimming clubs are not available for men, teenagers or children.

Children are the future and most children would like to avoid the obesity crisis which is plaguing their parents and grandparents.

In order to save the younger generation from the obesity crisis it is important to educate them about healthy eating and how to avoid becoming obese.

Many parents don't want to be slaving over a hot cooker these days and opt for convenience foods.

Eating a wrap, Panini or sandwich "on the go" will not put on weight. It is the additional pack of crisps and sugary drink which need to be avoided, as they are very high in calories.

Most Chinese food is not excessively high in calories except for the fried rice and chips. A much lower calorie option is to opt for boiled rice with Chinese main courses.

Again, it is the amounts we eat. Dividing a typical Chinese main course between two people, or refrigerating half of the portion for the next day is enough food.

The obesity crisis is caused mostly by people eating excessive amounts of food.

Italian food including take-away pizzas are not excessively high in calories. Again it is the amount obese people are eating at one time which is basically too much.

Indian food is high in calories and it needs to be eating in moderation.

So therefore, in order to lose weight, it is important to cut down on portion size not just while you are on a diet, but for life.

Depending on how much overweight you are, it can take some time to lose the weight.

It is a very difficult task, virtually impossible, for clinically and morbidly obese people to return to a healthy weight, but it is still worth trying to lose the weight in order to become healthier and slimmer.

It is best to change your eating habits for life and achieve a slow, steady weight loss of 2-3lb per week, instead of crash dieting. If you crash diet, you will put all the weight back on again as soon as you adopt your old habits of eating too much.

It is important to know that when you do reach your target weight, a woman can increase their calorific intake to approximately 2,000 calories per day and 2,500 calories per day for a man to maintain their target weight and stay a stable weight.

Included in this book is a portfolio of calorie counted recipes which will make losing weight enjoyable for those who enjoy cooking for their friends, family and themselves.

So in order to achieve optimum health, it is time to forget junk food, fad diets and take a brave step. Throw the deep fat fryer in the recycling bin, buy a blender or food processor, and a good quality steamer, get fit, get slim, enjoy life again, and let's crack the obesity crisis.

What is an Antioxidant?

The theory of the antioxidant is not generally accepted by orthodox medicine, but according to nutritionists, prevention is better than the cure.

Antioxidants are essential nutrients like vitamin A and beta carotene (The most active precursor of vitamin A), in other words vitamin A can be synthesized from beta carotene. Vitamin C and E, plus the minerals zinc and selenium constitute the antioxidants.

Oxygen which is one of the basic building blocks of life i.e. plant and animal life is so important it is needed by every cell for every second of every day. We breathe in oxygen and exhale carbon monoxide. But it is plants who take in carbon dioxide and produce the oxygen we breathe. This is why it is so important to preserve rain forests. Without oxygen, living organisms cannot release the energy in food which drives all biochemical processes.

Oxygen is chemically reactive and very dangerous. When oxygen becomes unstable, it can lead to cellular damage, which can trigger cancer, inflammation, arterial damage and premature ageing.

To leading nutritionists, unstable oxygen molecules in the body are known as free radicals – chemicals capable of disarray are called the antioxidants, but orthodox medicine does not yet accept this theory.

According to nutritionists, free radicals are made all combustion processes, including smoking, the burning of petrol creating exhaust fumes, radiation, frying or barbequing food, burnt food and normal body processes.

It is no longer a mystery how slowing down the aging process can be achieved. Experiments show that animals fed with diets low in calories and high in antioxidants, live up to 40 percent longer, and are much more likely to be active during their lives. It could be decades before these discoveries are accepted to apply to humans.

"Large scale surveys show that the risk of death is substantially reduced in those with high levels of antioxidant food supplements in their blood" (2000 Holford P)

What are the best sources of vitamin A?

Vitamin A and beta carotene are found in back liver, red liver, carrots, watercress, cabbage, sweet potatoes, melon, pumpkin, mangoes, tomatoes, broccoli, apricots, tangerines, and asparagus.

The function of vitamin A, retinol and beta carotene is that it is needed for healthy skin, not just on the outside but for tissues within as well. It also protects the body against infection. Vitamin A (Retinol and beta carotene) is not only an antioxidant but it is also an immune system booster. It is essential for night vision and it is claimed to protect against many forms of cancer by many nutritionists, but this evidence is not accepted by orthodox medicine generally.

"High levels of vitamin A in the blood had been associated with reduced risk of certain cancers. These include putting acute myeloid leukaemia into complete remission and suppressing carcinogens in the neck and head by the field of nutritional medicine."

Beta carotene which can be converted into vitamin A in the body is also anti-cancerous.

A Japanese study of 265,000 peope found a significant correlation between low beta carotene intake and lung cancer. Infact the risk of lung cancer is similar for those who smoke and have good antioxidant levels as it is for non-smokers with low antioxidant levels." (2000 Holford P)

The Benefits of Vitamin C

Vitamin C is without doubt been found to be master immune boosting nutrient amongst nutritionists. It has been found to improve the performance of antibodies and is antiviral and antibacterial as well as being able to destroy toxins produced by bacteria. It is also thought to lower blood pressure.

Sources of Vitamin C include:

Sweet potatoes, carrots, watercress, peas, broccoli, cauliflower, mangoes, melon, peppers, strawberries, tomatoes, kiwi fruit, grapefruit, oranges, lemons and limes.

The juice of a lemon and lime, in hot or cold water, with a teaspoon of honey is a healthy way of ensuring adequate amounts of vitamin C daily. Instead of boiling potatoes and vegetables, it is best to cook them in a steamer to preserve the vitamins as vitamins A, C and E are prone to oxidation reducing their nutritional benefit substantially, as the vitamins are destroyed through cooking.

Vitamin C supplements in tablet form are harmless as it is water soluble and is excreted daily in the urine.

Many doctors would say it is best to get your vitamin C in your five daily amounts of fresh fruits and vegetables and fruit juices per day. This is true, but in today's tough economic climate, it may be difficult for lower income families to provide fresh fruit, fruit juices and fresh vegetables daily. So sometimes it is not such a bad idea to top up your vitamin C levels in tablet form. It is also very true that in Britain and Ireland we often do not get a wide variety of fresh fruit especially in small supermarkets. Fruit and vegetables are often refrigerated and chilled before it reaches our shops and often had a short shelf life. The fruit we buy which comes from mainland Europe often "Goes off" before we even get the chance to eat it. We are not as lucky as our neighbours on the continent who have a fresh fruit supply daily.

It is recognised that in the field of human nutrition and diabeties, vitamin C is particularly lowered in smokers. A smoker who does not take vitamin C supplements is more likely to have premature wrinkles as vitamin C is depleted in smokers. Increased intakes of vitamin C visably reduces the signs of premature aging in smokers. Dietary sources are always most effective as well as being a good source of fibre.

"A ten year study of eleven thousand people completed in 1996 found that those who supplemented their diets with the antioxidants vitamin C and vitamin E halved their risk of death from cancers and heart disease. It was also found that vitamin E is a powerful anticancer agent, especially in combination with selenium" (2000 Holford P)

Vitamin E is commonly known as the beauty vitamin as it is an antioxidant which helps to protect the body's cells from oxidative stress, or free radicals.

In the 1960's two nutritional doctors, Dr Linux Pauling and Dr Ewan Cameron first demonstrated the amazing anticancerous properties of vitamin C. They gave terminally ill cancer patients 10grams of vitamin C per day and found that they lived four times longer than patients not on vitamin C. Many studies have been performed since, but it is not widely accepted in orthodox medicine. But a review of vitamin C for non hormone cancers is very strong."

A strong positive correlation has been revealed between high does of vitamin C and longevity of cancer patients.

Sources of Vitamin E include:

Sweet potatoes, peas, meat, seeds and nuts, tuna, mackerel, salmon, wheatgerm and beans.

A study of many thousands of nurses who supplemented their diet with vitamin C, vitamin E and beta carotene effectively reduced their risk of having a heart attack by 22 percent. This study also claimed that taking these antioxidants reduced the risk of having a stroke by 40 percent.

Selenium, iron, manganese, copper and zinc are minerals involved in boosting the immune system and are claimed to have protective powers against cancer and premature ageing. The best sources of selenium are to be found in sea food and sesame seeds. The best sources of zinc are oysters, ginger, lamb, nuts, peas, haddock, egg yolk, whole wheat grain, rye, oats, peanuts and almonds.

Zinc is also thought to be anticancerous and to prevent premature ageing. The main role zinc has is to protect the DNA. Zinc is the most important immune boosting mineral, and it helps fight infections. Zinc can be found easily in a well balanced diet of milk, cheese, meat, eggs, fish, whole grain cereals and pulses.

The antioxidants are no guarantee against cancer and heart disease, but theory and proven facts suggest that taking vitamins and minerals increase the chances of optimum health and a longer, healthier life.

It really does matter what time of the day or night you eat – it depends on the calorific value if you are a man you needn't take any more than 1500 calories per day and 1200 calories if you are a woman because some people cannot sleep on an empty stomach.

History of Food in Britain

Prehistoric hunters probably cooked some of their food before they knew how to make fire; they cooked over burning wood taken from fires that had started naturally. Men learned how to make fire by about 500,000 BC.

Roasting meat on splints was the earliest form of cookery and the roasting of animal heads, offal, dried blood and bone marrow mixed with fat provided variation in the diet.

Obviously the food choice of early Stone Age man was very limited but the change in lifestyle which the Neolithic farmers brought to England from Flanders in the 4th century BC greatly diversified the choice of food available. In the Neolithic period the lifestyle of man underwent a major change. Man progressed from the nomadic hunter-gatherer to the settled farmer, cultivating crops and domesticating animals. The change in lifestyle affected Neolithic man's eating habits in several ways. Since his food source was now more reliable, man wasn't as likely to experience long periods of hunger between meals. He therefore ate more regularly with the domestication of animals, the milk available from cows and goats became a popular drink. The Neolithic farmers were also the introducers of pottery to the British Isles. This had important influences on the development of cooking. With the introduction of pottery, fish and meat which previously could only be roasted could now be steamed or boiled. The advent of pottery greatly diversified the food choice because cereals and herbs could be added to stewing meat to add variety to the diet.

In the bronze age which began about 3000 BC the new innovation of cheese making evolved by adding rennet to sour milk.

Butter making was introduced by the Celts and involved the agitation of milk until the cream solidified to form butter. The Celts were the first invaders of Britain and Ireland and came in the 700's BC.

In pre-historic times cookery remained fairly simple and it was only when the Romans conquered Britain in 44AD that more sophisticated methods of acquiring and cooking food were introduced to Britain. They also introduced more sophisticated methods of acquiring and cooking food were introduced to Britain. They also introduced more sophisticated cookery equipment such as the metal tripod for supporting pans over the fire. This was useful for cooking dishes involving sauces which required controlled heat. The Greco-Roman form of cuisine introduced to Britain by the Romans involved the addition of many new foods to the standard diet, and it basically involved the addition of imported herbs to meat, fish, cereals, vegetables and nuts. The new foods introduced by the Romans to Britain included wine, olive oil, Mediterranean herbs, oriental spices, root vegetables including carrots, parsnips, turnips, onions, garlic and green vegetables including cabbage and lettuce. Roman cookery also introduced the addition of sauces which were highly seasoned with the herbs to a variety of meat and fish dishes. Of the variety of spices introduced by the Romans pepper from Indian and ginger from Asia Minor were the most popular. Pepper was very popular with the Romans and was added to almost every dish. Roman cookery also involved the use of a large amount of eggs especially as a thickening agent. A typical Roman recipe, using eggs was "Patna". This dish involved boiled beans pounded up in a mortar with seasoning, milk and eggs cooked over a low heat in a "Bain Marie."

It was the Romans who first introduced fruit and vegetables as a major constituent of the daily diet in Britain. They cultivated fruit trees in gardens and were the first to plant orchards.

However, the main impact of Roman cuisine was on rich British landowners and town dwellers of southeast England. The remoter Northern and Western peasants remained largely unaffected by the new culinary innovations introduced to Britain by the Romans.

The end of the Roman occupation of Britain in the 5th century AD due to the fall of the Roman Empire heralded many changes to the lifestyle of people in Britain. New Germanic tribes namely the Angles and the Saxons invaded Eastern Britain in the 5th century hence the name Anglo-Saxon. Following the withdrawal of the Romans from Britain, many of the sophisticated methods of Roman cookery methods fell into disuse in Britain and there were few new innovations in cookery in any part of Britain, in fact cookery methods became relatively simple compared to the previous highly sophisticated Roman methods. After the settlement of the Anglo-Saxon farmers, sheep, pigs and goats came to predominate over cattle, mainly for economic reasons. Sheep were very popular mainly because they were highly economic providing wool with milk as well as meat. Pigs were also popular because they provided bacon a favourite food among the Anglo-Saxons. During the early Middle Ages religion influenced the diet of the British Isles to a great extent. With the introduction of Christianity to Britain and Ireland in the 5th century AD fish became an important consistent of the diet because on fast days such as Friday in memory of Good Friday and during Lent the consumption of meat was forbidden and was therefore replaced by fish. This new trend had important economic implications because it economised on meat consumption and caused an expansion in the fishing industry. Herring and Mackerel fishing especially during the Viking conquests of the 8th Century AD and 9th century AD became an important factor in the British and Irish economies. One of the few new cookery innovations of the early

Middle Ages was the traditional British pie. This dish consisted of meat and vegetables sealed in a strong pastry crust and baked. The traditional cereal pottage also constituted a large part of the diet during the Middle Ages, especially among the common folk. The cereals included oatmeal, barley, rye meal and the green-leaved vegetables added to pottage consisted of beet, cabbage, peas and beans. During the Middle Ages the large variety of exotic herbs and spices imported to Britain during the Roman occupation were no longer available immediately after the 5th century AD because the Anglo Saxon piracy made the English channel dangerous for shipping, and the few oriental spices which did arrive provided rare luxuries for the wealthy. During the Middle Ages the elaborate forms of bread cookery practised by the Romans was also abandoned in favour of the simple methods employed by the Anglo Saxons and the popularity of wine as a favourite drink diminished in favour of ale and beer which were the popular drinks of the Anglo Saxons. The staple diet of the peasant society during the Anglo-Saxon period was very simple, consisting of pottage, bread and ale and it reflects the simple lifestyle of the Anglo-Saxons in contrast to the extravagant lifestyle and eating habits of the Romans.

When the Romans invaded Britain and Ireland marked by the conquest of William the Conqueror at Hastings in 1066, further changes in lifestyles and eating habits occurred in the British Isles. Under the Romans, the feudal system grew. Wealth was based on land owning which centred on the manor. The manor was seen almost as a self-sustaining economic unit consisting of a manor house in which the landlord dwelled.

The manor was surrounded by an estate which consisted of grazing lands, common fields, a mill and a village in which the tenants lived. Since roads were of a very poor quality in the Middle-Ages, very little food was transported from one place to another, and for this reason each manor was almost self sufficient in food.

Like the Romans the Normans introduced many new culinary skills to the British Isles but with the growth of the feudal system. It was mainly the aristocracy who enjoyed the new culinary innovations, while the staple diet of the peasantry remained to be then gruel accompanied by milk, cheese, butter, cream and eggs known collectively as white meats. Fresh meats and spices were the true mark of the rich man's diet. After the Norman Conquest, beef again became the most popular form of meat and the number of cattle on the manor rose considerably in the decades following the Norman Conquest. It was the custom among the rich during the medieval times to host huge banquets in the manor house. At one such banquet, the wedding feast of one of Edward III's sons "wine ran in water pipes and there were thirty courses with enough food to feed 10,000 men." The Norman aristocracy enjoyed a sophisticated cuisine based on that of Norman-France which had been inherited from the Roman era, and modified through the centuries. One striking similarity between Norman and Roman cookery was the liberal use of herbs and spices. The rich seasoned their main dishes with a wide variety of spices including cinnamon, ginger, saffron, cardamom and many new spices which were unknown in Roman times such as nutmeg, mace, cloves and galingale. Through trade with Southern Europe during the Norman period the first citrus fruits began to reach Britain and Ireland. These included oranges, lemons and grapefruits, as well as dried fruits such as prunes, figs and dates. Again these exotic fruits could only be enjoyed by the well to do other new commodities to be introduced to Britain and Ireland by the Normans included rice, refined sugar from the Middle East. Because of its initial rarity and costliness, sugar was highly valued and could be afforded only by the rich. But it gradually became more easily obtainable by all classes, slowly replacing honey as the medieval spice destined to have the greatest effect on Britain and Ireland's eating habits in future centuries.

During the Tudor and Stuart era from the 15th century to the 17th century lavish banqueting was still practised widely among the royalty. A typical banquet during Henry VIII's reign consisted of as many as seven main courses from a huge selection of beef, mutton, pork, veal, game, venison or fish delicacy of sturgeon, porpoise or whale. During Elizabeth I's reign from 1557 to 1603 the old custom of fish days continued, but now mainly for economic rather than religious reasons.

Meat animals in Britain became scarce and expensive during the late 1500s and for this reason; restrictions on meat eating amongst the peasant society were enforced. One of the new cookery innovations of the Elizabethan era was the introduction of eggs into the cookery of sponge and fruit cakes and biscuits. In Tudor times it was also common practise to cook fruit before eating it. Apple pies and pumpkin pies were popular Tudor dishes.

The various foreign explorations of the Tudor era also brought a variety of fruits and vegetables to Britain including tomatoes from Mexico, bananas from West Africa and the potato which was introduced from South America by Sir Walter Raleigh in 1586. During the 17th century the growing of potatoes was greatly encouraged in order to replace expensive imported grains as the staple food of the peasantry. However in Ireland the policy had disastrous consequences because crop failure from 1845 – 52 as a result of potato blight caused the death of millions during the Great Famine.

Amongst the royalty, eating habits changed quite dramatically in style in the 17th century. In Charles II's court, privacy was the big change: great public feasts lost favour and the lavishly cooked dishes which in previous centuries fed thousands at huge banquets were now confined to the private table of the King only. In the same period another major change in the eating habits of the rich was the slide of the dinner hour from noon to the evening hours. This new trend was due to the growing popularity of drinking beverages such as tea, coffee or chocolate and rolls at mid-day, the new fashion among the wealthy of that era. These new beverages were imported on merchant ships from countries like Jamaica, Brazil, Mexico and China. Tea and coffee when first introduced could only be afforded by the rich but with growing popularity these beverages were found even in the poorest homes, tea eventually replacing beer and ale as the common beverage of the peasantry. In addition to the new beverages mentioned above, new drinks to join the alcoholic range were hard spirits such as gin from Holland and whiskey from Ireland.

Dinner from the wealthy still involved a series of meat and fish dishes, and poultry, which was once considered to be a poor man's dish now became popular with the rich. Vegetables which previously appeared chiefly in soups began to join the meat in the main dish in the modern fashion. Market gardening was another new innovation of the 17th century diversifying the range of fruit and vegetables which could be grown. In the glass-houses of the big estates were grown such fruits as peaches, nectarines, oranges and lemons. New vegetables of the 17th century included artichokes, cucumbers, melons and pumpkins.

Although eating habits changed quite significantly for the rich in the 17th century, lifestyles and eating habits for the peasantry didn't change to any great extent. It was only at the beginning of the 18th century with the advent of the Industrial Revolution that drastic changes in lifestyle and eating habits occurred for the poor. The great change in the lifestyle of the poor was related to the phenomenon of rural or urban migration during which Britain was transformed from a rural-agricultural society to a predominantly urban-industrialised society. Rapid population growth was another phenomenon of the 18th century. A population increase of 5.5 million in 1702 to 9 million in 1801 meant that there was great pressure for space on the land and this was one of the main reasons for migration to towns. The fundamental change in lifestyle during the 18th century was that when people were driven off the land they were cut off from their natural food supply and were compelled for the first time to buy food.

The great change in eating habits which accompanied the Industrial Revolution was that, when removed from the arable land, people were compelled for the first time to buy food, making money a necessity for survival.

In order to provide food for the growing number of city dwellers, agricultural techniques needed to be improved substantially to establish increased productivity. This necessity was fulfilled by the agricultural revolution of the time. Mechanisation of agriculture, the practice of crop rotation and storage of fodder to keep animals alive during the winter months meant that land now produced much larger amounts and indeed better quality foods to satisfy the growing demands in expanding towns and cities. However the great influx of immigrants to towns contained with a fast population growth rate resulted inevitably in overcrowded living conditions which brought problems of poverty, food shortages and epidemics such as cholera from contaminated drinking water. The meagre diet of a typical British factory worker of the 18th century consisting of bread and butter for breakfast, broth and peas for dinner and bread and cheese for dinner reflects the poverty-stricken lifestyle of the working class in industrialised urban areas. However, for the very poor, the only means of substance apart from the soup kitchens which saved many from standard starvation in the 18th Century was scraps of food such as potato peeling and rotten vegetables thrown away by others.

Although the 18th century was a difficult period for the working class whose lives were affected by hardships, the lifestyles of the well to do were inevitably still extravagant. A typical dinner in a wealthy household consisted of a "large cod, a chine of mutton, some soup, a chicken pie, a fillet of veal with mushrooms, hot lobster, apricot tart, jellies and fresh fruit with port and wine to drink." The only significant change in the eating habits of the wealthy in the 18th century was the growing popularity of French and Italian foods in the diet.

In the 19ᵗʰ century living standards and hence food quality and choice improved considerably for the working class urban dwellers. The hardship which accompanied the Industrial Revolution was at last over and the British Commonwealth prospered in the Victorian era. The general rise in living standards could be attributed to two main factors. Firstly increasing importation of food from other Commonwealth countries through the free trade policy provided a plentiful supply of cheap food and prevented any shortages. Secondly, advances in technology produced increased agricultural yield by the use of chemical fertilisers and increasingly efficient farm machinery. Along with increased productivity improved transportation allowed fresh foods to be brought quickly to towns and cities from distant regions. At the beginning of the 19ᵗʰ century advancing technology developed new preservation methods such as bottling and tinning techniques, allowing perishable foods like meat, fruit, vegetables and milk to be conserved for long periods of time. The development of refrigeration in the 1870s allowed frozen meat to be imported to Britain from America and Australia, and the development of pasteurisation in 1890 allowed milk to be transported on long journeys without souring quickly.

All of these new technological innovations being particularly beneficial to the urban-dweller whose survival depended on how efficiently adequate food supplies could be transported to cities.

Although the English working class people suffered some degree of hardship during the 18ᵗʰ century, in the 19ᵗʰ century, living standards improved greatly in the Victorian Era.

Through-out the course of history it can easily be observed that as the lifestyles of the British and Irish people has changed as a result of a combination of closely related factors such as technological advances, socio-economic conditions and the influences of the various groups of settlers. There was an associated gradual change in the eating habits of the population. The degree of change however depended on social class. As the eating habits of the British and Irish people is traced down the centuries it becomes increasingly ore evident that food choice has diversified enormously from the scanty food supply of primitive man to the huge, complex variety of food available today, thanks to modern food technology.

In Old Stone Age time there was essentially no class distinction but down through the ages there gradually developed a clear distinction between rich and poor. In the 18th and 19th century especially since the advent of industrialisation, the differentiation between rich and poor became even more distinct.

In Stone Age times and when mankind survived in an agricultural society, there was basically no class distinction and everyone had equal wealth.

But in the 19th century especially when industrialisation gripped the western world it was not just the Irish, Scottish, Dutch, etc who suffered from the results of the potato blight. There was an underclass in England as well who were scavenging from bins.

In the late 20th century and the 21st century, there is a new underclass in the western world, single mothers especially single mothers who come from poor families. Those who lack in skills, education and the ability to earn a living to support their children are living at the bottom of the socio-economic heap on very low incomes.

Young women who should be part of the workforce are becoming a burden to their families and to society. Very often, they are unfit to even hold down jobs and are being supported meagrely by the government.

In the 21st in the UK there is a new underclass of black, white, Indian and mixed race young people, the prodigy of the 20th, single mothers, thieves, looters, deviants, not just unemployed but unemployable at least some of them.

Some in all classes especially the middle class and upper class are still able to hold together nuclear families i.e. the mother the father and their children. Even in these tough economic times both the mother and the father are working and they afford a healthily diet, and on average live a longer life span than working classes people and their children.

It is not just a matter of a healthy diet; there are deep socio-economic problems as well as obesity especially in the working classes.

There should be more rights regarding access to children for fathers, even if it takes a DNA test to prove they are the father of the child.

Single mothers in low socio- economic groups are not feeding themselves or their children properly.

As well as providing for their children fathers usually have a better disciplinary manner with children which should start from babyhood.

It does not matter whether the parents are married; co-habiting, separated, divorced or annulled the children are happy if they have both parents in their lives.

The conservative party, forecasts that by 2030 half the population of the U.K. will be obese.

The aim of this book is to try and slow down and for reverse this trend, as in Human Nutrition and Dietetics which is basically preventative medicine "you are what you eat".

Nutrition in the Past

What was so different about what we were eating in the past compared to since the Millennium when there has been an explosion of overweight, obese and clinically obese people, especially women, many teenagers and even children?

Overweight, obese and clinically obese people are rarely seen eating in public. So what are they eating, where and when? Are we really becoming a nation of lazy, obese people, too lazy to look up a recipe book to cook a substantial meal for the family, opting for takeaways out of the Chinese or the Fish & Chip shop and happily munching ourselves to death in front of the television with crisps and snacks?

On the other hand, alcoholics who are often secret drinkers usually are very thin and undernourished. There is a big taboo about smoking these days, making it illegal to smoke indoors in all public·places. The only place a smoker can "light up" is in their own house and this is often banned by other family members who may be non-smokers. But yet smokers are not afraid to be seen smoking in public places, outside shopping centres, cafés, and public houses, etc. But how often do you see an overweight person eating in a public place except for restaurants, hotels, etc.? How often do you see an overweight person munching a packet of crisps or a chocolate bar on the street or at a bus stop or even driving in their car? I say "never" as this behaviour is totally secret behaviour done in their own home. How much food do excessively overweight people eat? I say tonnes and tonnes of extra calories. In medical terms, the body must take in 3500 kilocalories to put on a pound of weight or use up 3500 kilocalories to lose a pound of weight. In total if you want to lose a stone weight which is 14 pounds, you must use up 49,000 kilocalories. A clinically obese person who needs to lose ten stone in weight therefore needs to use a rather whopping 490,000 kilocalories. How did our sophisticated society in the United Kingdom and the United States of America in particular get our diet and nutrition so wrong in the present times?

With rising food costs these days in the USA as well as Britain it is actually as inexpensive to eat out of a takeaway to avoid washing up saucepans and crockery, but only encourages lazy behaviour. As well as encouraging lazy housekeeping, homes which do not provide healthy well balanced meals for the family can result in a lack of vital nutrition for adults and children. It is not as people these days do not know what a healthy balanced diet is, it is just a lot of people really do not care about their health and they will eat what tastes nice but is not necessarily good for you.

Throughout past decades, there always were Takeaway Chip shops, Chinese Takeaways and Fast Food outlets, like Mc Donald's, Burger King and Kentucky Fried Chicken in the USA, throughout Britain and Europe. In past decades people did eat out of Fast Food outlets but not as often as in today's society. It seems that our diet has changed for the worse because people are basically overeating in the 21st Century taking in many more calories than is necessary.

Diseases of affluence means that people drive around in expensive, comfortable cars and consume comfort foods resulting in them getting into a cycle of overeating, lack of exercise and weight gain.

Many people blame feelings of depression for comfort eating. Doctors are also blamed for the fact that their medication for depression increases the appetite and results in a cycle of depression, medication for depression which patients claim increase the appetite and therefore overeating and gaining unnecessary weight.

Many things can trigger off depression, bereavement, divorce, a broken romance, debt crisis, unemployment or just becoming over the age of forty.

Many people would confess that they were always slim and trim until they turned forty. This time of your life can be critical in fighting the fat barrier.

It is just worrying that is no longer just over forties. Many young people, adolescents and even children can be classed as overweight. They now, additionally have the problem of fighting the fat barrier.

There is only one solution, lowering calorific intake as much as possible without having to go on a starvation diet, just a sensible low fat, low sugar diet, with vigorous exercise routines such as swimming, going to the gym, or brisk walking for at least 20 minutes at least three days a week.

Fasting is not a word many people want to hear these days. But in order to stay within an acceptable weight limits, it is necessary to eat nothing more than a piece of fruit between meals. Crisps, chocolates, sweets, bags of crisps, alcohol, are full of empty calories that are not needed for health.

Healthy living and a great figure or physique does not come naturally. It requires a lot of hard work and dedication as well as pride in you for achieving this goal.

Twenty or thirty years ago it was unusual to be obese. But these days it is quite normal and average to be overweight, obese or clinically obese.

The new profession of Heath Promotion was launched in 1945 by The World Health Organisation with the declaration "health is not merely the absence of disease, but a state of complete physical, mental and social wellbeing with the absence of disease or infirmity."

The obesity crisis which we are now experiencing in Britain and the USA most acutely is something which medicine and The Health Promotion Profession would not even have anticipated twenty years ago.

Instead of coming closer to complete health for the majority of the population we are moving further away from a state of complete physical and mental health and social wellbeing. Through Health Education children were taught hygiene principals and parents, in particular mothers, were instructed in hygiene, nutrition and childcare through home visiting.

(Lewis 1980)

Visits to the home are often done by a community dietician but there are just not enough qualified dieticians to fulfil this role in the wider community.

In the Republic of Ireland the Department of Health produced a consultative statement entitled Health – the Wider Dimension (Department 1986). This document stated that "the focus of health policy needs to be widened to take into account the many factors apart from the health service which impact on health." It also stated that emphasis should be placed on health promotion.

This suggests that health promotion needs to broaden its horizons and interact more with the general public on a wider scale and deal with health issues such as obesity and cardiovascular disease through more interaction with the general public by health promotion officers.

Food in the Bible

In today's harsh economic climate with rising food prices, people are tempted to buy the cheapest possible food; processed, tinned and many convenience foods. Working mothers often opt for convenience foods which can be reheated in the oven or the microwave.

It is difficult to research into the past to find where people ate healthy diets and lived long lives. But if you look in the Bible chapter 37 – chapter 50 in the Book of Genesis, you will find the famous story of Joseph and His Amazing Technicoloured Dream Coat as dramatized into a hit musical by Andrew Lloyd Webber and Tim Rice.

Some cynical people would regard what is written in The Bible as a fairy story.

But it is documented in chapter 50 v22 that Joseph lived to 110 years of age and his father Jacob also known as "Israel", whose twelve sons including Joseph constituted The Twelve Tribes of Israel. In Chapter 47, verse 28 it is recorded that Jacob lived to 147 years of age.

The question is what was it about these ancient people that they had such longevity thousands of years before the advent of modern orthodox medicine? Was it anything to do with the food they were eating? There are many references to what these Egyptians and Israelites were farming in this part of the Old Testament, and they were obviously farming cows, cattle, goats and sheep.

In Chapter 45, verse 10, there are references to herds (of cattle). In chapter 38 verse 13 there is reference to sheep and in chapter 38 verse 17 there is reference to a "kid" lamb. In chapter 41 verse 2 there is reference to cows, in chapter 49 verse 12, there is reference to milk. In chapter 37 verse 31, there is reference to a goat.

There is also reference to grapes in chapter 40 verse 10, fruits chapter 43 verse 11 baked food chapter 40 verse 17 and bread chapter 43 verse 32. In this part of the book of Genesis they also new how to make wine from grapes.

In chapter 43 verse 11 there is a special reference to honey, pistachio nuts and almonds.

This seems to have been the staple diet of Israelites and Egyptians in this Ancient Civilisation going back to about 4,000 years ago.

The first striking thing about their diet is that it is not an awful lot different in many ways to the diet we eat today in Britain, Ireland and all over The Western World. They would not have known about butter making or cheese making, and they did not eat chicken, eggs or any kind of poultry. They would also have not had the technology to preserve food, so they would have been relying on a fresh organic diet.

Does this not teach us something about our diet today? Most people know an organic diet is healthier than a diet that has had nothing added to it before it reaches the supermarket shelves.

Take a chicken for example. It is more expensive to buy free range eggs compared to battery eggs where a hen is kept in a cage indoors in the dark with hundreds of other hens to lay eggs. It is also more expensive to buy an organic chicken i.e. a chicken that lives outdoors on a farm. Outdoor chickens are happier and tastier chickens and free range eggs are healthier than battery produced eggs, as they are laid by happier, healthier hens.

It is more expensive to buy organic beef, lamb, pork, chicken, fruits and vegetables. Sometimes they are not even available in large supermarket chains.

With rising food prices, rising unemployment, a rise in the cost of living in general it may seem unrealistic to buy organic foods. But it depends on how much you value your health. As the old saying goes "Your Health is your Wealth". A big mortgage and a big car is no good if you haven't got your health.

It's not just about dieting. It's about what diet foods you are eating.

In this biblical story of Joseph there is very little mention of sickness or death, except for the death of Joseph's brother Judah who had two sons who died in the land of Canaan called Er and Onan.

But in the house of Jacob that came to Egypt included seventy of his descendents chapter 46 verse 27, the mortality rate seemed to be very low. Could there be a positive correlation between the plain, simple but totally organic diet these people in The Bible ate and their longevity.

Even for people who are not religious the Bible can be looked upon as a historical document of life in Ancient Times. Very few could argue that it is a fantasy story. It gives us a great insight into the lives of those Ancient peoples in one of the world's first known civilisations.

But Christians have the right to have a reservation, indeed a major objection against others telling lies about The Holy Bible in order to accumulate wealth for themselves. A classic example is when a company in Northern Ireland, here in the heart of South Armagh, calling themselves 'Linwoods' used the Bible as a sales gimmick pretending that people ate Flaxseed in the bible, to make them healthier and increase their longevity.

Hard sales techniques were used to try and convince uneducated people that flaxseed is good for health. It was said directly to me by the owner of this company, an old man now over 75 years of age that flaxseed was proved to be eaten by Tutankhamen as it was found in his mummified body by John Carter in 1922. If this is true, flaxseed didn't do him much good as he died aged 22 years.

Controversy continued as I began to ask questions in 2012. This businessman who was successfully using sales talk planted suspicion in my mind. I compared the calorific content for flaxseed in these food supplements to the calorific content of crisps and found them to be similar – approximately 550 kilocalories per 100g, the highest calorie food available on the market. I had a major reservation, unknown to so many people especially the victims in the USA; this food was and still is being sold as a health food, fuelling the obesity crisis in Britain and the USA, a very hard sell.

Again independently, I decided to do my own market research locally in Armagh City amongst shoppers. Housewives' major complaint was that flaxseed was too expensive to buy for a family as well as food for a large family.

I didn't get the opportunity to do any further investigations as I rang the office of this Linwoods company. The boss came on the phone and said to me "Don't read the bible! Do not read the Bible!" I immediately defiantly replied "And who are you to be such an expert on the Bible?" and hung up.

Two days later I received a nasty note in the post from the owner of the company. This biological uncle said to me:

> Veronica,
>
> Do not have anything more to do with the sales, promotion or advertisement of our seeds."
>
> John Woods

The envelope the name and address o this company was on the outside of the envelope so I just wrote "Return to sender" and put it in the post to him.

I was still searching for proof of my suspicions that this theory that flaxseed as a food was eaten by people in the bible.

It was only a hunch that humans should not be able to digest milled flax even if it is fortified with nutritious vitamins and minerals.

This hard sell was pushed on me by this old man closely related to me, an uncle along with a book titled "Flax your way to better health" by a licensed dietician in the USA – Mrs Martin. She made a sweeping statement that flaxseed was eaten in the bible thousands of years ago but she could not quote references from the bible.

So I consulted a qualified dietician called Wendy who was educated in Northern Ireland at the University of Ulster. I raised my concerns with Wendy who is a Born Again Christian and Wendy willingly search the bible over the computer and she quickly confirmed that "Yes", flax is referred to many times in the bible, but there is no reference to people eating it" It was probably used for the same reason in ancient times as it is for today, for producing linen.

This leads me to suspect that milled flax is unfit for human consumption.

I consulted a Born Again Christian preacher who is also a teacher by profession, said to me when I spoke to him about my findings, he said "This man will be made accountable for his actions in their world and the next"

In the meantime his products are still being transported by cargo ship to America, and this old man has travelled as far away as San Francisco to preach to fat, vulnerable Americans about the wonders of flaxseed which has twice the calorific content of chips, never mind any other food. There are easier ways of getting vitamins and minerals into your system through tablets which contain no calories at all, and are of course less expensive.

In the mean time I wish to present research which individuals can use to draw their only conclusions to give them autonomy about how to adhere total nutrition.

Flaxseed does contain many nutritious vitamins and minerals but not vitamin C because it is a white crystalline solid which cannot be added to flaxseed successfully but if you are not trying to lose weight it is suitable to eat in small amounts.

At equal the calories of crisps and double the calories of chips, this megalomania doesn't care how much his flaxseed contributes to the obesity crisis in Britain and the USA.

The wonderful properties of honey eaten in the book of Genesis suggests that this sweetener was one of the reasons that these people lived over 100 years of age on a completely organic diet, and the sweetener they used was honey.

NATURE'S WAY

There is more to worry about than just our diet. There is the future of mankind and planet earth. We can learn from the Bible as many people connect God and Nature closely.

It is evident in the New Testament that Jesus Christ was very knowledgeable about nature as he is the Son of God. Jesus said in a parable:

"Look at the fig tree and all the trees. As soon as they come out in leaf, you see for yourselves and know the summer is already near". Luke Chapter 21 V 29, 30.

Another example amongst many of Jesus Christ's references to nature is the parable of the sower.

"A sower went out to sow his seed. And as he sowed, some fell along the path and was trampled underfoot, and birds of the air devoured it. And some fell on the rock, and as it grew up, it withered away, because it had no moisture. And some fell among thorns and the thorns grew up with it and choked it. And some fell into good soil and grew and yielded a hundred fold." Luke Chapter 8 V 4-8.

During the heyday of scientific discoveries for medicine various scientists have made discoveries which can prolong life. These include Joseph Lister who discovered antiseptics in Glasgow in 1865. Pierre and Marie Curie isolated radium in 1911, and in 1928 Sir Alexander Fleming made a significant discovery as he isolated penicillin.

These discoveries amongst many others were major contributions towards saving lives in the developed world.

In 1946 when the new profession of Health Promotion was founded by the World Health Organisation, it wasn't anticipated that we would have modern problems such as heart disease and cancer.

It is not yet conclusive that cancer is diet related but certainly heart disease and complications.

By the end of World War II medicine had eradicated many killer diseases such as diphtheria, small pox and tuberculosis. There was great hope of a healthy future for the human race.

The World Health Organisation's initial definition in 1946 was:

"Health is a state of physical and mental and social well-being with the absence of diseases and infirmity."

But unfortunately they did not anticipate the emergence of today's killer diseases such as cancer and heart disease.

Nature has a way of controlling the World's population. A prime example is The Great Famine in Ireland between 1845-47 where millions died because of a failure of potato crops as a result of a potato blight which made potatoes unfit for human consumption. Ireland at the time was over populated and under resourced. The population of this small island of Ireland was 8.5 million. About 2 million people died of starvation and approximately another two million went on the coffin ships to the New World, and many did not survive the voyage to reach America alive. There was still food grown in Ireland at the time of the Great Famine especially grain. The English didn't come and confiscate Irish grown food. It was exported to England by the Irish Government to fund the wealthy in Ireland regardless of the poor, starving and destitute people in famine cottages at the time of the Great Famine.

One reason why the North of Ireland didn't suffer in the Great Famine was because they were industrious. One example was that they had a thriving flax industry which is used to make linen. The wealthy people with land made their money growing flax which is used to make linen, and the poor people in famine cottages often worked in factories for very low pay to produce the linen until the early 20th Century.

But Ireland was not the only country to be affected by the potato blight. Many people died in the Highlands of Scotland and also in Scandinavia as a result of the potato failure.

England seemed to have escaped the Great Potato Famine. They didn't cause the potato blight. But at the height of the British Empire, Queen Victoria donated £5 to Ireland for famine relief, and she gave the starving people in the Scottish Highlands no money at all.

In the destitute people who were living in famine cottages didn't have the inspiration or even have fishing rods to catch fish in the rivers, lakes or the Atlantic Ocean, to survive the Famine.

The Great Famine of 1845-47 is an example of how nature can bring about a population cull. We used to die of diseases of poverty. But now we are dying of diseases of affluence.

Orthodox Medicine today does not have a great deal of sympathy for people who are obese or are becoming clinically or morbidly obese.

In the 21st Century it is now England which is over populated, but not yet under resourced because of the clever way this current government is managing its finances.

A lot of people criticize the current health service in Britain. But in many cases illnesses are diet related, and people are not taking responsibility for their own health. With a healthy diet, many ailments can be prevented.

Nature has a way of controlling the World's population. Because of the environmental problems created in the 20th Century, resulting in the melting of the polar ice caps, the Open University thought in June 2015 that the World will come to an end by 2052 and we will all drown.

But it may not be so bleak. A few people and animals survived a major flood in the Bible, at the time of Noah's Ark according to Biblical history.

But the situation may not be critical. The premature death of the obese, clinically and morbidly obese people is likely however.

There could be another population cull as the world is over populated.

We are endangering our planet through our consumerism, but younger people are much more environmentally conscious than people were in the 20th Century, in an effort to save the planet through, for example, recycling glass, plastic and paper.

Previous generations including our elderly people today nearly destroyed Planet Earth. Never mind being on the brink of a nuclear war, they were cutting down the rainforest which produces the oxygen we breathe. But in recent decades our generation and the younger generation are planting a sapling for every tree they cut down in the rainforest.

Nobody knows what is going to happen. But nature itself can bring about population control such as it did with the death of millions in Europe in the 1400's remembered as the Black Death. AIDs or Ebola did not become a major epidemic, but it could be possible, a disease orthodox medicine cannot control any more than they did in the 1400's in Western Europe caused by the black rat, hence the name the Black Death, could happen even in the 21st Century and cause a pandemic again to result in a cull in the World's population on a scale never known before which religious people would call "an act of God".

It could be an obesity crisis which is part of our next pandemic. Those in the Western World who are clinically or morbidly obese are making no contribution to society at all except increasing the price of food, making life more difficult for those who are working hard to sustain the economy, as well as our ageing population.

A healthy diet and vitamin supplements can often save lives because it gives patients the strength to survive illness which would kill those not on a healthy diet. It is just expensive and inconvenient to cook healthy food for women especially who don't want to bother messing up their kitchen or wash dishes or saucepans. But there is an easy alternative, using a steamer to cook potatoes, vegetables, meat, chicken or fish, which can be left unattended for up to half an hour unless the water in the steamer evaporates. The benefit of using a steamer is that no additional calories are added to the food, which is of course why people gain weight, by eating more calories than they expend. It takes 3,500 kilocalories which is not expended in energy to gain a pound and 3,500 kilocalories needs to be expended to lose a pound, as recognized by state registered dieticians.

Medicine in the UK is coming down very hard on obesity at the moment. If you are even a stone over-weight you are told to lose weight.

But as long as you stay within your ideal weight range it is not dangerous to carry a few pounds in fat as a reserve, for example, if you become ill or need to go through an operation, to have energy reserves to speed up recovery.

People who need to lose a lot of weight can become despondent as it is a huge task in order to lose a huge amount of weight. It just takes determination and will power in order to save their own lives and morale can be increased for over-weight men and women in the same position, by helping each other to make us happier people.

FIGHTING THE FAT CRISIS

This weight reduction diet is not a crash diet of 1,000 calories per day or less. It is approximately designed to lose weight at a rate of 1-2lbs per week. A sudden crash diet of less than 1,000 calories per day will result in a weight loss of up to 5lbs per week, but this is not realistic. On the first week of a crash diet you only lose water, fluid and when your normal eating habits resume you go back to your previous fluid.

This reduction diet plan is good because:

1. It produces weight loss
2. It is good for your health
3. It is designed towards changing your eating habits for life.
4. It does not leave you hungry or lacking in physical strength
5. It is easy to follow
6. It is designed to bring you inside healthy weight limits.
7. It is tasty and nutritious
8. It is a well balanced mixture of complex carbohydrates, not too high in proteins and low in salt, sugar and saturated fat.

Exercise is vital in conjunction with a weight reduction diet, because if you don't exercise loose skin will develop where the weight has been lost and it costs £4,500 in this country for a tummy tuck where loose skin is likely to develop, around the abdomen. You can be active around the house, running up and down the stairs, floor exercises mowing lawns. All these activities use up calories. Go walking, swimming or to the gym. It doesn't matter how big you are. Most swimming pools have a hoist to lower and raise bigger people in and out of swimming pools. Aqua aerobics can be very enjoyable too. Contrary to popular belief, moderate exercise actually decreases your appetite. Physical activity is necessary for the appetite mechanism to work properly. People who don't take exercise actually have bigger appetites than those who take regular physical exercise. So if you are not physically active you are more likely to pile on the pounds. Those who take regular exercise such as walking, cycling, running or swimming including in a leisure centre, on bicycles or treadmills can generate their metabolic rates that are eight to ten times above their basal metabolic rate, i.e. resting metabolic rate. As discovered by Professor McArdle exercise physiologist at City University New York. He goes on to say that "vigorous exercise will raise metabolic rate for up to 15 hours after exercise."

This diet and any weight reduction plan should come with a health warning that exercise is crucial in a weight reduction plan to result in a perfectly toned figure/physique.

If you find it difficult to lose weight on your own join slimming club for support. Alternatively, you could join a gym where you could listen to music and exercise three times per week.

There is another advantage to exercising while dieting or even if you are happy with your size and weight and just exercise regularly to maintain a healthy weight and stay fit. During exercise the pituitary gland in the brain releases hormones called endorphins which create a "feel good" factor like a small shot of morphine into the bloodstream. It can be experienced by any physical activity, running, cycling, swimming for example or walking at a fast pace, or running on a treadmill in the gym. People think illegal substances are necessary to feel "high". But little do most people know illegal substances aren't necessary to feel high. You can get that high feeling from moderate to vigorous exercise.

Don't get paranoid about what the scales say when you are dieting and exercising. During a prolonged period of diet and exercise, you will become slimmer, but this may not register on the scales. The reason is during exercise, fat is converted into muscle and muscle is denser than fat. You may weigh heavier than is recommended regarding your ideal weight for your height ratio, but do not worry. Gauge your weight more by your size in clothes. If you are a woman of 5"4" aged about 40 and you wear a size 12 to 14 in clothes, but weight 11 stone weight, don't worry. This is not an unrealistic woman who has built muscle from prolonged periods of exercise. It is the same for men. A fit muscular man will always weigh heavier than a man of the same height and build who is not doing regular exercise.

Before starting this reduction diet, go to your G.P. to ask if there are any complications you might have particularly diabetes Type I and Type II. A diabetic diet is much more complicated than a normal diet and the specifications of a diabetic's diet cannot be changed unless it is sanctioned by a G.P or dietitian. Before starting this reduction diet ask your G.P. how much weight you should lose and what your body mass index is, how far you are from your ideal body mass index. All this information should be stored on computer for each patient.

Don't aim to be too thin. It is easy to lose too much weight once a weight loss programme is being successful. It is important not to diet to excess because too much calcium in particular can be lost from the skeleton resulting in bone fractures because of excessive dieting. The most dangerous being a fracture of the hip bone, resulting in the fact that the person, particularly women over 65 years of age, may never walk again. A diet rich in calcium and Vitamin D is crucial for everyone particularly women as women are more likely to suffer bone fractures than men.

Vitamin D is very important for the absorption of calcium phosphorus and magnesium into the bones. Zinc is important as well as it helps in the formation of new bone cells.

Prolonged slimming through-out life can result in osteoporosis. The result can be that a person can lose up to 25 percent of the skeleton by the age of fifty. Bone fracture is particularly prevalent in women after the menopause. Bone fractures occur in one in three women and one in twelve men by the age of seventy.

Scientists think that high protein diets which are acid forming results in a neutralising effect of two main alkaline agents sodium and calcium. When the body's reserves of sodium are used up calcium is taken from the bones. Therefore, the more protein you eat the more calcium you need. High protein diets therefore can lead to calcium deficiency. Some medical scientists now believe that a lifelong consumption of a high protein, acid forming diet may be a primary cause of osteoporosis.

Prolonged weight loss programmes, where the weight swings up and down according to how much food a person is eating or indeed how much alcohol they are consuming as alcoholic beverages contain a lot of calories, means that dieters could be damaging their health unless they achieve a sustainable, slow weight loss reaching their target weight and keeping their weight within healthy limits for life. This is not easy to achieve. But if you are serious about losing weight you need to stop comfort eating for every little problem that comes along which totally contradicts the whole purpose of going on a weight reduction diet. Major problems such as a death in the family, divorce, marital separation, moving house, financial problems especially debt these days can cause people to comfort eat.

It is not wrong to eat between meals. It just depends on what type of food you are eating. Fresh fruit of any kind excluding avocados as they are high in calories but suit as a main course are suitable for snacking in between meals. Suitable fruits include apples, oranges, plums, strawberries and raspberries for example. Some vegetables are suitable too such as carrots and celery. Avoid the usual snacking foods such as chocolate, sweets and crisps as they are very high in calories and you will never lose weight snacking on these types of food.

Avoid alcohol on a weight reduction diet as it is too high in calories and you will never lose weight. A couple of glasses of wine, beer or spirits at the weekend is as much as can be recommended, or you will not lose weight no matter how much you diet to try and lose weight.

Avoid fast food outlets or fish and chip shops. Avoid chips and fried rice with Chinese food. Eat boiled rice instead and Indian takeaways are only to be taken occasionally because Indian food is very high in. It may sound like bad medicine but the only way you are ever going to achieve a weight that is within your ideal weight range is to avoid the above temptations and throw out your deep fat fryer. Cook with a little extra virgin olive oil or ordinary olive oil in a frying pan or wok or just grill food in a George Foreman grill or under a normal grill. Barbequing in the summer time may produce free radicals which have damaging effects on your health. But occasional barbequing is still lower in calories than deep frying food.

Reward yourself for every 5 kilos you lose. Buy yourself something nice with the money you didn't spend on food. But don't buy yourself too many new clothes as you are losing weight. Don't buy designer clothes unless it is for something very special like a wedding, because a new wardrobe may lower your incentive to achieve your target weight ie between a normal range from size 8 to size 16. Aim for a target weight, but consider your bone structure. A person with a big bone structure can carry more weight than a person with a very small bone structure. Aim for a clothes size which flatters your figure/physique.

A young woman of 20 years of age may look good in a size 8 – 10 but generally the taller a person is, the more weight they can carry. Despite what some people might think it is not such a good idea to be ultra thin because organs like the heart, liver and kidneys for example need to be surrounded by a little fat to protect them from damage, e.g. in a car accident.

Don't necessarily aim to be too thin over the age of forty. If you had aimed to be a size 8-10 under forty years of age, it is ok to be a size 10-16 over forty years of depending upon height and bone structure. A little weight will help disguise unwanted wrinkles on your face and neck. An older person who is too thin can look gaunt in the face. If you are over forty and very thin wrinkles can become more visible.

Even if you find your weight is difficult to keep within reasonable limits, remember if you are a size 32 you are not beyond redemption. Losing weight is a very big challenge. But it is necessary to have positive mental attitude, mind over matter and think. "I used to be a size 12-14. I can get back there." Don't treat Christmas as an excuse for a Christmas binge of food and drink because it can be particularly difficult to lose the weight in the New Year. Have a Merry Christmas but try to avoid over indulging in sweet foods especially.

There is a science behind the number of calories needed to achieve weight loss. It is not recommended to go on a diet below 1,000 calories per day as when this is done the body starts to conserve fat and use muscle for energy. This philosophy is preached by many nutritionists and is widely accepted by medicine to be true. A diet low in saturated fat, higher in protein and higher in complex carbohydrates is much more successful, and losing weight should be less painful as the client should not be hungry on this type of a calorie controlled diet and gradually lose weight.

Healthy eating habits need to be taught to mothers of young children especially overweight, obese or clinically obese mothers who often produce overweight children. This is a very important issue because in the foreseeable future the rising number of obese children means that Social Services could consider childhood obesity as a form of child abuse. We do not want to be raising another generation of obese and clinically obese young people so mothers today need to be taking out the cooking pots and cooking well-balanced healthy meals. In this book there is many healthy meals to be cooked which will not put on weight, and if not for the family, for a single person living alone they can be portion sized, put into containers and frozen for future meals. Otherwise this reduction diet is guaranteed to lose weight as it is calorie controlled along with at least moderate exercise and the healthy eating recipes are guaranteed to keep your weight stable when a target weight is reached.

With many people who are obese, clinically or morbidly obese, weight gain can be because of medication resulting in the fact that the medication can slow down the metabolic rate i.e. the rate that the body uses up calories.

There is only one way to counteract the sleepiness and lack of energy a person is on for many ailments especially depression and heart problems for example this is to include caffeine in the diet. This can be in the form of coffee, diet coke or coke zero.

On many types of medication, it says if drowsy do not operate machinery or drive. If this is the case do not take alcohol as it is a depressant and will slow you down even more, but in the early part of the day take diet coke, coke zero or coffee. But not in abundance. These drinks are a stimulant and unless you want to be buzzing and cannot sleep it is recommended not to take caffeine after 6pm if you wish to have a good night's sleep. Caffeine is also a diuretic. It helps pass urine and prevents a bloated stomach. Some medication especially for depression, bipolar disorder and perhaps other psychiatric disorders can cause constipation and a bloated stomach making you feel as if you have put on even more weight which is depressing.

But when you drink a few cups of coffee especially in the morning it can naturally help your bowels move without having to take artificial powders from your G.P. to counteract constipation i.e. it is a natural laxative. Tea does work too but to a lesser extent. But don't get obsessed with drinking coffee because you could find yourself with severe bouts of diarrhoea.

Black coffee with a little artificial sweetener and skimmed milk if you are dieting, and if not just brown sugar or a teaspoon of honey is an appetite suppressant. In other words, coffee can actually help you diet. Coffee manufacturers will love me for giving my secret away about how to stay a size 10 -12 at the age of 51.

Losing weight can be an uphill struggle for people who are on medication which can cause drowsiness compared to people that are on no medication. But it can still be done with diet and specifically exercise. This basically means keeping "on the go". You can walk to the shops instead of driving the car and get a taxi home with your purchases. You can spring clean the house cleaning the insides of kitchen cupboards, for example, hoover, wash out floors, give your bathroom and kitchen a once over instead of sitting in front of the T.V. munching crisps and take pride in your nice clean house. You can also mow your lawns and weed flower beds and you can grow your own herbs which you can use in your healthy diet plan, such as parsley and thyme.

Even if you do have to stay on a strict diet to lose ten kilos in six months or a year it is better than gaining another ten kilos in six months or a year. Psychological disadvantages of being overweight, obese or clinically obese can result in a person feeling unattractive especially to the opposite sex and have low self-esteem. A woman may lose interest in getting her hair done or using make up, or a man may shave their head instead of going to the barber to get a haircut. A man or woman with a weight problem may pay a lot of money for a treadmill for their own house or garden shed or garage but soon lose motivation to use the object. Some dieters may admit to losing twenty stone in the last ten or twenty years and gaining nearly 25 stone weight.

Losing or gaining a few pounds on a regular basis does no harm but dramatic weight gain and loss, swaying from being fat and thin cannot be good for the heart.

Young women can be the most vulnerable. Size 8-10, even size zero is often portrayed in glossy magazines as the perfect physique for young women and if these stars put on a few pounds they are heavily criticised. Young women feel heavily pressurised by the media attention on Hollywood stars in particular. This is especially true of young mothers specifically single mothers of young children. They have so much responsibility regarding their child or children, they forget about themselves and their own health and welfare.

Many pregnant women are under the illusion that they are eating for two. But in reality they are not necessarily doing so. When you are pregnant you only need about 400 – 500 extra calories per day plus about a half a litre of milk. It is best not to put on excess weight during pregnancy because after the baby is born the mother has one less thing to worry about; rather than just getting back into shape. It is fine for a young mother to go back to a size 8-10 after having a baby. Glossy magazines portraying many Hollywood stars getting into perfect shape after having children. There is nothing wrong with this. It is a good example for young women.

But people forget the greatest sex symbol of the 20th was Marylyn Monroe and she was a size 14. It is ok to be anything from a size 8-16. Below a size 8 you are facing anorexia nervosa, the most lethal mental illness as one in six patients with this illness die. Over a size 16 you are facing obesity, clinical obesity and morbid obesity, one of the biggest problems the current government is facing because of its medical complications.

There are just not enough government funds available to the NHS to provide all the obese, clinically obese and morbidly obese people in society with a gastric bypass. There is only one solution; live with the pains of hunger in order to let the stomach shrink and adjust to living with less food and alcohol. In other words, moderation being the operative word. This means you will be healthier and feel much better if you keep the amount of food and liquids you put into your body within reasonable limits as well as taking a litre of water per day with a lemon and lime squeezed into it for a healthier glow of your skin because of its high Vitamin C content rather than just drinking water.

There is just one specific medical problem which affects weight gain or weight loss i.e. an underactive thyroid gland, which often causes weight gain. The thyroid gland contains the metabolic rate. An underactive gland can cause dramatic weight gain whereas an overactive thyroid gland can cause dramatic weight loss and if it is left untreated for too long it can cause a stroke or heart failure.

So if you are not eating very much and you are still gaining weight or to the contrary if you are eating a lot and cannot put on weight, you could have an overactive or an under active thyroid gland. This organ in the neck which controls the metabolic rate; i.e. the rate the body uses up energy could be malfunctioning; it is therefore a good idea to go to your GP to see if he/she thinks it is necessary to get a blood test done regarding the function of your thyroid gland.

In some cases, extra weight especially in women around their abdomen and stomach is not fat at all but fluid. In most people this fluid can easily be rectified with fluid retention tablets from your GP. If a patient is unfortunate enough to be on tablets like lithium to stabilise mood swings such as bi polar disorder, fluid tablets cannot be prescribed, and unfortunately the patient has to live with the fluid retention. But for others who are not on such medication it is worth visiting your GP to try taking fluid retention tablets. But this is not the answer to losing fat. This must be done with limited calorie intake.

The only solution to staying within a desirable weight range is to eat and drink in moderation and this includes tea or coffee. No more than five cups of tea or coffee is recommended in the day by Medicine, Dietetics and the Health Promotion Agency. Too much caffeine can cause heart palpitations and general over activity. Some young people like to drink energy drinks especially as it gives a feeling of being high. But this is not recommended as it may result in the temptation of going on to stronger drugs and can cause heart palpitations.

Using coffee as a stimulant and an appetite suppressant is however the lazy dieter's way to keep their weight under control. It is much better to eat three small meals and fruit between meals but you can include tea and coffee as well in moderation.

The worst thing you can do is starve yourself all day and eat a huge meal at night, because when you are asleep your body is only at its resting metabolic rate and the remaining energy is turned to fat. Make the main meal of the day a substantial lunch and you will not feel so hungry the rest of the day. Regular exercise, even if it is only walking the dog, a sensible diet; going through the pain of hunger pains to allow the stomach to shrink so you need less food, will eventually result in weight loss and a happier person.

"Most obese people have slower rates of metabolism than slim people. One of the big problems with crash diets of below 1,000 calories per day is that the body sees the reduction in food as a threat, and slows down the metabolic rate by as much as 45 per cent.

A gym instructor said "If the food intake is less than 1,000 calories per day the body starts to conserves fat and use protein as an energy source."

A sensible diet plan is designed to specifically be about 1,200 kcal for a woman and 1,500 kcal for a man to promote weight loss on a sensible calorie intake, which should not make the dieter feel hungry, with constant snacking which is actually thought to speed up the metabolic rate.

"The human body is designed to run on complex carbohydrates i.e. in other words slow releasing carbohydrates which means whole grains, beans, lentils, vegetables and fruit."

Modern diets are at last emphasising foods which release their sugar content slowly. Slow release of sugar produces a more consistent energy level and gives the body a better chance to use up the food rather than turning it into fat. (Holford. P 2000)

To expand your taste buds, eat beans including red kidney beans in a chilli con carne or for children adding baked beans in tomato sauce to a chilli con carne. Simple baked beans on toast can replace a meal on a diet without upsetting the calorie balance.

Some people find a high protein diet full of fish, chicken, lean meat, fruit and vegetables helps weight loss and a reduction in potatoes, rice and bread. Brown bread and brown rice are more suitable for a weight reduction plan, as they are high in fibre and are more slow releasing carbohydrates than take for example white bread and white polished rice.

These recipes are high in protein. It has a sensible balance of protein, fat and carbohydrate as well as fibre plus vitamins and minerals.

While on a weight reduction diet it is best to take supplements. These include vitamin C. A good source of vitamin C is the juice of a lemon or lime, and the B complex vitamins daily, as well as a good quality vitamin mineral supplement as well as cooking with olive oil, a good natural source of omega 9.

BEATING YOUTH OBESITY

Cracking the obesity crisis for the sake of the younger generation is of paramount importance.

Unhealthy traits, unfortunately pass down through the generations. An obese child generally does not have a slim mother and father. Usually their parents are overweight, and bad eating habits influence the child.

There is a very wide range of healthy, low calorie foods researched in this book which are full of healthy fats, vitamins and minerals. These foods need to be substituted for children, instead of giving them foods with empty calories such as crisps, soft drinks, sweets, cakes, chips, sausages and burgers which lack vital nutrition.

Healthy cooking is generally not lazy cooking.

It generally takes a special effort to cook a healthy diet. There is one piece of equipment which is a lazy option, but is very healthy. It is a steamer. You can cook fish or chicken and various vegetables of your choice in the steamer, filling it full of water and inside of half an hour the food is cooked and all the vitamins and minerals are preserved, such as the vitamin C in potatoes and the vitamin A in carrots.

Healthy eating needs to be introduced from babyhood, to educate a baby's palate towards liking healthy food. Most people start to spoon-feed babies at three months of age. It is best to avoid packet, tinned or baby food in a glass jar. Instead of this lazy option, it is recommended to steam vegetables such as carrots, broccoli, parsnips, celery, potatoes, or any type of vegetable, mash it and with a little gravy, spoonfed babies from three months of age, and start educating your children from infancy towards eating a healthy diet for life.

Obese children are not happy children. You can see the sadness in their eyes, that they are trapped inside a fat body that they don't like, and these children are looking for help.

Some parents think they are being kind, by giving their children comfort foods, but instead they are being very cruel.

Parents need to change their whole attitude to food for the sake of future generations. It is easier to reverse the obesity crisis with children in general, compared to some adults who may be clinically or morbidly obese, in which case it is very difficult to reverse the condition.

The N.A.C.N.E. Report by The National Advisory Committee for Nutritional Education issued in 1983, stated that we need to lower saturated fat, sugar, salt and increase fibre in our diets.

But unfortunately for some people this information has not been filtered through, and it is today's children and young people who are paying the price and are generally unhealthy.

This can include heart disease, diabetes, and high blood pressure.

Even in the 1980's it was identified that teenagers had fatty deposits inside their arteries, known as arthrosclerosis. This can lead to a blockage near the heart, and case a heart attack even in young people. This is caused mainly in children and young people eating too much saturated fat. Non-saturated or polyunsaturated fat is considered to be a healthy fat. But the tricky thing about it is, that once this healthy fat is used more than a few times, it's chemical structure changes into dangerous saturated fat and this can lead to heart disease including in children and young people.

By law fish & chip shops and all fast food outlets must change the oil they are cooking with every three days. Fast food outlets are obviously one of our main concerns regarding the obesity crisis. As long as they are not over used, by law they are safer than if you are cooking in a deep fat fryer at home, not knowing when the oil has changed into dangerous saturated fat or not.

If you do not eat occasionally out of fast food outlets and fish and chip shops, to reduce the chances of obesity and heart disease in children and young people, it is a good idea to buy a steamer and put the deep fat fryer in the recycling centre, if parents are serious about beating childhood obesity.

Buying your children food from a fish and chip shop or a fast food outlet is permissible occasionally but not as a staple diet, every day.

It is best to give children the healthy types of food rich in vitamins and minerals to keep the family in a high nutritional status as well as slim.

Using up excess calories through exercise is an important factor regarding physical health, and weight control. Children should be discouraged from spending too much time watching TV, playing their computer and mobile phones.

Weight control is achieved between a delicate balance of calorie intake and calorie usage.

In the field of Human Nutrition and Dietetics it is acknowledged that calorie usage comes down to simple mathematics. 4.2 kilojoules of energy = 1 kilo-calorie. You must use 3,500 kilo-calories of energy to lose a pound and you must take in 3,500 kilo-calories more than you need to gain a pound, and this excessive energy is converted into fat and stored under the skin known as adipose tissue.

It is this adipose tissue which is a major threat to westerners, and although slimming clubs wouldn't know it, losing weight is an exact science, known only in detail by State Registered Dieticians, who usually obtain a Bachelor of Science or a Bachelor of Science – Honours in Human Nutrition and Dietetics.

If parents can afford it, and they are worried about child obesity, it is advisable to attend clinics in which private dieticians work independently of the National Health Service, to gain 100% reliable information about weight loss and diet related diseases. The independent dieticians are advertised generally in Yellow Pages or over the internet.

In general it is advisable to give children multivitamin – mineral supplements. Visible signs will be seen in an improvement in their skin, nails, teeth and hair. It is however very important to give children who are on a weight reduction diet vitamin and mineral supplements as they could be missing out on vital nutrition while losing weight.

If you value your child's health, their self-esteem and their general appearance, their self awareness and their image, because we all want our children to be as attractive as possible and as successful in life as possible.

THE DANGERS OF WHITE CRYSTALLINE SOLIDS

Salt

There is two widely used white crystalline solids which the National Advisory Committee for Nutritional Education against since the publication of the N.A.C.N.E. Report in 1983. They were salt and sugar.

The reason why they advocated lowering salt intake is because it causes hypertension commonly known as high blood pressure.

It is advisable that children should be trained from babyhood to not eat much salt. It would not be harmful in very small amounts. If salt is used in cooking, then it should not be put on food before you eat as well. In other words this compound called sodium Chloride NaCL can lead to high blood pressure which is an irreversible condition and it can only be controlled by medication from the doctor, and it very often starts from parents being irresponsible by giving too much salt to their children. It is not east to do, but the palate needs to be educated to enjoy food which does not contain too much salt and this includes many tinned, packet and processed foods.

Sugar

Cheap, widely available white crystalline solids are very dangerous to Western Society. White cane sugar was considered harmless, but in reality it is much more dangerous to young people than hard drugs which are also white crystalline solids, such as cocaine and amphetamines. As they are expensive and most people can't afford them, sugar seems to be most dangerous in liquid form, especially in soft drinks. Children cannot be totally denied sweets. Children like sweets, but as any dentist would agree, it is the frequency of sugary substances in contact with the teeth which causes dental decay. Obviously if a child or young person is drinking minerals constantly, sugar is constantly in contact with the teeth and this can cause tooth decay. It is best for children and young people to decrease the time sugary foods are in the mouth and to clean their teeth at least twice a day and use mouthwash form as young as possible.

Other obvious aspects of health regarding the use of sugar labelled scientifically as sucrose is the danger it presents regarding the obesity crisis and links to insulin dependant diabetes which is prevalent amongst children and young people, whereas mature onset diabetes is known as non-insulin dependant diabetes which can be controlled by medication and dietary restrictions, regarding sugar intake.

Prevention is better than cure for many illnesses. In the budget of 2016, the Chancellor of the Exchequer Mr George Osborne, made one of the most clever decisions ever made in No.11 Downing Street by putting a taxation on sugar, and this new trend is set to continue long term in the UK.

It was a very clever move as it is tackling the problem at its source by increasing the price of this cheap, available and dangerous substance, sucrose, commonly known as cane sugar.

There is a healthy alternative for parents who are worried about their children becoming addicted to sugary drinks especially. It is old fashioned, but it is wise. If parents can't persuade children to drink bottled water, a healthy alternative is diluting squashes including Ribena which is a healthy alternative and also high in vitamin C.

The key is to train children as young as possible to enjoy healthy alternative foods and drinks which are not as dangerous for health, as young as possible because as they grow into older children and teenagers with the obesity problems and health complications, it is more difficult to change unhealthy eating habits. The most successful strategy is for parents to change unhealthy eating and drinking habits themselves and lead their children and the younger generation by setting a good example.

CARBON CHEMISTRY

Education is what is left when everything else we learned at school or University is forgotten. The chemistry of food is organic as it is based on carbon, as carbon is the chemistry of living things, or things that were once alive like a piece of meat, or a piece of cabbage. If it is not based on carbon we can't eat it such as a rock or a piece of metal or plastic as it was never alive and does not contain carbon which makes it an inorganic substance.

Chemistry is therefore divided into two groups, organic and inorganic chemistry.

Proteins are slightly different from carbohydrates, fats and alcohol as they are not based on just carbon, hydrogen and oxygen. Alcohol is known chemically as ethanol and its chemically formula is C_2H_5OOH which means it has two atoms of carbon, six atoms of hydrogen and two atoms of oxygen held together by chemical bonds.

Protein is different as it is based on, not just carbon, hydrogen and oxygen, but as so nitrogen and sometimes phosphorus and sulphur atoms joined together in very complicated chemical bonds.

At the moment of death the spirit leaves the body and all that is left behind in the corpse is these elements, carbon, hydrogen, oxygen, nitrogen, phosphorous, sulphur, iron, calcium and a few trace elements such as potassium, magnesium, manganese fluorine, selenium, zinc cobalt and molybdenum which are inorganic substances.

The most nutritious foods we can eat are usually low in calories and high in vitamin and minerals. A healthy diet including these vitamin and mineral rich foods will help you stay younger and healthier for much longer.

There are foods which are lower in calories that much of the food which is available, but it is not vitamin rich. You can eat these healthy foods in larger quantities without gaining weight to help achieve a healthy, slim physique.

Do You Know Your Vitamins?

VITAMINS

Vitamins are organic substances required by the body in small amounts. Since the body cannot make them, they have to be provided by the diet. They do not provide the body with energy.

The term Vitamin was first introduced in 1912. As the vitamins were discovered, they were identified by letters of the alphabet. Later, as each vitamin was isolated in pure form and its chemical structure was determined, it was given a chemical name.

Vitamins have been classified into two groups, water soluble and fat soluble and this helps us to understand the distribution of the vitamins in foods.

Any excess intake of the water soluble vitamins including the B complex and vitamin C are readily dissolved by the kidneys and excreted in the urine – therefore there should be no danger in being given an excess of these vitamins. Fat soluble vitamins including vitamin A, D, E, F and K cannot be excreted in this way and any excess beyond the immediate requirements is stored in solution in the liver. The amount that can be stored is not unlimited. In fact too much of these fat soluble vitamins can be toxic and make you feel very ill. If you are in any doubt about the strength of these vitamins and how much of them you should be taking, consult your pharmacist. But in general you cannot go wrong with a good quality multivitamin daily.

TABLE 1.1

This table is a list of the foods most commonly found in supermarkets which allow the dieter to cook their own recipes with the knowledge of the calorific content of various foods. This table illustrates which foods you can take in large quantities and also foods to avoid to lose weight. This information gives dieters the autonomy or independence to decide what to eat themselves instead of adhering to traditional diet plans. High intakes of fresh fruits and vegetables are recommended to create a feeling satiety, reducing the hunger pains, as well as being very highly nutritious weight loss optimum health is achievable through everyone creating their own diet plans.

RECEIPES

These healthy eating recipes are designed so that even if you are on a reduction diet, you can have a dinner party or a family meal enjoy beautiful food and yet lose weight.

If you are in a high nutritional status, healthy food, vitamin and mineral supplements will help you fight periods of illness and also prevent the onset of many killer diseases, particularly cardiovascular disease. Nutritional Medicine is a form of preventative medicine and if you have any queries about the benefits of these supplements you can consult your GP before commencing a weight reduction diet and attend your G P as you progressively lose weight.

Try not to have relapses by going back to your bad eating habits as this will slow down your progress.

Don't expect miracles overnight. If you need to lose several stones, you could look at a time span of a couple of years to achieve your target weight.

Achieving your ideal weight will not be easy. It will be a long arduous task involving a lot of determination and hard work, and sometimes you may feel that you are not making progress, but in the long term you really will be successful. You will feel a new self-confidence, look and feel years younger.

Zinc is also thought to be anticancerous and to prevent premature ageing. The main role zinc has to protect the DNA. Zinc is the most important immune boosting mineral and it helps fight infections. Zinc can be found easily in a well balanced diet of milk, cheese, meat, eggs, fish, wholegrain cereals and pulses.

The antioxidants are no guarantee against cancer and heart disease but theory and proven facts suggest that taking vitamins and minerals increase the chances of optimum health and a longer, healthier life.

WHAT ARE THE BEST SOURCES OF VITAMIN A?

Vitamin A and beta carotene are found in beef liver, red liver, carrots, watercress, cabbage, sweet potatoes, melon, pumpkin, mangoes, tomatoes, broccoli, apricots, tangerines and asparagus.

The function of Vitamin A, retinol and beta carotene is that is needed for healthy skin, not just on the outside but for tissues within as well. It also protects the body against infection. Vitamin A (retinal and beta carotene) is not only an antioxidant but it is also an immune system booster. It is essential for night vision and it is claimed to protect against many forms of cancer by my Nutritionists, but this evidence is not accepted by orthodox medicine generally.

High levels of Vitamin A in the blood has been associated with reduced risk of certain cancers. These include putting acute myeloid leukaemia into complete remission and suppressing carcinogens in the neck and head by the field of Nutritional Medicine.

Beta carotene which can be converted into Vitamin A in the body is also anti cancerous. "A Japanese study of 265,000 people found a significant correlation between low beta carotene intake and lung cancer. In fact the risk of lung cancer is similar for those who smoke and have good antioxidant levels as it is for non-smokers with low antioxidant levels." (2000 Holford P)

THE BENEFITS OF VITAMIN C

Vitamin C is without doubt been found to be the master immune boosting nutrient amongst Nutritionists. It has been found to improve the performance of antibodies and is antiviral and antibacterial as well as being able to destroy toxins produced by bacteria. It is alo thought to lower blood pressure.

Sources of Vitamin C include:

Sweet potatoes, carrots, watercress, peas, broccoli, cauliflower, mangoes, melon, peppers, strawberries, tomatoes, kiwi fruit, grapefruit, oranges, lemons and limes.

The juice of a lemon and lime in hot water or cold water with a teaspoon of honey is a healthy way of ensuring adequate amounts of Vitamin C daily.

Instead of boiling potatoes and vegetables it is best to cook them in a steamer to preserve thge vitamins as vitamins A, C and E are prone to oxidation reducing their nutritional benefit substantially as the vitamins are destroyed through cooking.

Vitamin C Supplements in tablet form are harmless as it is water soluble and is escreted daily in the urine.

Many doctors would say it is best to get your vitamin C in your five daily amounts of fresh fruits and vegetables and fruit juices per day.

This is true, but in today's tough economic climate, it may be difficult for lower income families to provide fresh vegetables daily. So sometimes it is not such a bad idea to top up your vitamin C levels in tablet form. It is also very true that in Britain and Ireland we often do not get a wide variety of fresh fruit especially in small supermarkets. Fruit and vegetables are often refrigerated and chilled before it reaches our shops and often has a short shelf life. The fruit we buy which comes from mainland Europe often 'goes off' before we even get a chance to eat it. We are not as lucky as our neighbours on the continent who have fresh fruit supply daily.

It is recognised that in the field of Human Nutrition and Dietitics, vitamin C is particularly lowered in smokers. A smoker who does not take vitamin C supplements is more likely to have premature wrinkles as vitamin iC is depleted in smokers. Increased intakes of vitamin C visibly reduces the signs of premature ageing in smokers. Dietary sources are always most effective as well as being a good source of fibre.

"A ten year study of eleven thousand people completed in 1996 found that those who supplemented their diets with the antioxidants vitamin C and vitamin E halved their risk of death from cancers and heart disease. It was also found that vitamin E is a powerful anticancer agent, especially in combination with selenium" (2000 Holford, P). Vitamin E is commonly known as the beauty vitamin as it is an antioxidant which helps to protect the body's cells from oxidative stress, or free radicals.

In the 1960's two nutritional doctors, Dr Linus Pauling and Dr Ewan Cameron first demonstrated the amazing anticancerous properties of vitamin C. They gave terminally ill cancer patients 10grams of vitamin C per day and found that they lived four times longer than patients not on vitamin C. Many studies have been performed since, but it is not widely accepted in orthodox medicine. But a review of vitamin C for non-hormone cancers is very strong: "A strong positive correlation has been revealed between high doses of vitamin C and longevity of cancer patients."

Sources or vitamin E include:

Sweet potatoes, peas, meat, seeds and nuts, tuna, mackeral, salmon, wheatgerm and beans.

A study of many thousands of nurses who supplemented their diet with vitamin C, vitamin E and beta carotene effectively reduced their risk of having a heart attack by 22 percent. This stufy also claimed that taking these antioxidants reduced the risk of having a stroke by 40 percent.

Selenium, iron, manganese, copper and zinc are minerals invloved in boosting the immune system and are claimed to have protective powers against cancer and premature ageing. The best sources of selenium are to be found in sea food and sesame seeds. The best sources of zinc are oysters, ginger, lamb, nuts, peas, haddock, egg yolk, whole wheat grain, rye, oats, peanuts and almonds.

Zinc is also thought to be anti-cancerous and to prevent premature ageing. The main role zinc has to protect the DNA. Zinc is the most important immune boosting mineral, and it helps fight infections. Zinc can be found easily in a well balanced diet of milk, cheese, meat, eggs, fish, whole grain, cereals and pulses.

The antioxidants are no guarantee against cancer and heart disease, but theory and proven facts suggest that taking vitamins and minerals increase the chances of optimum health and a longer, healthier life.

Do You Know Your Vitamins?

VITAMINS

Vitamins are organic substances required by the body in small amounts. Since the body cannot make them, they have to be provided by the diet. They do not provide the body with energy.

The term Vitamin was first introduced in 1912. As the vitamins were discovered, they were identified by letters of the alphabet. Later, as each vitamin was isolated in pure form and its chemical structure was determined, it was given a chemical name.

Vitamins have been classified into two groups, water soluble and fat soluble and this helps us to understand the distribution of the vitamins in foods.

Any excess intake of the water soluble vitamins including the B complex and vitamin C are readily dissolved by the kidneys and excreted in the urine – therefore there should be no danger in being given an excess of these vitamins. Fat soluble vitamins including vitamin A, D, E, F and K cannot be excreted in this way and any excess beyond the immediate requirements is stored in solution in the fat in the liver. The amount that can be stored is not unlimited. In fact too much of these fat soluble vitamins can be toxic and make you feel very ill. If you are in any doubt about the strength of these vitamins and how much of them you should be taking, consult your pharmacist. But in general you cannot go wrong with a good quality multivitamin daily.

Chemistry of Vitamin A

Vitamin A is a fat soluble range of compounds including retinol, retinal and retinoic acid.

Vitamin A is soluble in fat, insoluble in water and retinol itself only present in animal fats. In general Vitamin A isn't lost in cooking, steaming or baking. It is destroyed by exposure to oxygen as it is an antioxidant.

Vitamin A is also present in another form Beta carotene; which is found in plant foods which are yellow orange in colour like carrots and peppers and are known as carotenoids. Some of these carotenoids are converted back to Vitamin A, during the digestion.

Many of the most common diseases in the twenty first century are associated with a shortage of the antioxidants, and vitamin A is recognised as one of the major antioxidants, along with beta carotene including vitamin C, vitamin E, selenium and zinc.

Diseases which can develop because of a lack of the antioxidants including vitamin A are cancer cardiovascular disease, hypertension Alzheimer's disease, diabetes and even mental illness.

These claims are well documented by a nutritionist (P Holford 2000) in his book The Optimum Nutritional Bible, first published in 1997. These claims, however are completely rejected by orthodox medicine because there is no proof about these discoveries.

There is one piece of evidence about the therapeutic properties of vitamin A which does carry weight as a result of extensive research. Large scale studies show that the risk of death is substantially reduced in those with either high levels of antioxidants in their blood from high levels from supplements or high dietary intake of these vitamins. This information however comes with a health warning. The fat soluble vitamins including vitamin A are fat soluble and toxic levels can build up in the liver and this can cause a feeling of general malaise, In order to ensure general health and safety it is best not to take any extra vitamin A than is recommended in a daily multi vitamin on top of dietary sources of vitamin A, D E and K as they can build up to toxic levels But if this does happen your doctor will tell you that the effect will wear off in a few days. So it is safest to not overload your body with foods fortified with the fat soluble vitamins and vitamins and minerals as well, or you could be doing yourself harm. Evidence is emerging after many years of large scale studies in the field of nutrition that levels of vitamin A are consistently low in people with lung cancer. In fact, having a low vitamin A level doubles the risk of cancer, according to nutritional research. Similarly a high intake of beta carotene from raw fruit and vegetables reduces the risk of lung cancer in non-smokers. Vitamin A also helps to maintain the integrity of the digestive tract, lungs, and all cell membranes, preventing viruses from entering the cell. The major antioxidants have a major protective effect on the cell against certain types of cancer. Ongoing trials on humans support researchers into nutritional therapy about how nutrients work in synergy to protect the body against certain types of cancer. Sooner this will be accepted by orthodox medicine. Nutritionists have also discovered that beta carotene which is converted into vitamin A inside the body is also anti-cancerous. A Japanese study of 265,000 people as recorded by Patrick Holford, found a significant correlation between low beta carotene intake levels and the incidence of lung cancer. Research by nutritional therapists reveals that the risk of lung cancer is the same for people who smoke and have a good antioxidant level as it is for non-smokers.

With a low antioxidant level obviously it is better not to smoke because smoking can cause other types of cancers such as mouth and throat cancer and there is no evidence of antioxidants being of any benefit for these types of cancers.

But good health is not all about having high levels of antioxidants in the body it is about a healthy diet from infancy. There is one world famous family who consistently have very low levels of coronary heart disease, cancer and disease in general, and that is The British Royal Family.

Their general good health and longevity could be very closely linked to the fact that they eat an organic diet. The Royals would not eat any type of convenience foods including packet or tinned. People would say 'But they can afford it, and they have their own chefs. This is true, it depends on how high up on your list of priorities you put your health.

Unfortunately a totally healthy diet especially for a large family can be expensive but eating out of fast food takeaways and eating convenience foods is not really any cheaper and a false economy. Even for wealthier people where a mother is working full-time they can be very often too exhausted after a long day's work to even cook a healthy diet. They often take the easy option and rely on convenience foods and takeaways. For a woman with children especially part-time work or job sharing really could be beneficial to their family because they would have more time and energy to cook a healthy diet. It is especially difficult for single mothers or fathers trying to balance a career, finances and looking after their health and the health of their children.

Vitamin A Deficiency

Night blindness is one of the earliest symptoms of Vitamin A deficiency to occur. As the deficiency gets worse the epithetical cells which produce mucus tend to lose their sticky secretions in the cells become hard (keratinised). So the protective effects of these cells are diminished and this sometimes lays the person more open to infectious diseases.

If the lining of the epithelium (one or more layers of closely packed cells governing the external and internal surfaces of the body varying in structure according to their function), in the respiratory tract is dry, it becomes cracked where bacteria lodges and colds take longer to clear up. As cells dry up cilia (any of the short threads projecting from the surface of a cell, e.g. lung cell); Vitamin A is an anti infectious vitamin and it helps to clear up infection very quickly. Small lumps of keratin tend to clog pores of the body especially on hands, arms and thighs. People with a severe Vitamin A deficiency don't have sweat evaporated from the skin surface due to clogged pores and the body temperature builds up.

Exerothelimia

Exerothelimia affects the epithelial tissue of the eye. This involves the cornea and the conjunctiva. If this dries up the surface of the eye, it becomes very itchy and dry. A lot of this is due to the lack of tears. The cornea begins to get cloudy but if the person is treated at this stage they can be cured. If not, treated ulceration of the cornea occurs. If this begins, the lens is perforated and blindness occurs.

In the foetus and early childhood, if there is a Vitamin A deficiency, this can affect the teeth. The enamel is often poor. The enamel of the teeth is the hardest epithelium in the body. If the enamel of the teeth is poor, later on in life, the teeth are more susceptible to decay. This is primary deficiency of Vitamin A but an overdose of Vitamin A is possible and is toxic.

Secondary deficiency of Vitamin A doesn't occur until after the stores of Vitamin A are depleted and is most often a disease of poverty.

In underdeveloped countries, the staple diet is lacking, beta carotene the main precursor of retinal Vitamin A; and even where these vegetables are available e.g. carrots, red peppers babies are not given them.

Dietary Sources of Vitamin

Vitamin A is commonly found in the following food: Sweet potatoes, carrots, watercress, peas, broccoli, cauliflower, mangoes, meat, melon, peppers, pumpkin, tomatoes, cabbage and squash.

Diet and nutrition are influenced by economic status as well as by gender, with the highest income groups tending to have the healthiest diets (Townsend et al 1988). In all age and gender groups, good dietary habits are influenced by income but so-called healthy balanced diets are more common among women than men (Blaxter 1990).

Research indicates a correlation between gender and social position, diet and health status.

"Married males have lower death rates than those who have never married, and married man report better health than single men do. This may be due to the presence or absence of a significant female carer encouraging her male partner to seek help when needed and setting the tone for a healthy life. (Miles 1991)

This is reflective of a happy relationship. But amongst unhappy women they can choose to ignore their husband's health problems, perhaps in order to acquire large amounts of property or money in marriages based on money especially which does happen and certainly did happen in the past.

The same is true for women. A woman's health can be good with the support of a reasonable husband. In unreasonable relationship for example where the man is perpetrating domestic violence and or alcoholism, a woman will generally be healthier single and vice versa.

People in work generally enjoy better physical and mental health than those who are unemployed. Unemployment increases the risk of illness and premature death. A middle aged man who loses his job is twice as likely to die in the next five years as a man who remains employed. (DoH 1999).

B Complex Discovery

The B vitamins are vital for optimum health. They are found in in many foods as part of a well balanced diet to achieve maximum mental performance such as in whole grains, pork, beef, peas, beans, lentils, brown rice, fish, eggs, bananas, avocados, and some green leafy vegetables. In other words, the B complex can be found as part of a well balanced diet. The only problem is if you are on a weight reduction diet, and you are reducing your food intake, you can find yourself lacking in these vital vitamins. The same is true if you are physically ill and you have lost your appetite. In these situations, a vicious circle can begin. A lack of the B complex can result in a deterioration in your mental health. This could include anxiety, depression, and in severe cases this can lead to symptoms such as confusion and mental deterioration.

This can lead to dependence on medication for depression and complications. Such medications can lead to weight gain which defeats the purpose of dieting. This is because prescribed medication for nervous disorders can slow down the metabolic rate, and even limited food intake cannot prevent weight gain. This is one of medicines biggest challenges today. Doctors especially psychiatrists know that in many cases their prescribed medication can often result in weight gain. But sadly scientists have not yet invented medication which does not cause drowsiness and weight gain. This unfortunately is one of the main causes of the obesity crisis. In addition, depression can lead to comfort eating which often leads to weight gain. Stress and anxiety can also result in over indulgence in alcohol which is also high in calories. As a nutritional consultant limiting high calorie foods and alcohol as well as taking regular exercise is the best advice if you wish to achieve weight control. It's a matter of putting theory into practice. It is advisable to take a good quality B complex supplement daily. In a short time, you should experience an improvement in your mental health especially if you are the type of person who has a history of any type of anxiety or depression. But if you are on any type of prescribed medication it is risky to stop it against medical advice. The danger of taking any kind of tranquilisers is that after a period of time they can become addictive. But if you take the B vitamins on top of prescribed medication they will not interfere with prescribed substances as the B vitamins are a natural organic material in origin. There are thirteen vitamins in the B complex. If you value your health it is not advisable to buy very cheap B vitamins. It is evident that cheap brands are often not high enough in strength to be effective. But after about a month taking the B complex along with a good quality multi vitamin daily you should find yourself in much better physical and mental health.

B Complex Vitamins

The B group of vitamins is a collection of essential nutrients that have certain characteristics in common.

Firstly, they are all water soluble, and secondly they are found in similar food sources such as Brewers Yeast, animal meats, wholegrain cereals and vegetable proteins.

There are certain people who are particularly susceptible to Vitamin B deficiency. These include:

- Alcoholics, partly because of their poor diet and partly because of the effects of alcohol upon Vitamin B metabolism.
- Those with poor dietary intakes. For example, those who eat a lot of junk food, or the elderly.
- Those with increased requirements, e.g. pregnant and breast feeding women, growing children and adolescents.
- Those on long term drugs such as anticonvulsants, certain antibiotics and oral contraceptives.
- Those with a psychiatric history. Deficiencies of Vitamin B1; B6, folic acid and Vitamin B12 are particularly likely.

A chronic deficiency of the B Vitamins may result in mental changes without there ever being any physical signs.

Vitamin B1 Thiamine

Although Vitamin B_1 was one of the first vitamins ever recognised, known for thousands of years. It was not until the late nineteenth and early twentieth century that it was recognised as having a dietary role.

In the Far East consumption of "polished" or refined rice often led to Vitamin B1 deficiency. In the Second World War many European prisoners of war, held in the Far East developed B1 deficiency termed Beri Beri (extreme weakness), was a term used to describe Vitamin B1 deficiency.

The function of Vitamin B1

Vitamin B_1 is mainly found in skeletal muscle, heart muscle, brain, kidney and liver. It plays a crucial part in energy production and carbohydrate metabolism. Deficiency results in rapid deterioration in both skeletal muscle function as well as brain and nerve function. The absorption of thiamine from the diet requires the presence of folic acid and deficiency of folic acid may result in a thiamine deficiency.

Substances which destroy thiamine are found in tea, coffee, certain raw fresh water fish, a number of fruits and vegetables including blackberries, blackcurrants, beetroot, spinach and cabbage.

Dietary Requirements

The requirements for thiamine depend upon calorie intake. With high carbohydrate sugar or alcohol intakes, the requirements rise.

Deficiency symptoms and signs

The body has very little in the way of Vitamin B_1 stores and a deficiency can occur within a few weeks if intake is substantially reduced. Initial symptoms include depression, irritability, failure to concentrate, and deterioration in memory. In severe deficiency states (usually caused by alcoholism mental confusion with marked deterioration of short term memory is a feature. Such people confuse fact with fantasy particularly when explaining recent events that they cannot remember accurately.

Food sources: Watercress, squash, courgette, lamb, asparagus, mushrooms, peas, lettuce, peppers, cauliflower, cabbage, tomatoes, brussel sprouts, beans.

Vitamin B2 riboflavin

Riboflavin Vitamin B2 was first discovered in the 1930s when it was isolated from yeast extract.

Vitamin B2 plays a crucial role in the formation of a number of enzymes mainly found in the liver.

These enzymes allow the removal of molecules of hydrogen and the introduction of oxygen. By this process certain substances are metabolised and energy is released.

Vitamin B2 riboflavin enhances the metabolism of Vitamin B6. This is why some people with Vitamin B2 deficiency have Vitamin B6 deficiency symptoms and signs as well.

Those who might best benefit from riboflavin

- children during growth spurts
- pregnant and breast feeding women.
- Those who consume moderate to large amounts of alcohol
- The elderly
- Women on the pill or oestrogen replacement therapy.

Food sources: mushrooms, watercress, cabbage, asparagus, broccoli, pumpkin, beansprouts, mackerel, milk, bamboo shoots, tomatoes, wheat germ.

Vitamin B3
Nicotinic Acid and Nicotinide

There are several forms of Vitamin B3 Nicotinic Acid (which is known as Niacin) is very closely related to the other compounds

Nicotinide and niacin amide. Nicotinic Acid has specific effects on cholesterol metabolism and it actually thought to lower cholesterol levels. Although Vitamin B3 was discovered in 1911, its full role as a vitamin was not known until 1937.

Deficiency of Vitamin B3 produces pellagra, a condition characterised by dermatitis, diarrhoea and dementia. Other symptoms of Vitamin B3 deficiency include lack of energy, insomnia, headaches or migraine, poor memory, anxiety or tension, depression, irritability, bleeding or tender gums, acne, eczema and dermatitis.

Like many other B vitamins B3 was first isolated from yeast. B3 deficiency is more likely to develop in those with a low protein intake particularly if they have a high alcohol consumption.

Vitamin B3 plays an important role in the transport of hydrogen and in this respect it is similar to Vitamin B2, riboflavin. The majority of enzymes helped by Vitamin B3 are involved in glucose and carbohydrate metabolism and B3 help balance blood sugar. Vitamin B3 is also essential for brain function.

Food sources

The most common sources of Vitamin 3 include meat (particularly beef), milk, fish, especially salmon, tuna and mackerel, mushrooms, chicken, turkey, asparagus, cabbage, lamb, tomatoes, courgettes, cauliflower and whole wheat

The recommended daily amount of Niacin for children is 5-10mg and 13-17mg for adults.

Those who might best benefit from Nicotinic acid include:

Those who have moderate or large intakes of alcohol.

Those with a poor protein intake

Those with thyrotoxicosis (overactive thyroid gland, Crohn's disease)

High doses may be helpful in reducing elevated blood fat levels, schizophrenia and arthritis.

But this needs medical supervision.

VITAMIN B5

Pantothenic Acid

Pantothenic acid is one of the lesser known B vitamins. It plays a crucial role in many of the reactions involving carbohydrates, fats and amino acids. It is essential for brain and nerve function, helps make anti stress hormones steroids and maintains healthy skin and hair.

Food sources are found in eggs, wholegrain cereals and meats. Deficiency is only found in extreme conditions. Symptoms include fatigue, headaches, weakness, emotional swings, improved muscle co ordination, numbness and tingling, muscle cramps, nausea, vomiting and abdominal cramps, exhaustion after light exercise, anxiety and tension.

Pyridoxine

Vitamin B6

Vitamin B6 plays a major part in the metabolism of protein and its constituent amino acids. Vitamin B6 requirements are very much related to protein consumption: the more protein we eat, the higher our requirement for Vitamin B6.

Vitamin B6 is also involved in sugar metabolism and the metabolism of essential fatty acids which play an important role in inflammatory diseases, skin diseases and disorders of the immune and cardiovascular system.

Food sources include most meats, fish, egg, yolk, wholegrain cereals, bananas, avocadoes, nuts, seeds and some green, leafy vegetables, lentils, red kidney beans, onions

Deficiency Symptoms and Signs

It must be remembered that as with all the B vitamin people usually complain of mental changes, nervousness, insomnia and weakness before skin problems and other visible signs appear. The commonest physical sign of Vitamin B6 deficiency is the development of dermatitis in the areas of the nose, corners of the eyes and mouth and the development of an acne like rash particularly on the forehead as well as depression or nervousness, irritability, muscle tremors or cramp, lack of energy, tingling hands and water retention

Those who might best benefit from pyridoxine include:

- Women on oestrogen containing oral contraceptives.
- Women on hormone replacement therapy
- Pregnant women for nausea
- Women who suffer from premenstrual syndrome.
- Breast feeding women
- People suffering from psychological problems e.g. depression, anxiety, schizophrenia, insomnia.
- Hyperactive or autistic children.
- People with kidney diseases; kidney stones, kidney failure, bladder cancer
- Diabetes
- Those with increased need e.g. alcoholics: those with poor nutritional intake.
- Sufferers from cardiovascular disease to prevent excessive clotting of the blood.

Vitamin B12

In the late 1920s it was found the serious and often fatal disease of pernicious anaemia responded when victims ate massive quantities of liver or had injections of liver extracts. Vitamin B12 was finally isolated in the 1950s and was found to be the agent effective in the treatment of pernicious anaemia.

Vitamin B12 is found only in animal based foods. It is originally produced by bacteria but is essential to man if he is to be healthy. Vitamin B12 in the diet is absorbed by the small intestine but requires the presence of a compound known as intrinsic factor, produced in the stomach.

Those deficient in Vitamin B12 often have anaemia with symptoms such as exhaustion, shortness of breath on exertion, pale skin and mucus membrane. A lack of Vitamin B12 can also affect mental functions and elderly, confused, depressed or mentally deteriorating individuals could be suspected to have Vitamin B12 deficiency. Pernicious anaemia tends to run in families, and also to be associated with blue eyes and premature greying of the hair.

Those who might best benefit from Vitamin B12

- Those with pernicious anaemia
- People who have had their stomachs removed
- Vegan, pregnant or breast feeding women
- Those with small bowel disease e.g. Crohn's Disease or those who have had part of the small bowel removed.
- Those with bacterial bowel overgrowth.
- People complaining of tiredness, irritability, anxiety or tension, lack of energy, constipation, tender or sore muscles, pale skin.

Where there is impaired absorption of Vitamin B12 from the gastrointestinal tract Vitamin B12 is generally given by injection. The usual dosage is 1mg given at weekly or three monthly intervals depending on the clinical situation.

Food sources include oysters, sardines, tuna, lamb, eggs, shrimp, turkey, chicken, and cheese.

FOLIC ACID

Folic Acid is another member of the B vitamins group. Different forms of folic acid, the folates are found in food. The metabolism of folic acid is closely linked with that of Vitamin B12 and is vital for the function of the central nervous system. Folic acid is absorbed from the diet mainly from the first part of the small intestine. It is then transported to the liver where it is metabolised and stored. The body has approximately three to six months store of folic acid.

The best sources of folic acid include liver, green vegetables, kidneys, eggs and wholegrain cereals, peanuts, hazelnuts, cashew nuts, walnuts, avocado.

Mild deficiencies of folic acid may be very common in the general population. Increased levels are recommended to women who wish to become pregnant.

Any woman who has had a child with spina bifida or other severe abnormality of the nervous system should consult her G.P. before trying for a baby again.

Only the more severe folic acid deficiencies show up as anaemia. Those with a lack or either folic acid or Vitamin B12 will eventually become anaemic, which result in symptoms such as lethargy, tiredness, shortness of breath on exertion and paler of the skin or mucus membrane, poor memory, lack of energy, poor appetite, stomach pains, depression.

Increased requirements occur

- during pregnancy
- during breast feeding
- in premature infants.

It appears that a folic acid deficiency is especially common in those with a psychiatric illness. Those who are depressed or even schizophrenic can be markedly deficient, and correcting the folic acid deficiency has been shown not only to improve the patient's mood, but also to reduce his or her stay in hospital.

Biotin

Biotin is one of the lesser known B vitamins. It is widely distributed in meats, dairy produce, and whole grain cereals. In adults a deficiency of biotin may cause the development of a scaly dermatitis, with weakness and tiredness. Severe cradle cap in infants can also be due to biotin deficiency.

Biotin is particularly important in childhood. It helps the body use essential fatty acids and it helps promote healthy skin, hair and nerves.

Deficiency of Biotin in the diet also produces poor hair condition, premature greying of hair, tender or sore muscles, poor appetite or nausea, eczema or dermatitis.

Food sources include cauliflower, lettuce, peas, tomatoes, oysters, grapefruit, watermelon, sweetcorn, cabbage, almonds, cherries, herrings, milk and eggs.

INTRODUCTION TO VITAMIN C

Vitamin C has a number of important roles. These include maintenance of healthy connective tissue. A deficiency often leads to bleeding and poor wound healing. Vitamin C is involved in the normal metabolism of cholesterol and the production of the hormone cortisol by the adrenal gland in the brain. Vitamin C is biochemically active in the production of collagen found in both skin and bones, and it has powerful effects upon pulse rate and blood pressure. It is a powerful antioxidant and can be used as a food preservative. It also has anti-bacterial and anti-viral properties.

Vitamin C

In 1971, there was a study done of the effects of acute Vitamin C deficiency. Prisoners volunteered to live on a diet deprived of Vitamin C for nearly three months. The symptoms which emerged were:

Tiredness, fatigue
Rough skin
Haemorrhaging hair follicles
Change in the gums
Pains in the joints
A loss of dental filling
More teeth decay
Low level of Vitamin C in blood and urine.

Acute Scurvy

Degeneration of the tissues:- skin, teeth, gums, vascular walls, bone cartilage and muscle.

What leads up to Scurvy or Aetiology of Scurvy

Scurvy results from a long intake of a diet which is devoid of fresh fruit and vegetables. But diets which are lacking in food sources of Vitamin C are also lacking in other nutrients such as iron and folate. Another factor which can affect use of Vitamin C in the body is "stress".

Treatment

If severe scurvy is diagnosed synthetic Vitamin C in large doses should be given. To saturate cells with Vitamin C and when all cells are saturated with Vitamin C, there will be about 5 grams of Vitamin C in the body.

About 250mg by mouth 4 times daily and the worst symptoms should be past in a week. The groups of people in this country most at risk of developing scurvy are infants and the elderly.

Early Symptoms include:-

Listlessness, fatigue, weakness, breathlessness, muscle cramp, aching bones and joints, poor appetite, dry skin, red and rough covered with tiny haemorrhages gums affected, swollen and bleeding.

In men with excessive beer consumption, scurvy developed when the normal Vitamin C reserves of 1500mg in the body dropped to 300mg or less. Then petechial haemorrhages started to appear after 29 days. By that time no Vitamin C was excreted in the urine. By 90 days all of the subjects were showing many of the signs of scurvy.

Intakes of 6.5mg, 66.5mg and 130mg were all tried and all were effective in reversing the symptoms.

Infantile scurvy is likely to happen after 5 – 6 months to 24 months of age. Children can take symptoms quickly and die quite quickly. Delayed or infrequent wound healing and anaemia is very often present.

In Western Society however, scurvy would only occur in some self-inflicted dietary restrictions. But all over the world infantile scurvy develops fairly quickly.

In human experiments the main feature of clinical scurvy is anaemia. A number of factors are involved in the development of this anaemia. If green leafy vegetables are the main source of Vitamin C, and a person is deprived of green leafy vegetables they will also be deprived of folic acid and will develop folic acid anaemia.

Vitamin C and Iron

Vitamin C is needed to change ferric iron into ferrous iron to be absorbed into the bloodstream. Vitamin C is also needed to get Fe (Iron) into the heam of haemoglobin (the red blood corpuscle) to be absorbed into the bloodstream.

Lack of Vitamin C results in iron deficiency anaemia. Vitamin C also affects the stability of the membranes of the red blood corpuscle. If there are haemorrhages anywhere, iron will be lost, due to Vitamin C deficiency.

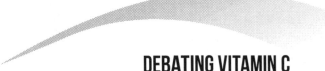

DEBATING VITAMIN C

The History of Vitamin C

Vitamin C, now known as Ascorbic Acid is a white crystalline simple sugar, which is water soluble. This means it cannot be stored in the liver and must be replaced daily in the diet.

Vitamin C is found naturally in fruits and vegetables, particularly citrus fruits and juice, blackcurrants, broccoli, cherries, kiwi fruit, mangoes, peppers, passion fruit, strawberries and green leafy vegetables.

Deficiency of Vitamin C is the cause of Scurvy. Ascorbic acid is widely distributed in the tissues of all plants and animals, with the notable exception of the dried seeds of cereals and pulses. Scurvy is not a disease that occurs in people on natural diets containing fresh foods.

Scurvy was classically a disease of sailors, as it frequently incapacitated the crews of sailing ships. It has a profound effect on the history of the colonization of the world by sea faring Europeans. When in 1497 Vasco Da Gama sailed round the Cape of Good Hope and established the first European Trading Colony on the coast of Malabar in India, 100 out of his crew of 160 men died of scurvy on the voyage. Although many sea captains, notably Jacques Cartier on a voyage in 1535 to Newfoundland, discovered the value of fresh fruits in the treatment and prevention of scurvy, it was not until about 1850 that scurvy ceased to occur in the merchant navies of the world. Scurvy has also determined the fate of many besieged cities.

Nowadays scurvy is uncommon but still an important disease. It is seen occasionally in socially deprived, mostly either old people living alone or people addicted to alcohol or other drugs, who live unsatisfactory diets containing no fresh foods. Outbreaks also occur in times of scarcity or famine in the populations of semi desert areas in Africa and Asia. In 1801 the Royal Navy insisted that every sailor got a daily ration of lemon juice. Fifty years later this was changed to lime juice. In 1865 this was extended to the British Navy.

In the 1920s Vitamin C was discovered to be the anti-scurvetic factor present in fruits and vegetables.

In 1928 Szent-Gyorgy had been studying natural reducing substances in Hopkins laboratory at Cambridge, and isolated ascorbic acid from the adrenal glands, oranges and cabbage leaves, but had not recognised its properties as a vitamin. But in 1932, Glen King who had started his work as a post graduate student in Sherman's laboratory in Columbia University completed his work in Hopkins laboratory at Cambridge and he identified Ascorbic Acid as Vitamin C.

A daily intake of 10mg of ascorbic acid is more than sufficient to prevent scurvy. Most people in Europe and North America get in their daily diet from three to ten times this amount.

Early symptoms of scurvy include tiredness, fatigue, rough skin, haemorrhagic hair follicles, and changes in the gums, pains in the joints, a loss of dental filling and more teeth decay.

Acute symptoms of scurvy include degeneration of the tissues including skin, teeth, gums, the vascular walls, bone, cartilage, and muscles.

Scurvy results from a long intake of a diet which is devoid of fresh fruit and vegetables. But diets which are lacking in food sources of

Vitamin C are also lacking in other nutrients such as iron and folate. Another factor which can affect use of Vitamin C in the body is "stress".

In the Western World scurvy would only occur in some self-inflicted dietary restrictions. Infantile scurvy occurs all over the world because it develops fairly rapidly. Very few animals get scurvy because most animals can make their own Vitamin C from glucose. Humans, bats and guinea pigs have to get a dietary source of Vitamin C as they cannot synthesise it from glucose.

There are many nutritionists who consider the high intakes of ascorbic acid are of benefit to health, and would reduce the prevalence of various diseases. It has been known for many years that Vitamin C is of benefit to health. Recent research shows that high intakes of Vitamin C are indeed of benefit to health.

Many Nutritionists believe that large doses of Vitamin C are of benefit in preventing and curing coughs and flus.

But this belief is not held by the medical profession.

Current research and knowledge is limited in that medical practitioners do not recognise that Vitamin C is of any benefit in preventing and curing colds and flu symptoms. Therefore Vitamin C is not widely used in society as it is not generally recognised as being of any benefit in the medical profession.

In the field of nutrition many documents have been written to say that Vitamin C supplements are of benefit to smokers "Taking daily vitamin supplements of 1000 milligrams won't cause any harm and may have some therapeutic effects. But it is difficult to measure the extent of these benefits. We know that Vitamin C is not a remedy for all diseases and will not cancel out the damage done by smoking. The best advice for smokers remains the same "quit".

Journal of American College of Nutrition (1999).

Reconciling the view of the medical field and that of the nutritional field to encourage doctors to accept that Vitamin C can really be of benefit to health is a difficult task.

"Some scientists believe your body's cells become saturated when Vitamin C supplementation reaches 1000 milligrams per day. Taking more than that could be like pouring water over an already saturated sponge, with the excess simply excreted in the urine.

(A case for Vitamin C copyright Weider Publications April 2000.)

The medical profession could indeed argue that this is true and that an excess of 100milligrams per day of Vitamin C is simply excreted in the urine.

There is therefore a great-deal of disagreement between the medical field and the nutritional field regarding the benefits of Vitamin C. Vitamin C in mega doses as a means of preventing the symptoms of cold and flu symptoms.is not a proven fact and is there disbelieved by orthodox medicine.

The fact that Vitamin C is a water soluble vitamin, and it needs to be replaced daily as it is not stored in the liver is a fact that is accepted within the medical profession.

But Vitamin C in mega doses administered before or after the appearance of cold or flu symptoms to relieve and prevent the symptoms of virus induced respiratory infections is not generally accepted by the medical profession. But the belief is strongly held by many nutritionists.

Considering that more people die of colds and flus in the Western World than of cancer, it is not safe to rely one hundred per cent on vitamin C as a cure for colds and especially flus even if this is claimed to be true by people who take vitamins to an extreme. Vitamin C on its own is one of the most harmless substances known on earth and it could have therapeutic benefits. If you have a cold or flu it wise to accept the doctor's cough medicine, antibiotics or the flu injection if it is recommended. Vitamin C will not interfere with pharmaceutical products. It is safe to take paracetemol in tablet form or in lemon drinks in addition to vitamin C if you have the cold or flu because vitamin C can only help speedy recovery in conjunction with what orthodox medicine recommends.

Prisoners engaged in an experiment, where they ate a diet totally devoid of vitamin C for nearly three months. The symptoms which emerged were:

- Tiredness, fatigue
- Rough skin
- Haemorrhaging hair follicles
- Change in the gums
- Pains in the joints
- A loss of dental filling
- More teeth decay
- Low level of Vitamin C in blood and urine.

Acute Scurvy

Degeneration of the tissues:- skin, teeth, gums, vascular walls, bone cartilage and muscle.

What leads up to Scurvy or Aetiology of Scurvy?

Scurvy results from a long intake of a diet which is devoid of fresh fruit and vegetables. But diets which are lacking in food sources of Vitamin C are also lacking in other nutrients such as iron and folate.

Another factor which can affect use of Vitamin C in the body is "stress".

Treatment

If severe scurvy is diagnosed synthetic Vitamin C in large doses should be given. To saturate cells with Vitamin C and when all cells are saturated with Vitamin C, there will be about 5 grams of Vitamin C in the body.

About 250mg by mouth 4 times daily and the worst symptoms should be past in a week. The groups of people in this country most at risk of developing scurvy are infants and the elderly.

Early Deficiency Symptoms include:-

Listlessness, fatigue, weakness, breathlessness, muscle cramp, aching bones and joints, poor appetite, dry skin, red and rough covered with tiny haemorrhages gums affected, swollen and bleeding.

In men with excessive beer consumption, scurvy developed when the normal Vitamin C reserves of 1500mg in the body dropped to 300mg or less. Then tiny haemorrhages on the surface of the skin started to appear after 29 days. By that time no Vitamin C was excreted in the urine. By 90 days all of the subjects were showing many of the signs of scurvy.

Intakes of 6.5mg, 66.5mg and 130mg were all tried and all were effective in reversing the symptoms.

Infantile scurvy is likely to happen after 5 – 6 months to 24 months of age. Children can take symptoms quickly and die quite quickly. Delayed or infrequent wound healing and anaemia is very often present.

In Western Society however, scurvy would only occur in some self-inflicted dietary restrictions. But all over the world infantile scurvy develops fairly quickly. As soon as infants are old enough to be spoon-fed usually at around three months of age they should be given fresh vegetables and fresh fruit mashed or pureed instead of packet food as it much higher in vitamins and minerals than packet food. This practice also educates an infant's palate so that they like the taste of fresh fruit and vegetables as they grow into adults. A typical drink which can be given to a small child is a smoothie which is rich in vitamin C. See recipes.

In human experiments the main feature of clinical scurvy is anaemia. A number of factors are involved in the development of this anaemia. If green leafy vegetables are the main source of Vitamin C, and a person is deprived of green leafy vegetables they will also be deprived of folic acid and will develop folic acid anaemia.

Vitamin C and Iron

Vitamin C is needed to change ferric iron into ferrous iron to be absorbed into the bloodstream. Vitamin C is also needed to get Fe (Iron) into the haem of haemoglobin (the red blood corpuscle) to be absorbed into the bloodstream.

The lack of Vitamin C results in iron deficiency anaemia. Vitamin C also affects the stability of the membrane of the red blood corpuscle. If there are haemorrhages anywhere, iron will be lost, due to Vitamin C deficiency.

Vitamin C: Fighting Infection.

There is a famous doctor of nutrition Dr Linus Pauling. His research has found that Vitamin C is important in the treatment and prevention of the common cold, which is a theory which is not accepted by orthodox medicine. But nutritionists claim that because the common cold kills more people than cancer each year in Britain, vitamin C can help prevent these deaths. Dr Pauling claims for the prevention of colds, doses in the region of 1-2g per day are needed when symptoms develop. There is no law against how much vitamin C anyone takes. A gram of vitamin C helps reduce the severity and incidences of colds. (P Holford 2000) It is claimed by nutritionists that when the body is high in vitamin C a virus cannot survive. Vitamin C is one of the least toxic substances known to man. With the onset of a cold taking vitamin C in conjunction with what the doctor recommends such as an antibiotic or a cough bottle could be beneficial according to some nutritionists. But this theory is disputed by most medical doctors as it is not a proven fact. For vulnerable groups who are advised to be administered the flu injection it is important to get this inoculation and taking a vitamin C supplement will do no harm. With the onset of a cold many people would not like taking vitamin C tablets, but they would be happy to take the juice of a lemon and lime with a teaspoonful of honey in hot water thus providing a natural source of vitamin, the juice of a fresh orange, a smoothie, or a good quality fruit juice.

Experiments done on whether Vitamin C really prevents colds show inconclusive results, but controlled studies show that some individuals benefit.

A number of other viral infections have been reported to respond to high doses of Vitamin C including measles, mumps, viral pneumonia, shingles and viral encephalitis. Again a lot of people would not wish to be heavily reliant on vitamin C tablets so it healthier to take fresh citrus fruits such as lemons, limes oranges and good quality fruit juices.

The Anti-ageing Properties of Vitamin C

The ageing process is thought to be due to Vitamin C deprivation itself, because poor diet or heavy smoking." In order to prevent and reverse arterial blockage, 1000mg vitamin C daily is thought that vitamin C helps to keep the arteries elastic making them flexible.

(P Holford 2000) Vitamin C is thought to reverse one of the major killers in the Western World, caused by hardening of the arteries or arterial disease.

Vitamin C is thought to prevent hardening of the arteries to the heart which can cause a heart attack, or myocardial infarction a stroke, a cardiovascular accident, hardening of the arteries in the brain which can lead to Alzheimer' s or possibly a thrombosis in the leg Holford claims that by increasing the elasticity of the major arteries in the body many of the major killers can possibly be prevented thus increasing the lifespan and leading to a longer healthier life. A daily supplement of 1000mg or a gram of vitamin C along with a good quality multi vitamin/mineral supplement can prevent many of today's killer diseases It is claimed that a healthy diet with, appropriate nutritional supplements, including vitamin C and regular exercise can defy the ageing process. Results are not instant. Patrick Holford maintains It can take a few years on a healthy diet and vitamin supplements before results are noticeable and the ageing process cannot be reversed only slowed down.

Scientifically this can only be done at a cellular level. The creams and lotions used on the skin are beneficial, especially to provide the skin with moisture But it is not the outer layer of the skin, the epidermis which determines health but the human body on a cellular level. The layer of skin underneath the epidermis called the dermis It consists mainly of collagen, interwoven with elastin which gives skin its elasticity and vitamin C is essential for the production of collagen which constitutes 70 per cent of the skin and 20 per cent of the entire body. The health of the skin also depends on other nutrients including vitamin A, E, selenium, and zinc. A lack of vitamin A can result in the over production of a protein called keratin which can result in dry, rough skin. Our skin is our natural outer clothing. A whole combination of nutrients determine the health of our skin, including essential fatty acids which provide natural moisture for the skin, and another major antioxidant, zinc which is needed for the production of new skin cells. (P Holford 2000) Women who spend a lot of money trying to maintain youthful skin would probably be interested in increasing their intake of vitamin C if it helps maintain beautiful skin. Beauty companies concentrate too much on putting creams on the epidermis of the skin but do not consider the significance of what you take into your body.

It is claimed by nutritionists that Vitamin C has many wonderful properties which prevent many killer diseases, and it is claimed to slow down the ageing process. Some of Holford's theories are accepted by some nutritionists.. But his theories are generally rejected by orthodox medicine mainly because Holford does not have any proof to back up his statements, and it all seems to be too wonderful to be true. However some people especially women believe that Vitamin C is good for their complexion and some women take the juice of a lemon and lime in hot or cold water every day instead of a Vitamin C tablet, and no doctor would criticise this as doctors recognise that any excess of Vitamin C is excreted daily in the urine, as it is a water soluble vitamin and it cannot be stored in the liver. It is right to put particular emphasis on Vitamin C but as most doctors would agree it is better for your health to obtain Vitamin C from natural sources such as citrus fruits and other fruits and vegetables, instead of a vitamin C tablet, Extra vitamin C is important for smokers as it is important for smokers as Vitamin C is depleted in smokers. It is wise to have Vitamin C in tablet form in the house in case you cannot get access to fresh Vitamin C every day. Otherwise it is best to take fresh vitamin C daily in the form of citrus fruit especially the juice of a lemon and lime.

Unfortunately for us in Britain and Ireland we don't have the cheap and varied access to citrus fruits and fruits and vegetable in general

.as they do in Mediterranean countries, and South East Australia Unfortunately for Northern Ireland and Scotland it has been recognised that we have the highest rate of coronary heart disease in the Western world. This is mainly because of a diet high in saturated fat, mainly food fried food. In contrast in Mediterranean countries they fry in olive oil, and their heart disease is much lower than in Northern Ireland and in Scotland

As Patrick Holford suggests, taking vitamin C and multivitamins are claimed by pharmacists and dieticians to be beneficial for health, but it is more important to look at our overall diet; in a holistic way

The Power of Antioxidants

It is at a cellular level that arterial damage and the ageing process can be prevented as suggested by Holford.. Oxygen is the basis of all plant and animal life and it is needed by every day to drive all biochemical processes which release energy from food. Oxygen is chemically reactive and very dangerous, and when unstable it is capable of oxidising other cells leading to cellular damage. These are known as free oxidising radicals, and they are the body's equivalent to nuclear waste. Free radicals are formed in all combustion processes including smoking, the burning of petrol which creates exhaust fumes, radiation from strong sunlight, sunbeds, frying or barbequing food. Chemicals capable of disarming free radicals are called the antioxidants. There are thousands of antioxidants, but the most common ones are found in essential nutrients. These include vitamin A beta-carotene, vitamin A and vitamin E.

The balance between your intake and exposure to free radicals may literally be the difference between life and death. You can tip the balance in favour of a long healthy life instead of possible death by making simple changes to your diet and lifestyle, and taking antioxidant supplements.

The ageing process cannot be reversed except temporarily with plastic surgery, but slowing down the ageing process is no longer a mystery. It is evident that the secret is to give the body the nutrition it needs from food and supplements and no more. The average man needs no more than 2500 calories per day and a woman no more than 2000 calories per day to maintain a healthy weight. A healthy diet should be low in saturated fat, salt, and sugar and high in fibre including plenty of fruit and vegetables. It is not an easy lifestyle if you wish to defy the ageing process. It requires hard work, sacrifice, dedication for life and giving up some of life's most enjoyed luxuries and taking a diet high in the antioxidants. This includes taking a generous amount of vitamin C and a multi vitamin –mineral daily on top of a healthy well balanced diet and regular exercise. It also involves limiting barbequing, sunbeds and avoiding strong sunlight.

By eliminating as many of these factors from your life which cause cellular damage from free radicals you will significantly be reducing damage to your body leading to

Cancer and arterial disease. It is claimed that antioxidants prevent:

Arterial damage
High blood pressure
Premature ageing
Myocardial infarction or a heart attack
A cardio vascular accident or a stroke
Alzheimer's disease
Cellular inflammation
(P Holford 2000)

The faculty of Health Promotion in the Open University substantiates some of these claims that: "Diet is a significant factor in determining health status (Blaxter 1990). Despite major health promotion campaigns demonstrating the link between inappropriate diet and most of the major diseases, for example cancers and heart disease, it is women who are making the most effort to change their diets. The Oxford Regional Health Authority Lifestyle Survey of 13,000 randomly selected adults living in Berkshire, Buckinghamshire and Northamptonshire provides helpful data relating to exercise, smoking, alcohol consumption and dietary habits (Roberts 1992). More female than male respondents described their health status as poor, although they reported fewer examples of health damaging behaviour.

The antioxidants particularly vitamin C are thought to prevent arterial blockage by keeping the arteries elasticated, basically cheating one of the main causes of heart disease, hardening of the arteries. For double protection drink about four glasses of red wine in the week to thin the blood. The French consume a lot of red wine and it is recognised by orthodox medicine that they have the lowest incidence of heart disease in the world even though they smoke as much as anywhere else in the Western World, and it is thought to be because they drink and often cook with red wine So in other words whether you smoke or not, if you eat a healthy diet, take vitamin C, and drink red wine, you are substantially reducing the risk of heart disease. Cheating hardening of the arteries, which happens naturally with age, known as arteriosclerosis. could be possible with a combination of a small quantity of red wine in the week and vitamin C preferably in its natural form concentrated particularly in citrus fruits. The juice of a lemon and lime in hot or cold water sweetened with a little honey is a healthy drink no doctor would criticize, Arteriosclerosis is not to be confused with atherosclerosis; the formation of fatty deposits inside of the artery walls in the presence of thick blood. One of our most lethal killers heart disease is preventable with a few changes in lifestyle. High blood pressure, caused by a combination of atherosclerosis, and thick blood can all raise blood pressure, putting you at greater risk of a thrombosis, angina, a heart attack or a stroke. Is also preventable with changes to the diet, especially by lowering the amount of salt in the diet, as it increases the amount of pressure on the heart muscle. According to Patrick Holford has also created an argument that increasing the dietary intake of magnesium, calcium and potassium in the diet and in the form of multivitamins can reduce muscular pressure on the heart. But most medical doctors would tend to disagree that simply taking a multi vitamin could make this possible.

Conventionally aspirin was used to lower blood pressure by thinning the blood, by reducing the risk of a heart attack by 20 per cent. But now vitamin E is considered to be four times more effective along with omega 3 fish oils as discovered in 1993 in

Cambridge University Medical School by Professor Morris Brown who discovered this finding.

Antioxidant protection is also thought to be proactive against at least some of the thousands of carcinogens. At least 75 per cent of cancers are thought to be associated with lifestyle including diet, smoking and alcohol consumption. Radiation and ultraviolet light, mainly from exposure to sunlight and sunbeds, environmental pollution food additives and drugs are thought to be additional carcinogenic risk factors by Patrick Holford. Orthodox Medicine would once again question his theories.

Vitamin C along with the other major antioxidants is thought once again by Holford to be very important as key player in the prevention of many killer diseases and is the key to achieving a long healthy life for many people. This diet therapy should be started as early in life as possible. Many parents give vitamins to their children and then stop this practice when they reach the teenage years. But vitamins and minerals are important for maintaining good health for all ages and should be started as young as possible.

Not just the Medical profession but many disciples allied to medicine such as pharmacy and human nutrition and dietetics and also many members of the general public would not take Patrick Holford's theories at face value and certainly not those in Government circles.

As a nutritional advisor an analytical approach indicates that at least some of what he says could be true, and some people would give him the benefit of the doubt. But in general it seems to be quite unbelievable that a vitamin C tablet could be the solution of killer diseases such as cancer and arterial disease.

The problem is that Patrick Holford's theories have not gone through clinical trials to prove conclusively if there is any truth in his claims about the benefits of vitamin C. At the minute his theories are futuristic. Clinical trials need to be done over a period of several decades to prove or disprove his theories. But vitamin C supplements are harmless, as it is water soluble and any excess is excreted in the urine. It is true that vitamin C is necessary on a daily basis, as it cannot be stored in the liver. No doctor pharmacist, dietician or other health professional would criticize taking vitamin C in the form of fresh citrus fruits but they would not recommend people to become heavily reliant on vitamin C in tablet form.

Patrick Holford's central ethos is essentially preventative medicine. His views are highly controversial. But if taking a multivitamin daily and other supplements of your choice plus generous amounts of vitamin C, this can only achieve a high nutritional status. If you can achieve total nutrition, it is sensible for people in good health to increase their nutritional status as a preventative measure prior to taking a heart attack or a stroke, high blood pressure or cancer instead of afterwards. In other words prevention is better than cure.

VITAMIN D

The scientific name for Vitamin D is cholecadciferol. It is widely accepted that Vitamin D is essential for normal calcium metabolism.

Vitamin D is said to be a vitamin as used to be thought that trace quantities were required in the diet. However, in people who are exposed to adequate amounts of sunlight, oral intake of Vitamin D is not needed to be taken as Vitamin D is synthesised naturally in the skin.

In less sunny regions of the world with decreased amounts of light, oral intake of Vitamin D is necessary. Eskimos are an exception. They still have medium – dark coloured skin, but their diet is very high in Vitamin D from fish oils.

Unlike other nationalities it is unnecessary for Eskimos to lose their skin pigmentation in order to maintain Vitamin D as they get enough Vitamin D in their diet.

Vitamin D has its main effects in bone and calcium metabolism.

Vitamin D is necessary

1. In the absorption of calcium and phosphate from the food we eat.
2. In the calcification of newly formed bone which is present at the growing ends of the bones in children and teenagers.

3. In kidney metabolism Vitamin D enhances the re absorption of calcium and phosphate from the urine so that it is not lost in the urine.

4. In bone marrow replacement the presence of Vitamin D appears to encourage the replacement of bone marrow tissues by fibrous tissue and the development of anaemia. This occurs in some children with rickets.

<hr>

Food sources of Vitamin D

The dietary sources of Vitamin D include fatty fish, cod-liver oil, eggs, milk, butter, cheese, halibut liver oil and food to which Vitamin D is added. In the UK vitamins A and D must by law be added to margarine.

Recommended daily intakes of Vitamin D

15.10µg for infants
and 2.5µg for adults and the rest is to be attained from sunlight

Vitamin D deficiency signs and symptoms.

Deficiency of Vitamin D depends upon the age of the individual involved and involves changes to the skeleton as a result of a loss of calcium.

Rickets is a disease which involves defective bone formation due to an inadequate deposition of calcium and phosphate in the bone. Where there is low calcium and phosphate plasma levels, new bone and cartilage won't mineralise and deformities in the skeleton develop. It affects young children and infants during the growing stage.

More energy is needed to produce Vitamin D in dark skinned people in Europe and Scandinavia in order for them to adapt to the climate. This may be the reason why Asians in Britain are more prone to rickets than white people.

Symptoms of rickets

Rickets (mainly seen in children)

Infants

1. bowed legs, due to child having to bear weight on poorly formed legs
2. chest and spinal deformities
3. softening of the skull bones
4. thickening of the top of the skull
5. delayed development of movements

Adolescent rickets

1. aching legs
2. swelling at the end of long bones
3. knee aches and pains
4. poor growth

Osteomalecia (mainly seen in adults)

1. bone pain
2. bone tenderness
3. weakness of certain bones especially the muscles attached to the hip bone meaning difficulty in getting out of a chair or climbing stairs.

Why does Adult Rickets occur?

Some Asian women develop adult rickets (osteomalacia) because of a lack of Vitamin D from sunshine as they are covered up so much by robes, and because of their diet.

Why are Asian women affected?

Asian women eat a vegetarian diet with no meat, fish or eggs. Others eat little meat with much chapatti and vegetables. Some go outside very little and avoid exposing their skin to the sun.

How can Adult Rickets be prevented?

By taking one tablet of Vitamin D daily if possible before breakfast. There is no need to change your diet.

Those who might benefit from Vitamin D include:
1. those who are exposed to little or no sunlight
2. the elderly
3. those who live in industrial urban communities
4. people living in institutions
5. dark skinned people living in a northern climate
6. Those who have a dietary deficiency of Vitamin D and calcium (e.g. vegetarians, Asian immigrants and Rastafarian).
7. those who do not absorb Vitamin D or calcium
8. Patients on long term drugs for epilepsy.

Toxicity of Vitamin D

Too much Vitamin D produces marked elevations in blood calcium levels. Symptoms of feeling generally unwell, drowsiness, abdominal pain, increased thirst, constipation and loss of appetite. In the long term it can cause calcification of the soft tissues, kidney damage and kidney stones. In severe cases it can be treated by taking steroids.

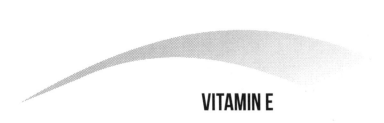

VITAMIN E

The existence of Vitamin E was discovered in 1922. About eight closely related substances known as tocopherols is known. Tocopherol comes from Greek meaning "to bear children", i.e. tocos childbirth and phoro to bring forth. Components of Vitamin E are light yellow in colour, heat stable and stable to acids and visible light. They are sensitive to alkalis, oxidation and ultraviolet light but is not destroyed by cooking temperatures. All tocopherols are anti oxidants, so they unite with oxygen within and outside the body.

Vitamin E is an essential nutrient for dogs, guinea pigs, rabbits, monkeys, young pigs, chickens, turkeys and rats. Results of deficiencies for them is known, e.g. rats fed on a highly purified diet of adequate energy value containing enough protein, minerals and vitamins, but totally lacking in vegetable fats containing Vitamin E these appear to grow and thrive tolerably well but they fail to reproduce.

The males become sterile and if the females do become pregnant, they tend to suffer spontaneous abortions and lose their young. It was probably due to this fact that Vitamin E was at one time known as the anti-sterility vitamin. Human reproduction is unlikely to be affected by a Vitamin E deficiency.

Functions

Vitamin E is an antioxidant and protects cells from damage, including against cancer. It also helps the body to use oxygen, preventing blood clots thrombosis and atherosclerosis. It improves healing and fertility as well as being good for the skin.

Deficiency signs include:

Lack of sex drive exhaustion, exhaustion after light exercise, easy bruising, slow would healing, varicose veins, loss of muscle tone and infertility. Diseases of the stomach, pancreas and liver can produce a Vitamin E deficiency just like other fat-soluble vitamins A, D, F and K as fat soluble vitamins are stored in the liver.

Living tissues are particularly sensitive to the damaging effects of oxygen and other oxidizing substances called Free Radicals which can seriously damage the structure of cell membranes as well as the contents of living cells; accelerated damage may lead to cell death. Vitamin E helps protect cells from this kind of damage.

It is now becoming evident that Free Radical reactions are responsible for such diverse physiological processes such as inflammation, ageing, drug induced damage, regenerative arthritis, alterations in immunity, cancer and cardiovascular disease.

Tipping the balance concerning how you may live a longer healthier life or die young depends very much on the levels of antioxidants in your blood. So far over a hundred antioxidant nutrients have been discovered. The most important are vitamins A, C and E, plus beta carotene, the precursor of vitamin A. Already large scale survey shows that the risk of death is substantially reduced in those with high levels of antioxidants in the blood including high dietary intakes or in the form of supplements.

Conversely, a low level of vitamin E is associated with Alzheimer's disease. Vitamin E supplements also reduce the risk of developing cataracts compared to those with high levels in the blood.

Vitamin C and E are powerful antioxidants combined working in synergy with each other, so that both vitamins work to their maximum potential. Supplementing vitamins C and E can actually reduce the risk of having a heart attack by up to 50%. (Holford. P 2000)

Vitamin A in the form of beta carotene has also been discovered to lower the risk of a heart attack by 40%. The risk of death from cardiovascular disease is substantially reduced by combining the major antioxidants, vitamins A, C and E On top of a healthy diet, it is best to take supplements in tablet form as you are guaranteed to get your RDA, recommended daily allowance, It is dangerous to take other food supplements highly fortified with especially vitamins A, D, E F and K as these vitamins are stored in the liver. An overdose of these fat soluble vitamins can be toxic and make you feel very ill.

Supplementing 1000mg of vitamin C has also been discovered to lower blood pressure. The essential antioxidant vitamins are found in red, orange and yellow coloured fruits and vegetables. The vitamins are rapidly destroyed during cooking especially during frying at high temperatures. Try to steam, not boil or fry vegetables such as carrots, broccoli, peppers, peas, cauliflower and cabbage are abundant sources of major antioxidants. Another great food is watermelon. The flesh is high in beta carotene and Vitamin C, while the seeds are high in Vitamin E, and the antioxidant minerals zinc and selenium. There are virtually no calories in watermelon, and it is a great diet food.

Try not to eat crisps, the highest calorie food on the market with an alcoholic drink. Eat any type of nuts instead; they are a good source of Vitamin E.

The suggested Optimal Allowance of Vitamin E is 70mg for children and 90-800mg for adults. For maximum antioxidant protection take 400-800mg per day. Well rounded nutrition, including generous amounts of Vitamin C and E can contribute substantially to extending the lifespan of those who are already middle-aged.

A ten-year study of eleven thousand people in 1996 found that a combination of Vitamin C and E halved the overall risk of death from all cancers and heart disease.

Vitamin E is a powerful anti cancer agent especially in combination with selenium. High blood levels of Vitamin E are associated with a significant reduction in the risk of developing cancer, while low levels of Vitamin E and selenium increase the risk of cancer by ten times.

In conjunction with selenium and zinc, Vitamin E increases the efficiency of the immune system. Hormonal imbalances including premenstrual syndrome and menopausal symptoms can be helped with Vitamin E as it is thought to protect the oxidation of essential and prostaglandins.

Vitamin E is best taken in synergy with the other major antioxidants especially Vitamin C.

To make sure you are taking your recommended daily allowances it best to supplement with all the major Vitamins A, B, C, D and F, but it is not necessary to supplement with Vitamin K as there is enough of it in the diet. It is also best to take a good multi-vitamin mineral supplement on top of a healthy diet to ensure optimum health. (Holford. P 2000)

Best Food Sources:

The range of sources is wide. Wheatgerm oil is one of the richest natural sources. Other good sources are: salad oils, polyunsaturated fats, margarines, whole grains, nuts and seeds especially peanuts or peanut butter, sunflower seeds, liver, egg yolk, meat, whole milk and butter. Seeds, nuts, tuna, mackerel and salmon are also good sources of Vitamin E.

Helpers:

Works well with Vitamin E and selenium.

Robbers:

High temperature cooking, especially frying, air pollution, birth control pills, and excessive intake of refined or processed fats and oils reduce the absorption of Vitamin E.

Vitamin E has anticoagulant properties. A very high Vitamin E intake may slow the blood clotting rate and this could be dangerous in some instances. Haemorrhaging is known to happen when excess Vitamin E coincides with a Vitamin K deficiency.

Diseases of the stomach, pancreas and liver can produce a Vitamin E deficiency, just like deficiencies of other fat-soluble vitamins A, D and K, as fat soluble vitamins are stored in the liver.

Vitamin E Sources

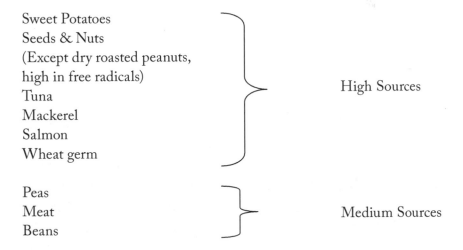

Sweet Potatoes
Seeds & Nuts
(Except dry roasted peanuts,
high in free radicals)
Tuna
Mackerel
Salmon
Wheat germ
} High Sources

Peas
Meat
Beans
} Medium Sources

ESSENTIAL FATTY ACIDS – VITAMIN F

Low Fat Diets

Low fat or even no fat diets have become increasingly more popular and media attention focuses on the danger of high fat intake and the apparent benefits of those trying to lose weight. However, have you ever considered that there might be such a thing as good fat?

Good Fats

Good fats, or essential fatty acids as they are technically known, are an important part of a healthy diet. They are found in fish, nuts, seeds and their cold pressed oils. It can be difficult to achieve the minimum requirement of essential fatty acids through diet, particularly those people who are not eating nuts, seeds and fish on a regular basis. In this situation it may be advisable to use supplements to compensate for low dietary intake.

Groups of essential fatty acids

Essential fatty acids play an important role in the health of the nervous system, immune system, skin, brain and have an anti inflammatory action as well as helping to improve metabolic rate, an action that could actually help with weight loss! Essential fats are also vital for hormone balance and there is also evidence to suggest that supplementing with Omega 3 fatty acids may be helpful in the prevention of cardiovascular disease, a major killer in Western Society.

Supplementation

Supplements of essential fatty acids are available as fish oil and linseed oil capsules to provide mainly Omega 3 fatty acids and evening primrose, borage and sunflower oil capsules to provide mainly Omega 6 fatty acids. There are also combination products which provide both Omega 3 and Omega 6 and Omega 9 fatty acids in one capsule. Omega 9 can easily be found by cooking with olive oil.

When supplementing with essential fatty acids it may be advisable to increase anti oxidant intake. The antioxidant nutrients include Vitamins A, C, E, and minerals selenium and zinc. These nutrients help to protect essential fatty acids from oxidation, a process where fatty acids are damaged by the effects of oxygen. Oxidised fats are potentially harmful to the body in the absence of sufficient antioxidants. A good overall vitamin and mineral supplement should mean that there will not be a deficiency of the antioxidants, as well as a daily supplement of Vitamin C as it is water soluble, cannot be stored in the liver, and must be replaced daily in the diet.

Sources of Essential Fatty Acids

Fat contains the essential fatty acids (EFAs) Omega 3 group linoleic acid, Omega 6 group linoleic acid and Omega 9 oleic acid group.

The essential fatty acids are specific types of polyunsaturated fats that can only be obtained from the diet.

Good dietary sources of Omega 3 are oily fish such as salmon, mackerel, herring, tuna and sardines. It is present in human breast milk and small amounts are found in green leafy vegetables and rapeseed, canola oils and avocadoes. Functions in the body include nervous system and retina development in young infants. It maintains the structure of the cell walls and plays a role in controlling of high cholesterol levels.

Good dietary sources of Omega 6, linoleic acid are plant seed oils, e.g. sunflower, safflower, soya, corn maize oils and Evening Primrose Oil.

The Omega 6 family also plays an important part in the structural role in all the cell membranes and have a cholesterol lowering effect; as well as a blood thinning effect at high intakes. It is converted to hormone like compounds called prostaglandins, some of which can benefit immune health, hormone health, skin health, blood pressure and platelet aggregation ("clumping") and pre menstrual syndrome.

The Omega 9 family is an important group of monounsaturated fatty acids, which include the fatty acid oleic acid.

Olive oil contains about 70 percent oleic acid. It is also found in rapeseed, canola and nut seed oil. Rapeseed oil was discovered, is grown, and is manufactured in Ireland. It is high in oleic acid and it is a monounsaturated fat. It contributes to reducing the rate of heart disease but it is not know internationally. According to the Department of Health up to 12 percent of total calories should come from monounsaturates. It is important to change cooking oil after using more than 3 times, or else healthy monounsaturated and polyunsaturated oils break down chemically to dangerous saturated fats, which can cause heart disease.

Research has shown that there appears to be a link between a high dietary intake of oleic acid with reduced levels of LDL blood cholesterol. This is one of the reasons for encouraging people to follow the "Mediterranean type" diet consisting of high levels of olive oil and anti oxidant rich fresh fruit and vegetables. Reduced rates of heart disease and other diseases are associated with this type of diet.

Research shows that LDL (low density lipoprotein) if found in large proportions in an individual's cholesterol is likely to be deposited in the artery walls. So the lower the LDL levels, the healthier the heart will be.

High density lipoprotein (HDL) has a beneficial effect. It can transport cholesterol out of the arteries, and back to the liver.

1. Source of Energy

Fat serves as a concentrated source of energy.

1g fat provides 9 kcal (37kj)

For women with an average intake of 8100kj per day, 35 percent of food energy intake would be:

35/100 x 8100 = 2835kj

Since 37kj are provided by 1g of fat, 2835kj are provided by:

2835/37 = 76g of fat

Therefore to meet COMA (Committee on Medical Aspects of Food and Nutrition Policy) recommendations total fat intake should average around 76/day for women. For a group of men with daily intakes of 10,600kj the average fat intake should be 100g/day.

2. Satiety Value

Fat tends to leave the stomach relatively slowly being released approximately three and a half hours after digestion. This delay in the emptying time of the stomach helps to delay the onset of hunger pangs and contributes to a feeling of satiety after a meal. The presence of fat on the duodenum stimulates the release of a hormone in the stomach, which in turn inhibits hunger contractions.

3. Fat Soluble Vitamins

Fat is therefore necessary for the absorption of the Vitamins A, D, E, F and K.

4. Sources of Essential Fatty Acids

Fat contains the essential fatty acids (EFAs) Omega 3, group linoleic acid, Omega 6 group linoleic acid and Omega 9 oleic acid group known as Vitamin F. The essential fatty acids are specific types of polyunsaturated fats that can only be obtained from the diet.

1. It is important to note that on a weight reduction diet there is no need to worry about losing essential fatty acids while losing fat. It is always the non-essential fatty acids which are used up first. But it is still necessary to keep topping up on essential fatty acids from the diet as EFAs cannot be synthesised in the body.

2. The COMA Committee have made recommendations about the percentage of energy provided by the various types of fatty acids.

Monounsaturated Fatty Acids	12%
Polyunsaturated Fatty Acids	1% minimum and
Linoleic Acid	0.2% minimum
Trans Fatty Acids	2%
Saturated Fatty Acids	10%

3. According to the COMA report it is ok to take 2 percent of the fat intake from the trans fatty acids. But Patrick Holford disagrees. He claims that because refining and processing vegetable oils changes the nature of any unsaturated oil,

for example in making margarine turning it into a hard fat through a process called hydrogenation. Holford claims that although the fat is still technically polyunsaturated the body can not make use of it. Even worse, it blocks the body's ability to use healthy polyunsaturated oils. This kind of fat is called a trans fat because its nature has been changed. Most margarines contain these so-called hydrogenated polyunsaturated oils. It is best to use a small amount of butter skimmed on bread or toast and to fry in olive oil.

4. The amount of fat in foods is often shown on food labels; in many cases there is also information about the saturated fatty acid (saturates) content in food. Most people in the UK eat more total fat and more saturated fat than COMA recommend.

There are many ways to reduce the total amount of fat in the diet:

- Use lower fat meats, e.g. chicken (without skin) and lean cuts of meat
- Use less fat in cooking and use low fat spreads for bread
- Grill and bake foods instead of frying and roasting.

To reduce the amount of saturated fatty acids in the diet, lower fat options should be chosen and fats richer in polyunsaturated fatty acids (e.g. sunflower oil, corn oil) should sometimes be used as substitutes.

5. Insulation

Deposits of fat beneath the skin (subcutaneous fat) serve as insulating materials so that the body is protected against shock e.g. in a car accident and from changes in environmental temperatures.

6. Food Sources of Fat

The percentages of calories contributed by fat tends to be relatively high in most animal foods e.g. whole milk has 3.2% fat which means 53% of the calories in whole milk come from the fat.

Ordinary cheddar cheese has 32% fat which means 68% of the calories in cheddar cheese come from fat.

Vegetable foods contain less fat. Wholegrain cereals have from 2% to 9% fat mainly in the germ.

7. The contribution of fat made by different foods to the diet as a whole depends both on the amount of any particular food eaten and the percentage of fat in the food.

The total amount of fat that people eat depends to some extent on their wealth. In richer countries and by more prosperous people, more fat is eaten than poorer people.

So a well balanced diet not too high in fat, sugar, salt, as low in these as possible and a diet high in fibre i.e. fresh fruit and vegetables, is recommended by the National Advisory Committee for Nutritional Education i.e. the N.A.C.N.E. Report 1983.

8. The essential fatty acids are needed for normal growth and behaviour and help with healthy cell membranes, a well balanced hormone level and a properly working immune system.

9. They are essential for the synthesis of tissue lipids (fats), play an important role in the regulation of cholesterol levels and are precursors of prostaglandins. These are hormone like

compounds which produce various metabolic reactions in tissues.

10. The essential fatty acids are important for the health of the skin bringing suppleness and a youthful appearance. Hair becomes shinier when the essential fatty acids, vitamin F are in good supply. Vitamin F is also important in the manufacture of sex and adrenal hormones. It also stimulates the growth of the beneficial intestinal bacteria.

11. Arthritis is said to benefit from Vitamin F and it also aids in the transmission of nerve impulses. A shortage of Vitamin F may lead to learning disabilities and poor memory.

Deficiency Symptoms

One obvious sign of Essential Fatty Acid or Vitamin F deficiency is dry skin. If Vitamin F is sufficient then the skin on the back of the hand should feel moist and when pinched should quickly return to normal. Hair loss and eczema may be a result of Vitamin F deficiency and may cause damage to the kidneys, heart and liver. Behavioural disturbances are also noted if there is a deficiency of Vitamin F. There is also evidence that the immune system can become less efficient with resultant slow wound healing and susceptibility to infections. Tear glands may also not work effectively and may dry up. With Vitamin F deficiency blood pressure and cholesterol levels may be higher and blood is more likely to form clots.

It is best to combine The Essential Fatty Acid with a good multivitamin containing Vitamin A, B3, B6, E, zinc, magnesium and selenium and 1000mg of Vitamin C daily. Omega 3, Omega 6 and Omega 9 are now available in a single capsule. But it is best to find dietary sources.

Dosage

The recommended Dietary allowance (RDA) is the minimum that you require per day, to avoid serious deficiency of this particular nutrient.

In therapeutic use of this nutrient the dosage is usually increased considerably, but the toxicity level must be kept in mind.

To prevent deficiency the required intake of essential fatty acids lies within a range of 1 to 2 percent of total calories although supplementation suggest 10 – 20 percent.

Toxicity and symptoms of High Intake

Toxicity has not been determined. Toxicity does not seem a problem but consult your doctor before adding fatty acid supplementation if you have a medical condition.

When more EFAs may be needed.

People who are overweight, obese, clinically or morbidly obese, have dry eyes, bruise easily and have frequent infections may consider increasing their intake of essential fatty acids, as well as those on a low fat diet or with dry skin, dandruff or brittle nails.

Vitamin F is sensitive to heat and air. Heating fatty acids can result in free radicals being formed.

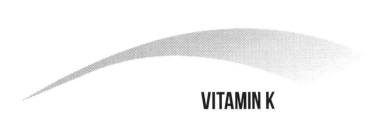

VITAMIN K

Vitamin K was first discovered in 1934 by a Danish Scientist who identified it as the fat soluble factor necessary for the coagulation of the blood. The Danish word for this process is KOAGULATION, so the factor was called Vitamin K, and was isolated in 1939.

Vitamin K is used to designate a group of substances belonging to a chemical group known as quinones.

Like the other fat soluble vitamins, vitamin K has a number of forms some is found in food and the remainder is synthesised by the bacterial flora in the human intestinal tract. It is toxic in large amounts.

Vitamin K is a fat soluble vitamin and is insoluble in water, stable to heat and reducing agents. It is prone to chemical change regarding alkalis, oxidising agents, strong acids and light.

Sources

In the diet, vitamin K is found in green leaves e.g. cabbage, broccoli, lettuce, green tea as well as egg yolk, soya bean oil, liver, cauliflower and tomatoes. Cows milk is also a source of vitamin K and is a richer source than human milk", and the remainder is synthesised by micro organisms in the intestinal tract. For absorption bile salts are necessary to store vitamin K in the liver.

Vitamin K has one major function, the synthesis of the enzyme prothrombin which is synthesised by the liver and is required for the clotting of blood.

Much of the intestinal synthesis occurs in the lower intestine and only a small portion of what is synthesised may actually be absorbed.

Deficiency of Vitamin K is manifested by a prolonged blood clotting time and the increased incidence of haemorrhage.

Vitamins and Surgery

In order to come through major surgery with minimum physical pain, and to achieve a speedy recovery it is best to be in a high nutritional status. In order to be in the peak of physical and mental health before an operation, three months prior to surgery it is advisable to take a cocktail of vitamins to be in the peak of physical and mental health. These vitamins include:

1. Vitamin B complex daily.
2. 1000mg vitamin C daily.
3. 1000mg cod liver oil once a week.
4. 1000mg omega 3 fish oil once a week
5. 500mg evening primrose oil once a week.
6. 1 multi-vitamin multi-mineral tablet daily.

After surgery

Take the above vitamins along with a capsule of zinc with vitamin C to speed up wound healing.

Recovery from surgery is speedy in people who are in a high nutritional status prior to surgery.

If you don't believe this theory or you do not have the money to buy vitamin supplements there is a general theme through this book of a cheap nutritious food which has caused much debate and controversy in orthodox medicine in recent decades

This food is the humble egg, a hen's egg, a duck's egg or a goose egg, whichever you prefer. The reason is if you look at the consistent number of times the egg yolk is identified as containing many vitamins and minerals, eggs are obviously a cheap nutritious food and is often used in baking, as well as eaten boiled, scrambled, poached, fried or in an omelette.

But orthodox medicine does not recommend that you eat more than six eggs per week as for many decades it was believed that eggs cause high cholesterol. This theory is now disproven by some nutritionists but to be cautious it is better not to eat more than six eggs per week preferably organic eggs which are also a good source of protein.

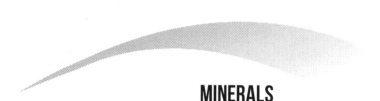

MINERALS

What are minerals?

Minerals are inorganic substances required by the body for a variety of functions such as:

- Formation of bones and teeth; essential constituents of body fluids and tissues; components of enzymes and nerve function.

Some minerals are needed in larger amounts than others, e.g. calcium, phosphorous, magnesium, sodium, potassium and chlorine. Others are required in smaller quantities and are called trace minerals e.g. iron, zinc, iodine, fluoride, selenium and copper. Despite being required in smaller amounts trace minerals are no less important than other minerals.

Different foods supply different amounts of most minerals for healthy people. In the UK, iron and calcium intakes are gradually decreasing, but most people don't show signs of deficiency. Some adolescent girls and women of child bearing age may be deficient in iron, and this may have implications for their future health. There is also concern about the calcium intake of some adolescent girls and young women.

IRON

The adult body contains about 4 grammes of iron, about the same as a 3" inch nail. It is the most important mineral element because it enables us to take the oxygen from the air and use it in the oxidation process involved in releasing energy from food. Iron is an essential part of the compound haemoglobin which makes red blood cells red in colour.

Functions of Red Blood Cells: To carry oxygen from the lungs to the tissues where it is needed for releasing energy from sugars. RBCs don't last forever but have a life span of about four months. The body is very thrifty with iron contained in old red blood cells. It reuses the old ones to make new ones. Some additional iron is needed especially when the volume of blood is increased i.e. when a child is growing.

It is very important to have sufficient iron in the diet, but it is however unfortunate that it is one of the minerals that is often lacking in the diet. To prevent this iron is now added to flour in the U.K., except for wholemeal flour.

Iron is stored in tissues such as the liver, spleen and bone marrow of a well fed adult.

Only a small amount of iron is absorbed from the diet and since the body conserves its own iron very efficiently, only a small amount is lost.

The daily tosses of iron amount to 0.5mg or 14mg per kg of body weight about 0.5mg is lost daily through sweating in the skin cells. Menstrually women lose on average 0.5 – 1mg daily.

An average diet contains about 10-15mg of iron per day.

Anaemia

The classical iron deficiency disease is (iron deficiency anaemia). As a result there is a reduction of the total amount of haemoglobin circulating in the bloodstream. As a result in iron deficiency the blood cells are usually pale and small in size (microcytic). They are also (hypocromic) decreased haemoglobin in these red blood corpuscles.

The aetiology of Iron deficiency.

Blood Loss

- Accidental haemorrhage, or through some disease, usually a chronic disease where there is bleeding e.g. peptic ulcers. Tuberculosis, excessive menstruation, people donating a lot of blood or parasites e.g. hookworm.
- Lack of iron in the diet or a shortage of iron increases demand. e.g. during adolescence, pregnancy, lactation and infancy.
- Inadequate absorption of iron can happen, usually from some villi in the small intestine common in the elderly.
- Lack of Hydrochloric acid in the stomach meaning that ferric iron is not absorbed readily.
- Protein Energy malnutrition.

Symptoms

Pale skin, dizziness, faintness, headaches, depression, poor appetite, breathlessness, palpitations, tiredness, weakness, fatigue, lowered resistance to infection, tongue and mouth affected, tongue gets ting slits, mainly in adolescence and women of child bearing age.

With the elderly, they sometimes get swelling of the ankles exaggerated angina and tingling of the fingers and toes.

Treatment

Medication is always needed, plus a diet with high iron content. Small meals at regular intervals are usually better. Medication is usually used from a G.P. and if absolutely necessary an intermuscular injection.

Sulphur

It occurs in a lot of body structures, more towards organic than inorganic compounds i.e. chemistry associated with the carbon atom.

Iodine

Goitre is an illness resulting from iodine deficiency. It is caused by an abnormal growth of the thyroid gland. Five thousand years ago in China people ate seaweed or burnt sponge to cure Goitre.

In 1820 it was discovered that goitre was a result of iodine deficiency. Simple goitre which is often endemic (prevalent or regularly found in an area) is due to a lack of iodine. The thyroid gland grows in an endeavour to produce enough of the hormone thyroxine which the body requires to regulate the metabolic rate and is obvious to medical practitioners. In 1895 it appeared to be that goitre was present where the iodine content of the water and soil was very low, and where the inhabitants lived entirely on local produce. In contrast, in countries where is a sea shore or where the soil or its produce are relatively high in iodine, goitre was unknown. In regions susceptible to goitre; the animals suffered from the same deficiency symptoms as humans. The animals produced weak or still born offspring. An iodine deficiency in a mothers pregnancy (humans); during the first trimester of pregnancy or even before conception can result in children to be born with a deficiency (cretinism).

Once goitre has developed in an adult it is useless to take iodine to reduce the over-developed gland.

The formation of goitre can also be found in some plants – cabbages, turnips, onions and garlic. Studies in some parts of Australia have shown that the slight growth of the thyroid gland can be due to goitrogenic substances in milk where animals are fed lots of the above plants e.g. turnip.

Absorption

Absorption of iodine seems to be from the upper part of the intestine probably between 15-30mg is in the body. 3/5 of this found in the thyroid gland, the rest is in the bloodstream.

The hormones in the thyroid gland thyroxin and triodothyronine discovered respectively in 1915 and 1952, both regulate basal metabolic rate. They influence protein, synthesis and cholesterol production. Excessive amounts of thyroxin accelerate the oxidative process, called hyperthyroidism in other words it increases the basal metabolic rate. In contrast people with hyperthyroidism decrease the basal metabolic rate.

Two days supply of iron represents a years supply of iodine. To replace iodine losses the iodine is obtained from the food found in water and soil.

Sometime iodinised salts are given to animals and people get iodine from milk and beef.

Refined foods don't usually contain much iodine but too much iodine is toxic called thyrotoxicosis so it is definitely not recommended to take iodine supplements in the diet.

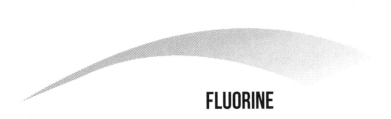

FLUORINE

Fluorine is essential to man, but some people believe that it is toxic in any amounts no matter how small. But it has been known since the 1930s that fluorine can be beneficial in preventing dental cares. During the 1960s, it was reported that fluorine in the form of sodium fluoride could have positive effects on patients afflicted with osteoporosis and other demineralisation problems. Epidermal studies have shown that there are fewer cases of osteoporosis in regions rich in fluorine, than elsewhere. Thus fluorine is not only important for dental health, but also for the maintenance of a normal skeleton in the adult.

The problem with fluorine is in finding a concentration which protects the teeth without causing harm. If the concentration in the water exceeds two parts per million, small brown marks appear on the teeth. They are unattractive but not dangerous. A concentration of 1 part per million i.e. 1mg per litre results in no marks on the teeth and the incidence of dental cares in children is decreased by 50 per cent or more. Some places adopt a fluoridation level between 0.7 and 1.2mg per litre as a sure, cheap, and effective measure against dental cares but is not done in Britain or Ireland.

Functions of Fluorine

It is the structural component of normal teeth. It is thought to activate some enzymes and inhibit others. Scientists have found that rats, when given a diet very low in fluorine in laboratories don't grow properly.

Fluorine is a mineral which is absorbed quickly. There are high levels of fluorine in the bones and teeth. Excess fluorine is excreted through the urine.

80 per cent of ingested fluorine is excreted in the urine by children and this can rise to as much as 98 per cent in adults.

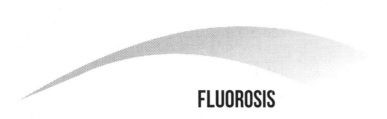

FLUOROSIS

Fluorosis is poisoning by fluorine. The grass, hay and grain usually eaten by domestic animals are rarely the cause of fluorine poisoning. Tea is an exceptional plant and can concentrate up to 100ppm of fluorine. In normal conditions, animal foodstuffs contain too little to constitute a danger to life. In some mining areas fluorine is given off. Lethal doses of fluorine produce a rapid loss of appetite, weight loss, gastroenteritis, muscular weakness, pulmonary congestion, cardiac, and respiratory arrest, seen mostly in animals.

Very few foods contain more than 1-2ppm of fluorine. Most of them contain less. The richest sources are seafoods and tea. One cup of tea gives 0.2 – 0.3mg of fluorine. It's impossible to give exact fluorine levels in foods as they depend so much on the environment. Concentrations can change. They can vary from 1-4ppm (parts per million). A level of 6-10 ppm means that there are risks of fluorosis for humans and animals.

Selenium

It is an essential element, but high levels could produce poisoning. The amount available in food is very much related to the protein content. Foods such as meat, fish, offal, cheese, eggs and cereals have high levels selenium, plus seeds.

There is some evidence that selenium has some influence on dental cares and dental decay. The frequency of dental decay and gum problems is much higher than when the soil is poor in selenium. Selenium was known for its toxic effects before it was known that it is an essential anti-oxidant. Around the 1930s it was found that blind staggers, a disease in animals was caused when the animals were grazing on pastures which were very high in selenium. In the early 1970s an organic derevative of selenium was found to be part of a particular enzyme glutathynone peroxidase. This particular enzyme GTP helps to protect red blood cells from oxidature damage caused by hydrogen peroxide and other peroxides formed during the oxidation of Glucose b-phosphate. See Patrick Holford's interpretation of selenium as an anti-oxidant. Holford P, The Optimum Nutrition Bible, Chp 27 p 170-171.

Selenium is present in a number of forms in food. It seems to be associated with proteins. In 1977 the average diet provided 244mg of selenium per day. There was a significant loss on cooking, but the concentration in the diet showed that results were quite high compared to other research work. Infants on artificial milk feeds had a selenium intake equivalent to that of adults about 3mg per kg of body weight. For those on natural milk, or prepared food the intake was 6mg per kg. It doesn't build up in the tissue and sudden infant death syndrome cannot be related to selenium levels in human tissue. Too much excess in the diet, according to some authorities might result in poisoning. Symptoms include depression, giddiness, gastro-intestinal disorders and dermatitis.

Selenium, as an antioxidant, especially referred to in Patrick Holford's Book "The Optimum Nutrition Bible" loosely associated selenium with conquering cancer. He associates a synergy of Vitamins A and E along with selenium to be able to fight cancer.

But it is very important for a cancer patient not to be overdosing on any vitamin or mineral associated with being an antioxidant i.e. Vitamins A or E or the minerals zinc or selenium as they could build up in the body and become toxic making the cancer condition worse, instead of better, maybe even fatal.

The only antioxidant that can be taken excessively is Vitamin C as it is water soluble and once the body reaches saturation point, the excess is excreted in the urine. As the profession of Human Nutrition and Dietetics recommends do not be taking an excess of 250mg daily in the diet. The easiest way to do this is not to eat protein to excess or the body could poison itself with excess selenium.

The Macro Minerals

Calcium, phosphorus, magnesium, sodium, potassium and chlorine are the bulk elements that are required in quantities of several hundred milligrams per day. They are involved in structural functions in bones and cells as well as metabolic functions.

Calcium

Calcium is one of the bulk minerals required by the body. Of the body's total calcium needs ninety nine percent is required for the bones and teeth. The remaining one percent is in solution and helps biochemical functions of various kinds.

Good dietary sources are: milk, cheese, broccoli, legumes, green leafy vegetables, nuts, seeds, peas, beans and lentils.

Excess Calcium

Too much calcium, as a result of metabolic or nutritional disorders can give to kidney failure and a number of other problems. For this reason, it is important to have the condition diagnosed early, even when mild. It can lead to kidney stones, poor muscle, constipation, abnormal pains, and loss of appetite, nausea, vomiting and deposition of calcium in sites outside the bone.

Phosphorus

Phosphorus is involved with calcium in the formation of bones and teeth, and like calcium, has a number of other functions as well. It is necessary for the working of every cell in the body, and is involved in energy production, storage and release. Calcium is the only mineral that we require in greater quantities than phosphorus. B vitamins are only effective when combined with phosphate in the body. A very important phosphorus containing compound is adosine triphosphate (ATP) which is involved in energy production and storage.

Good food sources of phosphorus include milk and milk products, nuts, and wholegrain cereals, poultry, eggs, meat, fish and legumes.

Potassium

Potassium is important in a wide range of bodily functions and is present in every cell in the body. It is essential for the correct working of the heart the muscles and nervous system and the maintenance of normal blood glucose levels.

Strict vegetarians have a high potassium, low salt diet if they do not add salt to their food. This is because fresh fruits, vegetables and whole grains are rich in potassium. On the other hand, meat eaters tend to eat too much sodium in relation to the potassium in their diet.

Sodium

The average adult has 70 – 100 grams of sodium in his or her blood. It is mainly outside the cells, in contrast to potassium which is mainly inside the cells.

Sodium is intimately related to the maintenance of the body's fluid balance and blood pressure, so the higher the level of blood sodium, the higher the blood pressure and vice versa.

Most of our dietary sodium is in the form of table salt, but a certain amount is derived from sodium nitrate which is used as a preservative in meats, and mono sodium glutamate, a flavour enhancer.

Excessive sweating results in a loss of sodium simply because the sodium content of sweat is high (hence the salty taste).

Working in hot environments, vigorous exercise or the excessive use of saunas can cause a considerate sodium loss and a resulting sodium deficiency.

The manifestations of sodium deficiency include nausea, vomiting, dizziness, cramps, exhaustion, apathy and extreme circulatory failure. Most of these symptoms can be corrected by replacing the water that has been lost along with the salt. Ideally you should replace salt with the next meal. Excessive sodium can increase blood pressure, and shortage of sodium can produce a low blood pressure.

Magnesium

Magnesium has been known for a long time as a treatment for high blood pressure in pregnancy and as an anticonvulsant.

A diet high in refined and processed foods is often deficient in magnesium, and this is made more significant if bran is added to such a diet because it binds what little magnesium is present, so rendering it less easily absorbed.

Magnesium is essential for many metabolic processes especially the cellular "pumps" which maintain the correct distribution of sodium, potassium, and calcium across cell membranes. Magnesium deficiency is associated with muscle cramps, or in extreme cases continuous cramps, especially of the hands and feet.

Sources rich in magnesium include nuts, shrimps, soya beans, whole grains and leafy vegetables. Tap water in hard water areas is also an important source of dietary magnesium.

How much of each mineral do we need?

The body requires different amounts of each mineral. Each person has different requirements according to their age, sex and state of health. The Department of Health has drawn up Dietary Balance Values (DRVs) of minerals for different groups of healthy people. The Reference Nutrient Intake (RNI) is the amount of a nutrient that will satisfy the needs of presently all the population.

Certain groups of people may have higher requirements for specific minerals, e.g. those suffering from certain medical conditions, those recovering from illness or some athletes. These people need to ensure they obtain adequate intakes by eating foods rich in the mineral concerned; sometimes supplements may be useful.

The bioavailability and absorption of minerals.

The bioavailability of a mineral (i.e. how readily it can be absorbed – used in the body) may be influential by a variety of factors. Phylate and oxalate found in some foods, reduce the absorption of calcium, iron and zinc. Iodine absorption may be hindered by nitrates. An excess of one mineral may hinder the absorption of another, e.g. excess iron reduces zinc absorption. In contrast, iron absorption may be increased when Vitamin C is consumed in the same meal. The amount of a mineral people actually absorb can vary and will depend upon their own needs, and how much they already have of that nutrient in the body. Minerals are fairly stable in normal food processing conditions.

Minerals and diseases

Iron deficiency anaemia is a common problem, often affecting women and young children throughout the world. Deficiencies of other minerals are rare in the U.K. and excess intakes are sometimes a concern e.g. sodium chloride (salt). Recent research has suggested that selenium and zinc may form substances produced in the body because of frying, barbequing, roasting food, environmental pollution and smoking. There is evidence suggesting that minerals such as zinc and Selenium, as well as Vitamins A, C and E, known as the anti oxidants protect against free radical initiated diseases possibly including many types of cancer and heart disease. Ageing is not a disease as such but the anti oxidant protection can possibly slow down the ageing process, There has not been enough experiments done yet on humans but results will come through in time as being conclusive.

I agree that Patrick Holford's synopsis of how beneficial the antioxidants can be to optimum health. There is just the worry that some people could carry this idea too far and result in a situation where vitamins A and E: plus the heavy metals Patrick Holford encourages, could result in toxicity, rather than improving the health of the human body and longevity, and defying the ageing process.

What are minerals?

Minerals are inorganic substances, i.e. substances that do not contain carbon, required by the body for a variety of functions such as:

They are essential for the formation of bones and teeth; are essential constituents of body fluids and tissues; and are components of enzymes and nerve function.

Some minerals are needed in larger amounts than others, e.g. calcium, phosphorus, magnesium, sodium, potassium and chlorine. Others are required in smaller quantities and are called trace minerals e.g. iron, zinc, iodine, fluoride, selenium and copper. Despite being required in smaller amounts trace minerals are no less important than other minerals.

The Macro Minerals

Calcium, phosphorus, magnesium, sodium, potassium and chlorine are the bulk elements that are required in quantities of several hundred milligrams per day. They are involved in structural functions in bones and cells as well as metabolic functions.

Calcium

Calcium is one of the bulk minerals required by the body. Of the body's total calcium needs ninety nine percent is required for the bones and teeth. The remaining one percent is in solution and helps biochemical functions of various kinds.

Good dietary sources are: milk, cheese, broccoli, legumes, green leafy vegetables, nuts, seeds, peas, beans, lentils, watercress and spinach.

Excess Calcium

Too much calcium, as a result of metabolic or nutritional disorders can give to kidney failure and a number of other problems. For this reason, it is important to have the condition diagnosed early, even when mild. It can lead to kidney stones, poor muscle, constipation, abnormal pains, loss of appetite, nausea, vomiting and deposition of calcium in sites outside the bone.

99% of the calcium in the body is stored in the bones and teeth, as calcium is needed to build the skeleton.

In childhood, calcium is particularly important when the bones are growing. Calcium is important for the elderly as the body's ability to absorb calcium becomes impaired with age.

The remaining few grams of calcium which is not in the bones and skeleton is in the nerves, muscles and blood.

Along with magnesium, calcium helps the nervous system to function as it works like "A pump system". Along with the main players in the nervous system, sodium and potassium, known as "The sodium-potassium pump".

Calcium also assists the blood to clot, and it also helps maintain the right acid / alkaline balance in the body known as the pH balance.

Too much parathyroid hormone levels is associated with bone pains, psychiatric symptoms and constipation.

An excess of parathyroid hormone can successfully be corrected surgically however calcium insufficiency is also associated with a wide range of mental disturbances. Defective calcium metabolism can respond to calcium supplementation to alleviate a wide range of psychiatric conditions. The most common are depression, anxiety, panic attacks, nervous twitches, insomnia and hyperactivity.

Heart attacks are usually associated with an unhealthy diet, high in saturated fat, but calcium also promotes a healthy heart. Symptoms of deficiency include muscle cramps, tremors or spasms, insomnia, nervousness, joint pain, osteoarthritis, tooth decay and high blood pressure. Severe deficiency causes osteoporosis.

Vitamin D is very important for the absorption of calcium and apart from dietary sources, one of the most important sources of vitamin D comes from exposure to sunlight.

Phosphorus

Phosphorus is involved with calcium in the formation of bones and teeth, and like calcium, has a number of other functions as well. It is necessary for the working of every cell in the body, and is involved in energy production, storage and release. Calcium is the only mineral that we require in greater quantities than phosphorus. B vitamins are only effective when combined with phosphate in the body. A very important phosphorus containing compound is adosine triphosphate (ATP) which is involved in energy production and storage. Phosphorus is also a component. Of DNA and RNA, and helps maintain the pH of the body, aids metabolism and energy production.

Deficiency Signs: Dietary deficiencies are unlikely since it is present in almost all foods. But they may occur with stresses such as bone fracture. Deficiency signs include general mucle weakness, loss of appetite, bone pain, rikets and osteomalacie.

Good food sources of phosphorus include milk and milk products, nuts, and wholegrain cereals, poultry, eggs, meat, fish and legumes.

Potassium

Potassium is important in a wide range of bodily functions and is present in every cell in the body. It is essential for the correct working of the heart the muscles and nervous system and the maintenance of normal blood glucose levels. Potassium enables nutrients to move into the cell, and waste products to move out of cells. It promotes healthy nerves and muscles, maintains fluid to balance in the body. Potassium helps relax muscles and also in the secretion of insulin for blood sugar control to produce constant energy, involved in metabolism. It maintains heart functioning, stimulates gut movements to encourage proper elimination.

Deficiency Signs: Dietary deficiencies include a rapid irregular heartbeat, muscle weakness, pins and needles, irritability, nausea, vomiting, diarrhoea, swollen abdomen, imbalance of potassium, sudden confusion and mental apathy.

Dietary Sources include: Watercress, cabbage, celery, parsley, courgettes, radishes, cauliflower, mushrooms and pumpkin.

Strict vegetarians have a high potassium, low salt diet if they do not add salt to their food. This is because fresh fruits, vegetables and whole grains are rich in potassium. On the other hand, meat eaters tend to eat too much sodium in relation to the potassium in their diet.

Sodium

The average adult has 70 – 100 grams of sodium in his or her blood. It is mainly outside the cells, in contrast to potassium which is mainly inside the cells.

Sodium is intimately related to the maintenance of the body's fluid balance and blood pressure, so the higher the level of blood sodium, the higher the blood pressure and vice versa.

Most of our dietary sodium is in the form of table salt, but a certain amount is derived from sodium nitrate which is used as a preservative in meats, and mono sodium glutamate, a flavour enhancer.

Excessive sweating results in a loss of sodium simply because the sodium content of sweat is high (hence the salty taste).

Working in hot environments, vigorous exercise or the excessive use of saunas can cause a considerable sodium loss and a resulting sodium deficiency which can lead to dehydration, nerve functioning, muscle contraction including the heart muscle and in energy production.

The manifestations of sodium deficiency include nausea, vomiting, dizziness, low blood pressure, rapid pulse, loss of appetite, muscle cramps, weight loss, exhaustion, apathy and extreme circulatory failure. Most of these symptoms can be corrected by replacing the water that has been lost along with the salt. Ideally you should replace salt with the next meal. Excessive sodium can increase blood pressure, and shortage of sodium can produce a low blood pressure.

Magnesium

Magnesium has been known for a long time as a treatment for high blood pressure in pregnancy and as an anticonvulsant.

A diet high in refined and processed foods is often deficient in magnesium, and this is made more significant if bran is added to such a diet because it binds what little magnesium is present, so rendering it less easily absorbed.

Magnesium is essential for many metabolic processes especially the cellular "pumps" which maintain the correct distribution of sodium, potassium, and calcium across cell membranes. Magnesium deficiency is associated with muscle cramps, or in extreme cases continuous cramps, especially of the hands and feet.

Sources rich in magnesium include nuts, shrimps, soya beans, whole grains and leafy vegetables. Tap water in hard water areas is also an important source of dietary magnesium.

Magnesium works with calcium in maintaining both bone density and nerve and muscle impulses. The average western diet is relatively high in calcium but often deficient in magnesium because milk, our major source of calcium is not a very good source of magnesium.

But both calcium and magnesium are present in green leafy vegetables, nuts and seeds.

Chlorophyll gives plants their green colour and magnesium is a vital component of chlorophyll. But only a small proportion of the magnesium within plants is in the form of this green pigment, chlorophyll.

Magnesium is essential for many enzymes in the body which are the catalysts which speed up biochemical reactions within the body.

Many enzymes involving magnesium work together with vitamins B1 and B6 to speed u the complex biochemical reactions which happen in the body.

Magnesium is also involved in protein synthesis and is vital for the production of some hormones. A lack of magnesium is strongly associated with cardiovascular disease. It has been discovered that abnormally low levels of magnesium in the heart can lead to muscles going into spasm, cramping of the heart muscle can result in the heart being deprived of oxygen, not by the usual obstruction of the coronary arteries.

Because magnesium is important in strengthening bones and teeth, promoting healthy muscles including the heart and also a healthy nervous system, and also is essential for energy production. It is important that the body has adequate intakes of magnesium.

Deficiency Signs include: Muscle spasms, muscle weakness, insomnia, nervousness, high blood pressure, irregular heartbeat, lack of appetite and kidney stones.

Good source of magnesium include: Wheat germ, almonds, cashew nuts, brewer's yeast, brazil nuts, peanuts, beans, garlic, raisins, green peppers, potato skin and crab meat.

The Trace Minerals

Iron

Iron is a constituent part of the proteins which act as oxygen transporters in red blood cells and in muscles. These proteins are called haemoglobin and myoglobin. In a healthy adult male about two thirds of the total of 4-6 grams of iron in the body consists of haemoglobin. The adult body contains about the same amount of iron as a 3" nail. Iron is the most important mineral element because it enables us to take the oxygen from the air and use it in oxidation processes involved in releasing energy from food.

Haemoglobin is found in the red blood cells. Haemoglobin carries oxygen from the lungs to the tissues where it is needed for releasing energy from sugars. Red blood cells don't last forever but have a life of about four months. The body is very thrifty with iron contained in the old red blood cells. It reuses the old ones to make new ones. Some additional is needed – especially when the volume of blood is increased e.g. in pregnancy or when a child is growing.

It is very important to have sufficient iron in the diet but it is unfortunate that iron is one of the minerals that is lacking in the diet. To prevent this iron is now added to all flour in this country except for wholemeal flour.

Second to the red blood cells the next largest amount of iron is found in the liver, spleen, and bone marrow, about 1g. Only a small amount of iron is absorbed from the diet. Since the body conserves its iron very well, only a small amount is lost.

Rich sources of iron include organ meats including liver, kidney and heart, egg yolk, legumes, cocoa, cane molasses, shellfish and parsley. Intermediate containing foods include muscle meats, fish, poultry, nuts, green vegetables and wholemeal bread.

Iron Deficiency Anaemia

Iron deficiency can cause many symptoms most of which are linked to the anaemia it produces. The symptoms of anaemia resulting from iron deficiency include listliness, fatigue, a very obvious heartbeat on exertion sometimes a sore tongue, tongue gets tiny slits, cracks on the corner of the mouth, difficulty with swallowing and concave nails.

In children, poor appetite, poor growth and decreased resistance to infection are common. Abnormalities of the gastrointestinal tract including the production of too little stomach acid have long been observed in iron deficiency anaemia.

Iron deficiency is very common in the UK and the USA. Those most at risk are children, pregnant women, women with heavy periods, strict vegetarians and people from low socio economic groups who have poor diet. Others who may be at risk are those with mal absorption problems, those with very little gastric acid following the removal of part of the stomach in an operation for ulcers or removal of the whole stomach because of cancer.

Tea and coffee has been shown to reduce iron absorption from food. Coffee has been found to reduce iron absorption by 39 percent compared to 64 percent with tea, when taken with a meal. So if you are at risk from iron deficiency do not take tea or coffee with meals, one hour before meals and half to two hours after a meal.

SULPHUR

It occurs in a lot of structures, more towards organic than inorganic compounds. The major function, in the body-usually found in the active tissue compounds. Deficiencies – related to intake of the sulphur containing amino acids.

IODINE

Goitre is an illness resulting from iodine deficiency. It is caused by an abnormal growth of the thyroid gland. Five thousand years ago in China people ate seaweed or burnt sponge to cure goitre. In 1520 it was discovered that goitre was a result of iodine deficiency.

Simple goitre which is often evelemic is due to a lack of iodine. To compensate for the lack of iodine, the thyroid gland grows in an endeavour to produce enough of the hormones which the body requires.

In 1895, it was found that the thyroid gland was particularly rich in iodine. Thyroxine and Tridothyromine are the hormones produced by the thyroid gland. It appeared to be that goitre was present where the iodine content of the water and soil was very low. The inhabitants lived entirely on local products. In countries where there is a sea-shore or where the soil or its produce are relatively high in iodine goitre was unknown. In regions susceptible to goitre the animals suffered from the same deficiency symptoms as humans. The animals produced weak or stillborn offspring.

An iodine deficiency in a mother (humans) during the first semester of pregnancy or even before conception can cause children to be born with a deficiency – cretinism, a condition which is characterised by dwarfism and mental retardation.

In some countries there is a lot of iodised salt sold. Once goitre has developed in an adult its useless to take iodine to reduce the over developed gland. The formation of goitre can also be provoked by certain goitragenic substances found in some plants: - cabbages, turnips, onions and garlic. Studies in some parts of Australia have shown that the slightest growth of the thyroid gland can be due to goitrogana in milk where animals are feed lots of the above plants e.g. turnip. Absorption of iodine seems to be from the upper part of the intestine probably between 15 – 30mg. About 3/5 of this is found in the thyroid gland; the rest is in the bloodstream.

Thyroxine was discovered in 1915. It regulates the basal metabolic rate, influences protein synthesis and cholesterol production. Thyroxine increases the metabolic rate of tissues and also controls growth. Excessive amounts of thyroxine being secreted from the thyroid gland, which consists of two lobes near the base of the neck, results in a process called hyperthyroidism. This causes nervousness, insomnia, sweating, palpitations and sensitivity to heat. Hyperthyroidism results in insufficient production of thyroid hormones by the thyroid gland and this can result in disorders such as cretinism or myxoedema, characterised by puffy eyes, face, hands and mental sluggishness.

Two days of iron supply represents a year's supply of iodine. To replace iodine losses, the iodine is obtained from food, in water and the soil. Sometimes iodised salts are given to animals and people obtain iodine from milk and beef. Refined foods don't usually contain much iodine. Too much iodine is toxic. Too much iodine is called thyrotoxicosis.

Fluorine

Fluorine is essential to man, but some people believe that it is toxic in whatever amounts. It's been known since the 30's that fluorine can be beneficial in preventing dental caries. During the 60's it was reported that fluorine in the form of osteoporosis and other demineralisation problems Epidemiological studies have shown that there are fewer cases of osteoporosis in regions rich in fluorine than elsewhere. This fluorine is not only important for dental health but also for the maintenance of a normal skeleton in the adult.

The problem with fluorine is finding an amount which protects the teeth without causing harm. If the fluorine in the water exceeds two parts per million small brown marks appear on the teeth. They are unattractive but aren't dangerous. 1 part per million, 1mg per litre results in no marks on teeth and the dental caries in children is down by 50% or more. Some places adopt a fluoridation level between 0.7 and 1.2mg per litre as a sure, cheap and effective measure against dental caries but fluoridation of water is not available in Britain or Ireland.

Functions of Fluorine

It is a structured component of normal teeth. It is thought to activate some enzymes and inhabits others. It has been found that rats when given a diet very low in fluorine don't grow properly. It is a mineral which is absorbed quickly. There are high levels in the bones and the teeth. Excess is excreted through the urine. 80% of ingested fluorine is excreted by children and this can rise to as much as 98% in adults.

Fluorosis – poisoning by fluorine. The grass, hay and grain usually eaten by domestic animals are rarely the cause of fluorine poisoning. Unless these substances are contaminated by substances containing very large amounts of fluorine. Even if fertilizer containing a lot of fluorine is used. Tea is an exceptional plant and can concentrate up to 100ppm of fluorine. In normal conditions, animal foodstuffs contain too little to constitute a danger. In some mining areas fluorine is given off. Lethal doses of fluorine produce a rapid loss of appetite and weight, and gastroenteritis, muscular weakness, pulmonary congestion, cardiac and respiratory arrest. Seen mostly in animals.

Very few foods contain more than 1-2ppm of fluorine. Most of them contain less. The richest sources are seafood and tea. One cup of tea gives .2 - .3mg of fluorine. It's impossible to give exact fluorine levels in foods as they depend so much on the environment. Concentrations can change. They can vary from 1-4ppm. Once you get to 6-10 ppm, there are risks of fluorosis for humans and animals.

SELENIUM

Selenium is an essential antioxidant but high levels could produce poisoning. The amount available in food is very much related to it's protein content and the geographical origin of the food. Selenium is depleted in refined foods and with modern farming techniques.

Selenium's antioxidant properties help to protect the body against attack by free radicals and carcinogens. It also reduces inflammation and stimulates the immune system to fight infections. It helps promote a healthy heart and selenium helps vitamin E function – necessary for the health of the male reproductive system.

Selenium is an immune enhancing mineral and it is abundant in seafoods and seeds especially sesame seeds. Other sources include tuna, oysters, molasses, mushrooms, herrings, cottage cheese, cabbage, beef liver and chicken.

There is some evidence that there is a link between selenium and vitamin E metabolism. Selenium also has some influence on dental caries. The frequency of dental decay and gum problems is much higher where the soil is poor in selenium.

Selenium was known for it's toxic effects before it was kknown as an essential antioxidant.

In the 1930's it was discovered that the blind staggers was a disease in animals who were grazing in pastures very high in selenium. It was found to be part of a particular enzyme glutathione peroxide. This particular enzyme GTP helps protect red blood cells from oxidative damage caused by hydrogen peroxide and other proxides formed during oxidization of glucose phosphate. Therefore it is necessary to take selenium supplements in small amounts as excessive use of supplements could be dangerous for health and they could be toxic.

MANGANESE

Some enzymes contain manganese. Man doesn't usually suffer from manganese deficiencies sometimes drugs combine with manganese and prevent absorption. Manganese is concerned with the formation of collagen in connective tissue. It has an enzymatic role. It is essential for human beings because it is necessary for formation of some of the complex polysaccharides. There are about 10mg in the body. Mg is widely distributed in food. It is found abundantly in tea. I cup can contain 1.3mg. Mg is not very toxic. Tea is the major source of mg in the diet. The average intake for the adult per day is 5.4mg. About 37% of mg in diet came from tea. 18% from bread and 13mg from other cereal products and 13% from vegetables. A cup of coffee contains about 1/12 the amount of mg as tea. The retention of mg in the body is known to be universally proportional to the calcium content of the diet. Human milk is very low in mg since mg is not stored in the foetus, this shows that there is a very broad tolerance range for manganese in the human body.

CHROMIUM

There is an early theory that chromium is linked to glucose, tolerance factor. It could be important in normal carbohydrate metabolism because of its insulin enhancing capabilities. It is now certain that chromium does play an important part in glucose tolerance. The GTF is the time required for the glycaemia level to return to normal in a fasting subject book who has ingested sugar only. It is estimated, Chromium trichloride appears to act successfully on glucose intolerance and it has been shown that the amount of chromium in the tissue decreases as people get older.

Giving glucose normally raises the levels of chromium in the serum and it increases the urinary excretion of chromium, except in old people.

In chemical trials some middle-aged and older people who have mature onset diabetes have shown an improved tolerance to glucose. A severe chromium deficiency has been noted in humans after prolonged parental feeding. In those cases glucose intolerance developed which was resistant to insulin. The process of refining decreases the amount of chromium. People in Western countries probably need less chromium and other refined carbohydrates.

The result of this could be a marginal chromium deficiency which might just be the factor to trigger sensitive adults into mature onset diabetes.

Spices and wheat and raw sugar, yeast and peanut butter.

Molybdenum

There seem to be two enzyme systems which depend on this particular mineral. The requirements aren't known. The amount the people get depends a lot on location because the mineral is found in the ground where the food is grown. High sulphate could interfere with the transport of molybdenum across the cell membranes. The inter relations are likely to be complicated but the overall consequence of increasing the dietary sulphate is to enhance the intake of molybdenum. If you increase the intake of molybdenum then you seem to excrete more copper.

COBALT

We know that it is a dietary essential for human beings because it is a component of Vitamin B12. Human beings must consume cobalt in the pre formed vitamin.

Cobalt is the only trace element which in human beings is physiologically active in one particular form i.e. in Vitamin B12. However man and non-rumnant animals are incapable of making Vitamin B12 from a cobalt rich diet and so a final chain is required. This is called the cobalt chain.

It passes via the rumnant animals such as a cow and due to their intestinal organisms; they use the cobalt to make Vitamin B12. Then human beings ingest the Vitamin B12 by milk and meat. There is a large safety margin between what is safe and what is toxic.

Zinc

Zinc is recognised as a very important nutrient involved in a wide range of metabolic processes. It is a component of over two hundred enzymes in the body. It is a component of DNA and RNA essential for growth, important for healing; it controls hormones which are messengers from organs such as testes and ovaries. It aids ability to cope with stress effectively. It also promotes a healthy nervous system and brain especially in the growing foetus and aids bones and teeth.

Zinc's main role is in the protection and repair of DNA, and for this reason it is found in higher levels in animals and fish than in plants. A vegetarian diet may therefore be low in zinc. Stress, smoking and alcohol deplete zinc, as does frequent sex as at least for a men, since semen contains very high concentrations of zinc. Oysters are popularly said to be aphrodesiacs. They are also the highest dietary source of zinc, and for both men and women, zinc is essential for fertility. (Holford P, 2000)

The availability of zinc to the body's cells is influenced by other nutrients, iron, manganese, selenium and copper. Excess zinc inhibits the absorption of copper and this can lead to copper deficiency anaemia.

Deficiency Signs

Poor sense of taste and smell; white marks on more than two fingernails, frequent infections, stretch marks, acne or greasy skin, low fertility, pale skin, tendency for depression, loss of appetite.

The availability of zinc from human milk is greater than from cows milk, soya milk and combined formulae. More attention should be paid to the trace elements in infant formulae.

A woman's zinc requirements increase during pregnancy and lactation and this means dietary zinc may be borderline or indeed inadequate at the best of times. Vitamin C tablets with zinc, 1000mg are required daily by pregnant and lactating women to avoid Vitamin C and zinc deficiency.

For many years it has been known from animal studies that zinc deficiency is associated with decreased fertility, increased rates of miscarriage and increased rates of congenital malformations.

Zinc Deficiency Symptoms and Signs

Slow growth
Infertility/delayed sexual maturation
Low sperm count
Hair loss
Skin conditions of various kinds
Diarrhoea

Immune deficiencies
Behavioural and sleep disturbances
Night blindness
Impaired taste or smell
Impaired wound healing
White spots on finger nails
Impotence, infertility, low sperm count, reduced sex drive
Psychiatric problems
Connective tissue disease
Reduced appetite

Those who might have an inadequate dietary intake of zinc are:

Those with anorexia nervosa, on fad diets and those on weight reducing diet.

Those on exclusion diets for food allergies

Strict vegetarians

Those on reduced protein diets

People who eat meal substitutes (soya "meat" etc)

The elderly

Alcoholics

Food sources

The best dietary sources of zinc are fresh oysters, ginger root, muscle meats such as lamb chops and steak, split peas, brazil nuts, beef liver, egg yolk, whole wheat, rye, oats, peanuts, almonds, walnuts, chicken, green pea shrimps, turnips, parsley, potatoes, garlic, hazelnuts, carrots, beans, milk, whole wheat bread, pork chops and corn.

Summary – Micro minerals

Manganese – co factor for some enzyme systems particularly in bone formation.

Selenium – part of the enzyme glutathione peroxide which protects membranes from lipid oxidation by destroying hydrogen peroxide.

Molybdenium – a co-factor for some enzymes.

Chromium – facilitates the function of insulin and favours normal glucose tolerance.

Cobalt – Part of Vitamin B12

Zinc – component of DNA and RNA. Important for healing. Controls hormones.

WHAT IS AN ANTI OXIDANT?

Antioxidants are essential nutrients like Vitamin A and beta-carotene (the most active precursor of Vitamin A). Vitamins C and E, plus the minerals zinc and selenium.

Oxygen which is one of the basic building blocks of life i.e. plant and animal life is so important it is needed by every cell for every second of every day. We breathe in oxygen and exhale carbon dioxide. But it is plants who take in carbon dioxide and produce oxygen for us to breathe. This is why it is so important to preserve the rainforests. Without oxygen, living organisms cannot release the energy in food which drives all biochemical processes.

Oxygen is chemically reactive and very dangerous: In normal biochemical reactions oxygen can become unstable and is capable of "oxidising" neighbouring molecules i.e. the removal of electrons or the addition of oxygen to a molecule. This can lead to cellular damage which can trigger cancer, inflammation, arterial damage and premature ageing. The bodily equivalent of nuclear waste known as free oxidising radicals must be disarmed to remove this danger.

Chemicals capable of disarming free radicals are called antioxidants. Free radicals are made in all combustion processes including smoking, the burning of petrol to create exhaust fumes, radiation, frying or barbequing food and normal body processes.

It is no longer a mystery about how slowing down the ageing process can be achieved. According to evidence gathered by Patrick Holford "Animals with diets low in calories and high in anti oxidant nutrients live longer infact up to 40 percent longer and are also much more likely to be active during their life. Long term studies have yet to be completed on humans but there is every reason to assume that the same principle apples to humans.

Large scale surveys show that the risk of death is substantially reduced in those with high levels of anti-oxidant food supplements in their blood."

What are the best sources of antioxidants?

Vitamin A and beta carotene are found in beef liver, veal liver, carrots, watercress, cabbage, sweet potatoes, melon, pumpkin, mangoes, tomatoes, broccoli, apricots, papayas, tangerines and asparagus.

What is the function of Vitamin A, retinol and beta carotene?

It is needed for healthy skin, not just on the outside but for tissues within as well. It also protects the body against infection. Vitamin A (retinol and beta carotene) is not only an anti-oxidant, but an immune system booster. It is claimed to protect against many forms of cancer and is essential for night vision.

Research has discovered some amazingly positive cures for cancer through taking the anti-oxidants.

"High levels of Vitamin A in the blood has been associated with reduced risks of certain cancers. These include putting acute myeloid leukaemia into complete remission and suppressing carcinomas of the neck and head.

Beta-carotene which can be converted into Vitamin A is also anti cancerous.

"A Japanese study of 265,000 people found a significant correlation between low beta carotene intake and lung cancer. In fact, the risk of lung cancer is the same for those who smoke and have good anti-oxidant levels as it is for non-smokers with low anti-oxidant levels."

Llolpod's ideas are not all just a theory without evidence to back his theories up. In some cases, clinical trials have been done but a lot of his work is inconclusive.

Vitamin C is without a doubt been found to be the master immune boosting nutrient. Vitamin C has been found to improve the performance of antibodies and is anti viral and anti bacterial as well as being able to destroy toxins produced by bacteria.

Sources of Vitamin C include:

Sweet potatoes, carrots, watercress, peas, broccoli, cauliflower, lemons, mangoes, melon, pepper, strawberries, tomatoes, grapefruit, kiwi fruit and oranges.

There is one major problem for the anti-oxidants. Vitamins A, C and E are prone to oxidation. Beta Carotene the vegetable form of Vitamin A is water soluble and highly prone to oxidation. Instead of boiling potatoes and vegetables it is best to steam them to preserve the vitamins.

In addition to dietary intakes of Vitamin C, it is best to take 1000mg of Vitamin C, as a supplement daily. Even if large doses of Vitamin C is not recommended by the medical profession, it can at least be accepted that an unlimited amount can be taken at any one time as the body will only absorb what it needs and the rest is excreted in the urine, as it is a water soluble vitamin, needed in the diet daily anyway.

Most doctors would say it is best to get your Vitamin C in your five daily amounts of fresh fruits and vegetables and fruit juice per day. This is true, but in today's tough economic climate, it may be difficult for lower income families to provide fresh fruit, fruit juices and fresh vegetables daily. So sometimes it is not such a bad idea to top up your Vitamin C levels in tablet form. It is also very true that in the British Isles we do not often get fresh fruit on our supermarket shelves. It is often refrigerated and chilled before it reaches our shops and often has a short shelf life, so often fruit we buy "goes off" before we even get the chance to eat it. We are not as lucky as our friends on the continent who have a fresh fruit supply daily.

It is recognised in the field of Nutrition and Dietetics that Vitamin C is particularly lowered in smokers. This fits in with Patrick Holford's theory of antioxidants disarming free radicals. A smoker who does not take Vitamin C supplements in their diet will have dry, wrinkly skin by the time they are in their 40s. But a smoker who takes Vitamin C supplements will have the same complexion of a non-smoker and the lungs of a non-smoker as the anti-oxidants disarm free radicals not just on the outside but on our inner organs too.

There is a famous doctor called Dr Linus Pauling who is a cancer expert, who along with another doctor, Dr Ewan Cameron first demonstrated Vitamin C's amazing anti cancerous properties in the 1960s.

"The gave terminally ill cancer patients 10grams a day and showed that they lived four times longer than patients not on Vitamin C. Many studies have since been performed. A review of Vitamin C research concluded that "evidence of a protective effect of Vitamin C for non-hormone cancers is very strong."

Dr Pauling and Dr Cameron's work is evidence based practise which has not been rejected by Orthodox Medicine but a strong positive correlation has been revealed between high doses of Vitamin C and longevity of cancer patients. It is a practice not widely used in Medicine. Chemotherapy and radio therapy are still the most widely used treatments for cancer, but if the individual wishes to use Vitamin therapy, then it is up to their own discretion.

"A ten-year study on eleven thousand people completed in 1996 found that those who supplemented both the anti-oxidants Vitamin C and Vitamins E halved their overall risk of death from all cancers and heart disease. It was also found that Vitamin E is a powerful anticancer agent, especially in combination with Selenium."

Research also shows that "in a massive study on nurses, supplementing Vitamin E and C effectively halves the risk of ever having a heart attack if they consumed 15 – 20mg of beta-carotene as well daily. It is claimed that this reduced by 40 percent the risk of having a stroke; and 22 per cent lowering the risk of having a heart attack.

Sources of Vitamin E.

The best sources of Vitamin E include:

Sweet potatoes, peas, meat, seeds and nuts, tuna, mackerel and salmon. Wheat germ and beans.

Selenium, iron, manganese, copper and zinc are all involved in the anti-oxidation process and boost immune power positively. Of these minerals selenium and zinc are probably the most important. The best sources of Selenium is said to be found in sea-food and sesame seeds and again it is claimed to have protective powers against cancer and premature ageing. The best sources of zinc are oysters, ginger root, lamb, pecan nuts, dry split peas, haddock, egg yolk, whole wheat grain, rice, oats, peanuts and almonds.

Zinc is thought to be anti-cancerous and to prevent pre-mature ageing. Zinc's main role is in the protection of DNA and it plays a major role in nearly every disease from cancer to diabetes as it is needed to make insulin, to boost the immune system and to make an enzyme called SOD (super oxide dismutase) which is a very important antioxidant, which helps disarm free radicals.

There is however a danger regarding intake of too much zinc. It is recommended to take 25-50mg of a zinc supplement per day. It increases your libido and your vitality.

Zinc is the most important immune boosting mineral. There is no doubt it helps fight infections." Zinc lozenges are available for sore throats. But the field of nutrition would again contradict this theory as too much zinc can interfere with copper metabolism.

Zinc can be found easily in a well balanced diet of milk, cheese, meat, eggs and fish, whole grain cereals and pulses.

"A lower level of Vitamin A and Vitamin E and beta-carotene is associated with Alzheimer's disease. The blood levels of Vitamin E and beta-carotene in sufferers are half those of elderly people who do not have Alzheimer's.

This theory has been rejected by orthodox medicine. Instead medical research has found conclusive that the B complex vitamins can prevent Alzheimer's disease by preventing the brain from shrinking by 50 percent as it does in the elderly who develop Alzheimer's.

As a Nutritional Consultant with a background in Human Nutrition and Dietetics I would not expect Orthodox Medicine to accept everything nutritionists claim to be true as I myself would find it difficult to accept all his theories without medical research proving such theories to be true. However especially regarding the power of the anti-oxidants there is no reason to believe that it is not realistic, and possibly will be accepted by orthodox medicine in the future.

The anti-oxidants taken either in the diet or as a dietary supplement will certainly do no harm.

A nutritional supplement including Vitamins, A, C and E Selenium and zinc is beneficial to overall health. It is often particularly difficult to eat enough foods containing Vitamin C so it is beneficial to take 1000mg of Vitamin C daily as a nutritional supplement.

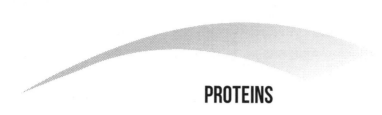

PROTEINS

What is protein?

A protein is a nutrient which builds body tissue and repairs as well as maintaining tissue. It can also be broken down to provide energy. The composition of proteins includes elements such as carbon, hydrogen, nitrogen, sulphur and phosphorus which combine to form amino acids which build proteins.

<u>Composition</u>

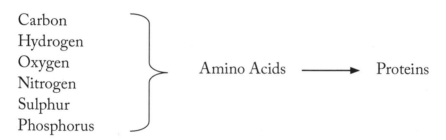

Carbon
Hydrogen
Oxygen
Nitrogen
Sulphur
Phosphorus

Amino Acids ⟶ Proteins

Essential Amino Acids are those which the body cannot manufacture itself. Adult essential amino include valine, lysine, leticine, isoleucine, methionine, phenylalanine, and tryptophan. There is one essential amino acid required for growing infants called Histidine.

The above amino acids are essential in food because the body can't build proteins without them. They can only be synthesized from the food eaten.

The main sources of the essential amino acids are found in meat and meat products, milk, cheese, eggs, and fish. Other sources include beans, lentils, quinoa, soya, runner beans, peas, corn and broccoli which is an important source of protein for vegetarians and vegans.

The disadvantage of animal protein is that they contain a lot of undesirable saturated fat which can lead to heart disease.

Protein Quality

Protein quality is determined by biological value, i.e. the ability to build new tissue when broken down to amino acids. If protein quality is high, then less protein is needed in the diet. Many essential amino acids are a high biological value. Fewer essential fatty acids are a high biological value.

High biological value protein is able to build tissue on their own. The chief sources are meat, fish, and eggs, i.e. animal foods. This is because animal protein resembles the amino acid content of human tissue.

Low biological value proteins i.e. plant don't contain enough amino acids to build human tissue because they are poor in essential amino acids.

An example of a high biological value plant food is soya, eaten a lot by vegetarians and vegans. The amount and proportion of essential amino acid is similar to those in proteins of animal origin. Sometimes a combination of two proteins will provide enough essential amino acids i.e. known as complementary value or supplementary value, combining foods to give better value protein. An average of 70 grams of protein should be eaten daily.

Nitrogen Balance

The nitrogen balance technique is used by physiologists to determine the minimum protein required for a person at any one time.

If the amount of nitrogen consumed in food balances the amount excreted from the body, then they are said to have nitrogen equilibrium. The lowest amount of protein needed in the diet which can maintain a nitrogen equilibrium is considered to suit the base amount of protein the body needs.

When a person is building new body tissues they excrete nitrogen and is said to be in Positive Nitrogen Balance (Anabolism). This situation exists during growth, infancy, childhood, adolescence, during pregnancy and lactation so obviously at these times the individual needs extra protein in their diet.

When a person excretes more nitrogen than they take in they are said to be in negative nitrogen balance (catabolism). This situation happens when the diet is so deficient in protein that the body's need for amino acids are not met. Negative Nitrogen Balance can result when the body's proteins are breaking down at an excessive rate. This can happen after major surgery, severe burns, during fevers and especially the under nourished infants and children in under developed countries.

Functions of Protein in the Body

Protein is needed for: -
1. Haemoglobin which is the red carpulses in the blood which carries oxygen around the body known as oxyhaemoglobin, the globin part consisting of protein.
2. Hormones which perform vital regulatory processes in the body are made from protein, for example, adrenaline. Insulin cannot be taken orally or it would be digested, so therefore it has to be injected straight into the bloodstream.

Proteins have many functions
1. They are the building blocks for new tissue protein which is the basic structure of many of the body's tissues.
2. Proteins constitute the chief solid matter of muscles, organs and endocrine glands.
3. They are the major constituent of the matrix of bones, teeth, nails, hair, blood cells and serum.
4. Enzymes which are catalysts for metabolic processes are also proteins.

Regulation of Water Balance in The Body

Protein helps in the movement of fluid between intracellular and intercellular parts of the body across the semi-permeable membrane in all cells by simple diffusion. The movement of this fluid within cells is known as intracellular diffusion and between cells is known as intracellular diffusion.

Protein as an Energy Source

1 gram of dietary protein equals 4 kilocalories or 17 kilojoules. Energy needs are the first priority for the body because the body must have fuel to provide energy. If there is not enough fat or carbohydrate in the diet, protein will be used for energy.

Protein and Body Compounds

Protein is the basic structure of many body tissues. In blood clotting fibrin strands form a mesh to cause the blood to clot and this is made from protein. Protein is also essential for the beginning of tissue repair, for example, in wound healing or recovery from surgery.

All cells and most fluids in the body contain protein. But bile does not contain protein and normal urine doesn't contain protein.

When protein is broken down initially it is deaminized. When protein is broken down in the liver, nitrogen is broken off from the protein molecule and carbohydrate hydrogen and oxygen is oxidized for energy or can be converted to fat for storage firstly in the liver and then in the adipose tissue.

It is a fallacy that if you eat a high protein diet you will lose weight faster. This is not true because any excess protein above and beyond what the body actually needs in the form of protein will automatically be stored as fat in the body.

Each species including man has its own characteristic proteins, for example, the protein in human muscle is different from beef muscle in cattle, but at the same time similar.

Protein in the Maintenance of Body Nutrients

Protein also maintains the body's neutrality, i.e. the control of the acid base balance in the tissues. During normal metabolism acids and bases are being formed due to chemical reactions of metabolism. Acids predominate, but proteins are capable reacting with acids or bases and are considered to be amphoteric substances or buffers capable of reacting with acids or bases, also known as alkalis, and are therefore capable of neutralising stronger acid or base/alkaline solutions which help keep body fluids neutral which is necessary for normal cell functioning.

Protein energy malnutrition (PEM) describes a range of disorders occurring mainly in under developed countries. It mainly affects young children and is the result of too little energy and too little protein in the diet. The two most common forms of PEM are marasmus and kwashiorkor.

During the 19th Century in the industrial towns in Europe and North America, marasmus, resulting from poor diets and numerous infections, took a toll on infant lives similarly as it does on many Asian, African and South American towns today, resulting in the death of many children.

Marasmus often occurs in infants under one year of age who have weaned off breast milk onto a diet usually of cereal which contains inadequate amounts of energy and protein. In underdeveloped countries today a rapid succession of pregnancies and early abrupt weaning, followed by dirty dilute milk or milk products along with poor housing, and a lack of equipment to make clean food result in repeated infections developing which can often result in the death of children.

Kwashiorkor arises in under developed countries after a prolonged period of breast feeding and the child is weaned onto the traditional family diet. But because of poverty their diet may be insufficient in protein. This is linked to poor land and bad agricultural practice.

Custom sometimes reinforced by taboos, determines that the limited supply of foods of animal origin is mainly given mainly to the men of the family. In many rural areas in under developed countries where Kwashiorkor in endemic, the food supply becomes scarce each year before the harvest. At this 'Hungry Season' the incidence of Kwashiorkor and other nutritional diseases increases.

(1983 Davidson Sir S, Passmore R, Brock J.F. Truswell A.S).

In 19th Century Ireland, Scotland, The Netherlands and Scandinavia at the time of the Great Famine from 1845-47, protein energy malnutrition would have been a classic example in 19th Century Western Europe.

However, because of starvation as a result of a potato blight, any fat reserves these people had would have been metabolized, and then the muscle and internal organs in their bodies would have been metabolized in order to provide energy. This resulted in skeletal bodies, not just thin and emaciated but the total starvation these men, women and children experienced ultimately caused their death amongst the poor in countries who experienced the potato blight as they had no other food sources because they were dependant on the potato.

During this era those who found themselves in the Workhouse were the lucky people because at least they got fed. But in places like the West of Ireland there would not have been such a place as a Workhouse. Those from the West of Ireland who were lucky enough to survive the journey on the 'Coffin Ships' to America at this tragic time in Irish history, just perished, but about a million Irish people did survive the journey to the New World.

In modern Irish history there is another group of people who died of starvation purposely as a political protest. These were a group of Irish Republican terrorists who went on a starvation protest in 1981 in a former prison in Northern Ireland called H-Block. There were about a dozen men and they all died of starvation inside a period of approximately forty days in jail.

There is a group of people who deliberately try to starve themselves to death as a result of believing that they are overweight when in fact they are seriously malnourished and underweight. This is known as

Anorexia Nervosa. It is the most life threatening of all mental health problems as one in six of these people die from a self-inflicted form of protein energy malnutrition. Anorexia Nervosa is often compounded with Bulimia. These people are often deluded that in their own image, that they are too fat. Orthodox medicine tries to save the lives of anorexia but often are unsuccessful.

Protein energy malnutrition is a term used to describe when the body reaches the stage of metabolizing its own muscle and especially its internal organs, the body becomes like a parasite, eating itself until starvation leads to the point of death.

CARBOHYDRATES

Carbohydrates are primarily an energy source. Complex carbohydrates, such as fruits, vegetables and whole grains also provide fibre in the diet. Simple carbohydrates are found in sugars and starches.

Carbohydrates provide most of the energy in almost all human diets. In the diets of poor people, especially in the tropics, up to 90 percent of the energy may come from this source.

Carbohydrates in food are divided into two categories. The first comprises available carbohydrates which can be digested in the upper gastrointestinal tract of man, absorbed and utilized as energy. These are the sugars, and certain polysaccharides such as starch.

Honey is a pleasant attractive food. At many times in the past it has acquired a special reputation either as a medicine or as a nutritious food. Most honeys consist of about 20 percent water and about 75 percent sugars, mostly fructose and glucose, with only traces of other nutrients and it is appreciated by all who enjoy a pleasant and attractive food.

The second category of carbohydrates is unavailable carbohydrates consists of fibrous polymers like cellulose that do not provide significant nourishment to man.

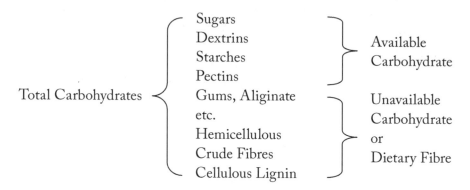

1983 Davidson, Passmore, Brock, Truswell

Available carbohydrates are fast releasing energy sources, such as sugar, honey, malt, sweets and most refined foods. Unavailable carbohydrates are slow releasing energy sources, commonly known as dietary fibre. These contain more complex carbohydrate and/or more fibre which helps to slow down the release of sugar.

Fast releasing carbohydrates give a sudden burst of energy followed with a 'crash' or slump in energy, while slow release carbohydrates provide a slower more sustainable release of energy which is preferable.

It is best to avoid refined foods such as sugar and white flour as they lack the vitamins and minerals needed for health, and they are one of the main contributors to the obesity crisis.

Instead you need to change your diet so that 70% of your calorie intake consists of slow releasing carbohydrates foods such as fresh fruit, vegetables, pulses and whole grain. Red kidney beans and baked beans are commonly eaten foods and they are a healthy source of slow releasing carbohydrates. Children often like simple beans on toast and this dietary habit should be encouraged for children and young people. Red kidney beans can be incorporated in various recipes such as chilli con carne, chilli fiesta or Mexican beef stew (See recipes).

Cheap, available or fast releasing carbohydrates is one of the major causes of the obesity problem which is becoming critical verging of an epidemic. It is difficult to change the habits of a lifetime, but it's a good start to avoid white sugar and white flour in the form of cakes, biscuits, white bread, white sugar in tea or coffee and sugary soft drinks.

Some people would think that this would be more difficult than giving up smoking. It certainly is challenging, but the obesity crisis has become such a challenge that it is becoming a choice of life or death. Doctors will not perform routine operations such as a hysterectomy or a hip replacement unless the patient loses the weight first.

In rural African society they have the lower incidence of bowel diseases such as appendicitis, colitis, diverticulitis and bowel cancer in the world as they eat 55 grams of unavailable carbohydrate per day compared to the U.K. average of only 22 grams per day.

If a clinically or morbidly obese person developed bowel cancer or related bowel disorders, surgeons would simply not operate on these people and this is why thousands are dying in hospitals in the U.K. today.

TABLE 2.1

Activity and Exercise Calorie-Usage Chart

It has been determined that, to keep fit, the average individual should expend at least 300 calories in some activity such as walking, golf or tennis. It is extremely difficult to lose significant weight through exercise. A half-hour of energetic bicycling, for instance uses up 200 – 280 calories which you put right back on by eating an ice cream.

Activity/Exercise	120 pound Woman (Calories)	160 pound Man (Calories)
Badminton	180-220	220-260
Baseball	160-200	200-240
Basketball	300-400	400-600
Bicycling moderately	100-120	120-140
Bicycling energetically	200 – 230	280 – 320
Bowling	80-120	100-140
Canoeing	100-150	130-180
Carpentry, workbench	120 – 140	140 – 180
Climbing stairs	130 – 160	160 – 190
Cooking, active	60 – 90	80 – 110
Dancing moderately	100 – 130	130 – 170
Dancing energetically, disco	200 – 400	250 – 500
Dishwashing by hand	60 – 90	80 – 110
Dressing, undressing	30 – 50	30 – 60
Driving auto	50 – 60	60 – 75
Dusting energetically	80 – 100	80 – 110
Exercising moderately	140 – 170	180 – 220
Football	250 – 300	300 – 400
Gardening, active	120 – 140	140 – 180

Golf, no cart	100 – 140	130 – 170
Golf, with cart	70 – 90	80 – 110
Handball	200 – 350	300 – 400
Hockey field ice	250 – 350	300 – 400
Horseback riding	140 – 160	160 – 220
Housework active	80 – 130	110 – 160
Ironing	60 – 80	70 – 90
Jogging, light	200 – 250	250 – 300
Lying, sitting at rest	15 – 20	20 – 25
Office work, active	70 – 130	90 – 150
Painting walls, furniture	130 – 150	150 – 180
Piano Playing	80 – 130	100 – 150
Polishing furniture, auto	80 – 120	90 – 150
Reading	15 – 20	20 – 25
Rowing vigorously	300 – 400	400 – 500
Running	300 – 400	400 – 500
Sawing wood	250 – 300	300 – 400
Sewing	25 -30	30 – 35
Singing	35 – 40	40 – 60
Skating energetically	200 – 300	250 – 350
Skiing energetically	200 – 300	250 – 350
Soccer	250 – 350	350 – 400
Squash	180 – 240	250 – 400
Standing, relaxed	20 – 25	25 – 30
Sweeping floor	80 – 100	90 – 110
Swimming steadily	200 – 300	300 – 400
Table tennis	150 – 180	200 – 250
Tennis amateur	180 – 220	250 – 280
Typing	80 – 100	90 – 110
Violin playing	70 – 100	90 – 130
Volleyball	180 – 220	220 – 280
Walking moderately	80 – 100	90 – 120
Walking energetically	140 – 160	160 – 180
Writing	25-80	30 – 100

Sugar Measuring Activity

On average we all eat about 100g of sugar a day which is well above the recommended target of 11 teaspoons a day set by the National Advisory Committee on Nutritional Education.

Table 2.1 illustrates calorie usage to help lose weight through activity and exercise.

Losing weight requires dedicated calorie reduction and regular exercise. If you use up 500 calories per day inside two weeks you will easily have used the 3,500 calories needed to lose a pound and even if you only lose a pound per week, inside a year this is 52 pound, about three and a half stones in weight.

Don't be despondent if you only lose a pound every one or two weeks – over time it is a significant amount it lose in fat.

A slow steady weight loss and a new relationship with food will result in a significant and lasting slim figure or physique rather than crash dieting, losing a lot of weight very quickly and regaining the weight if you go back to an unhealthy diet consisting of sugar and saturated fat. Slow, steady, significant weight loss is much more recommended to beat the obesity crisis. If we don't do something immediately about the epidemic on our hands - the obesity crisis, it literally could become a pandemic and kill half of the Western World.

Moderate changes in lifestyle involving reductions in calorific intake and increases in physical activity are the key to slow steady weight loss, as well as reassessing our relationship with food.

HONEY VS CANE SUGAR

In his budget on Tuesday 12th March 2016 in II Downing Street, The Chancellor of the Exchequer Mr George Osborne, did the wisest thing he ever did by increasing the price of sugar. Cane sugar is one of the most dangerous substances available on the market, and one of the main causes of the obesity crisis because it was cheap and widely available. The more he increases the price of white sugar especially, the better it will be for the Health of the Nation.

The British Government used to think that smoking was the most dangerous factor contributing to premature death. Now they are beginning to realize that obesity is as dangerous to general health and well-being as smoking. If an obese person needs emergency surgery such as an operation; for example, if a surgeon had to remove an obese person's appendix in order to save their life, a doctor would be forgiven if they could not save this person's life, as it is so difficult to operate through many layers of fat.

In fact, in recent years, surgeons will not perform routine operations until the patient loses the weight first.

White sugar is cane sugar grown in foreign countries such as China. It is very difficult to enjoy the taste of artificial sweeteners and most people don't like them. There is also the major problem of so many hidden sugars in our food today which most people are not aware of as illustrated in the table 1.1.

In the Biblical times, people did not have cane sugar or any kind of artificial sweeteners available to them so they used honey instead. These people who were descendants of Abraham lived much longer healthier lives, long before the dawn of orthodox medicine, than we do today and this could be very possibly to do with their diet.

Today honey is expensive compared to cane sugar which is very cheap. But for those who can afford it, it is a very nice alternative to cane sugar, for example, as a sweetener in coffee. A small teaspoon of honey in a good quality coffee brand is very tasty for a pleasant cup of coffee.

The science of why honey is so healthy compared to cane sugar is not yet known. It is a new challenge for scientists.

THE FACTS ABOUT FATS

There are two basic kinds of fat: saturated (hard fat) and unsaturated fat. It is not essential to eat hard fat, or ideal to eat too much of it. The main sources of saturated fat are meat and dairy products. There are two kinds of unsaturated fats; monosaturated fats of which olive oil is a rich source and polyunsaturated fats found in nuts, seed oils and fish.

Fats are a class of nutrients within the group of plants and animal substances called lipids, which do not dissolve in water. The lipid group includes fats, fatty acids, phosphides, waxes, and non-phosphorylated lipids. Most dietary lipids are fats or fatty acids.

Dietary fats are found in a wide range of foods which we eat. In nature, fats are contained within animal and vegetable tissues and man has known for a long time how to extract them to produce: -

Visible Fats: - such as butter, margarine, cream, lard, other table and cooking fats and vegetable oils.

About 60% of the fat in the diet consists of:

Invisible Fat: - which is less obvious such as that marbled throughout meat fibres in egg yolk, milk, herrings, nuts and wholegrain cereals.

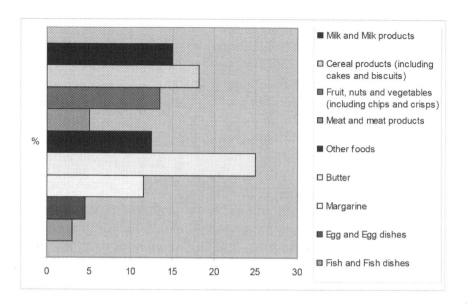

Chemical Composition

Fats are composed of three elements, carbon, hydrogen and oxygen, but the ratio of oxygen to carbon and hydrogen is much lower than it is in a carbohydrate. This means that less of the carbon and hydrogen in the fat molecule is oxidised as it occurs in food, therefore, there is a greater potential for the release of energy when these elements are oxidised within the body cells.

Structure of Fat

All fats are not alike. Each animal has a fat that is characteristic of its own species e.g. chicken fat is distinguishable from more solid beef fat and beef fat from mutton fat. The different characteristics of fats are the result of the kinds and numbers of fatty acids and their chemical arrangement in the fat.

Over 98 percent of the fat found in food is composed of triglycerides where the glycerol molecules have fatty acids attached to all three possible positions.

Saturated fats are solid at room temperature. Most animal fats are saturated. The exceptions are poultry and fish. This means animal fats are relatively high in saturated fatty acids.

Unsaturated Fats tend to be liquid at room temperature. Most vegetable fats are unsaturated (except for coconut oil). This means that most vegetable oils are relatively high in monounsaturated and polyunsaturated fatty acids.

Unsaturated fatty acids tend to produce a fat with a lower melting point, than a fat containing a high proportion of saturated fatty acids which has a higher melting point.and is therefore a saturated fat such as meat.

Fats are less dense than water so, when mixed with water fats rise to the surface.

Emulsified fats cannot form separate globules as the fat globules are in a finely divided form and are kept saturated from one another by an emulsifying agent, e.g. egg yolk fat is a naturally emulsified fat.

Function of Fat in the Diet

In 1994 the Committee on Medical Aspects of Food and Nutrition Policy (COMA) published a report on Nutritional Aspects of Cardiovascular Disease. It is recommended that no more than 35% of energy intake should come from fat and no more than 10% of energy intake should come from saturated fatty acids. These figures are intended as population averages, not as targets for individuals.

Protein Sparer

Fat in the diet supplies the body with a source of energy and so allows proteins to be used in the building and repair of tissues

Function of Fat in the Body

Energy Reserve

All tissue contains some fat. Excess fat is stored in specialised cells, the adipose cells. It is the fat in these cells which can be used for energy when required, and sometimes replaced later, so this is known as the Variable Fat Element in the body. The fat which is an essential constituent of cells is not used for energy and is known as the Constant Fat Element. The fats which are not used for energy are called Essential Fatty Acids.

Body Regulator

Fat is an essential constituent of the cell membrane of each individual cell and so helps to regulate the uptake and excretion of nutrients by the cells.

Insulation

Deposits of fat beneath the skin (subcutaneous fat) serve as insulating material for the body, protecting it against shock from changes in environmental temperature.

Protection of Vital Organs

Certain organs are surrounded by a pad of fat to protect them from physical shock e.g. kidneys and heart.

Digestion of fats

Fat tends to leave the stomach relatively slowly being released approximately three and a half hours after digestion. This delay in the emptying time of the stomach helps to delay the onset of hunger pangs and contributes to a feeling of satiety after a meal. The presence of fat in the duodenum stimulates the release of a hormone in the stomach, which in turn inhibits hunger contractions. Before fat can enter the general circulation to be transported to the tissues must be broken down chemically into molecules sufficiently small enough to pass into the cells of the membranes in the gastrointestinal tract.

Lipids in the Diet

Increase amounts of polyunsaturated fat in the diet and lower saturated fat in the diet in order to lower the incidence of heart disease.

Lowering cholesterol levels lower cholesterol in the blood, but replacing polyunsaturated fats for saturated fats in the diet does lower blood cholesterol.

Saturated and mono unsaturated fat are not nutrients: you do not need them, although they can be used by the body to make energy but poly unsaturated fats or oils are essential.

There is an increase in the incidence of heart disease where there is a high level of saturated fat and cholesterol in the diet.

Where there is an increased level of glucose in the diet there is an increase level of triglycerides in the blood and this is associated with an increase an blood cholesterol in order to reduce the chances of heart disease i.e. high blood cholesterol with high blood triglycerides pay attention to the following three points:

1. Reduce sugar level in the diet
2. Keep the fat contents in the diet to approximately 35% of the total calorie intake.
3. Use some poly unsaturated fats to replace some saturated fats.

Fat Soluble Vitamins

Vitamins A, D, E, F and K are soluble in fat solutions but are not soluble in water, and are usually found in fatty foods. They are found in plant foods too but this is not so obvious even some of these vitamins are derived from the leaves of plants, in seeds and nuts for example some of best source of vitamin E is in peanuts, sesame seeds and sunflower seeds.

In general fat soluble vitamins are not affected by cooking and processing. To enable us to absorb the fat soluble vitamins well we need some lipid material, and fat is needed in the diet for the absorption and storage of the fat soluble vitamins.

Because they are fat soluble they are not excreted readily in urine: they tend to be stored in the body, in the liver to be precise, because they are fat soluble vitamins if too much is stored in the body there can be toxic effects. Wee seldom take too much of any vitamin from natural food. When nutrients are used in large amounts they go beyond the stage of acting as a nutrient and really become a drug.

Cholesterol

It is not just a matter of high and low cholesterol. There is low density lipoproteins (LDL's) that carry cholesterol to the cells and can act like free radices and oxidizes and damage the arteries leaving deposits on the artery walls which can contribute to heart disease.

Good cholesterol refers to high density lipoproteins (HDL's) which transport cholesterol out of the arteries back to the liver where they can be reused or eliminated from the body. Cholesterol is not the problem. It is the ratio of HDL to LDL that is important. So the higher the HDL compared to the LDL cholesterol the lower the risk of heart disease.

The most dangerous piece of equipment we can have in our kitchen is more that dangerous it can mean the difference between life and death. It is the Deep Fat Fryer.

Fish and chip shops and all past food outlets are legally bound to change their frying oil every three days.

After using the deep fat fryer at home, more than three times, the unsaturated fat in the fryer, chemically changes into saturated fat which can clog the arteries known as arthreosclerosis which can lead to a heart attack or the need for a coronary artery bypass.

It is permissible to eat chips and other fried foods from a restaurant or take-away occasionally, but it is very dangerous to continuously use the deep fat fryer at home without frequently changing the oil, or you are asking not only for weight gain, but also cardiovascular disease.

HOW TO ACHIEVE A HEALTHIER HEART

Cardiovascular disease is a group of conditions affecting the heart, blood vessels and blood. They include coronary heart disease (a heart attack or sometimes known as a cardiac arrest and angina) hypertension (high blood pressure) blood clotting (excessive stickiness of the blood) peripheral, vascular disease (narrowing of the blood vessels, especially in the legs) strokes (obstructing or bleeding from a blood vessel in the brain) and high blood fat levels, poor circulation, varicose veins, chilblains and oedema (fluid retention).

Coronary heart disease is a major cause of death in Western Society. In the UK it accounts for nearly thirty percent of all deaths. Associated strokes (cardiovascular disease) accounts for a further twelve percent of deaths. A considerable amount of research has revealed that smoking and a high animal fat consumption (saturated fat) are associated with an increase in coronary heart disease.

Coronary heart disease usually manifests itself as angina (chest pain on exertion), a heart attack or cardiac arrest, also known as a myocardial infarction.

High blood pressure (hypertension) is a common condition, and it is linked to strokes, kidney disease, and to a lesser extent heart attacks. Research into possible association between dietary saturated fat intake reduction", and an increase in polyunsaturated fat in the diet has shown to reduce high blood pressure.

Hypertension or high blood pressure can be caused by atherosclerosis (a narrowing and thickening of the arteries) arterial tension or thicker blood. Arterial tension is controlled by the balance of calcium, magnesium and potassium in relation to sodium (salt). It is also thought Vitamin C and E and fish oils help to keep blood thin.

The risk of developing coronary heart disease can be reduced by:-

1. Stopping smoking
2. Reducing salt intake
3. Losing weight until you are no more than ten percent above your ideal weight.
4. Reduce consumption of animal fats such as cheese, butter, fatty meats, cakes, pastries, pies, processed cook chilled and frozen foods.
5. Take a good supply of green vegetables and fruit, at least five portions daily.
6. Use margarine and cooking oils high in polyunsaturated fats such as sunflower oil and safflower seed oil or a monounsaturated oil such as olive oil or extra virgin olive oil.
7. Reduce your consumption of refined carbohydrates and keep sugar to a minimum.
8. Do not exceed 14 units of alcohol per week for a woman, or 21 units for a man. I unit = ½ pint beer, lager or cider, 1 glass of wine, 1 measure of spirits or 1 measure of sherry/vermouth or 1 bottle of Alco pops.
9. Eat at least 3 portions of fish per week particularly oily fish such as tuna, salmon, mackerel, herring or sardines are recommended as they are high in Omega 3 fish oils.
10. Take regular exercise but consult your doctor before commencing any type of fitness plan.

This information has been known for the last twenty five years by medicine, the field of Nutritional Medicine and Human Nutrition and Dietetics, but it has been ignored by a wide section of society who may develop coronary heart disease as a consequence. Two main factors are responsible for heart disease:- atherosclerosis (the formation of deposits) or furring of the arteries and the presence of blood clots (thick blood).

Arteriosclerosis is hardening of the arteries. Arteries are elastic whether or not atherosclerosis is present; they tend to lose their elasticity and harden with age. One reason is lack of Vitamin C which is needed to make collagen, the intercellular "give" that keeps skin and arteries supple. Arteriosclerosis, atherosclerosis and thick blood can all raise blood pressure, putting you at a greater risk of thrombosis, angina, a heart attack (cardiac arrest myocardial infarction) or a stroke (cardiovascular disease).

Increasing the intake of Vitamin C in middle aged and older people restores artery walls. Another important part of his theory is lack of Vitamin C plus excessive levels of blood cholesterol and triglycerides (fats in the blood) causes severe arterial blockage leading to death.

It is advisable to take fish oil supplements, avoid fried food, limit intake of meat and foods high in saturated fat, and eat more foods high in Omega 3 such as salmon, tuna, herring, mackerel or sardines.

If you are a smoker or if you feel you are not getting enough Vitamin C, then a supplement of Vitamin C is necessary daily as smoking depletes Vitamin C levels in the body and leads to wrinkling of the skin. A supplement of 1000mg daily is recommended. This fact has been known in the field of Human Nutrition and Dietetics for the past thirty years and anyone over forty years of age needs a daily supplement of Vitamin C.

There are benefits of red wine for the heart. The field of medicine knows about "The French Paradox". The French are sensible users of red wine. They even give it to their children and France has the lowest rate of coronary heart disease in the world, and medicine is recognising this fact. As lay people would say:- "Red wine keeps the blood thin" Red wine basically prevents blood clots forming because if a blood clot becomes lodged in a main artery such as the aorta near to the heart, the result is a heart attack.

Alcohol in moderation is thought to help lower the risk of heart disease and increase levels of HDL cholesterol. 'Red wine is thought to be particularly good for you because of contains compounds which help lower bad (HDL) cholesterol thus affording greater heart disease protection'. Other nutrients in wine also have antioxidant effects, helping increase levels of good HDL cholesterol and lowering blood pressure'

(Kelly L 2009)

Diets high in soluble fibre have been shown in some studies to lower LDL cholesterol and total cholesterol by 30 per cent. Food sources of soluble fibre include oats, broccoli and asparagus. Vitamin B3 helps decrease the body's production of cholesterol.

High blood pressure is one of the complications associated with cardio-vascular disease.

Garlic consumption on a regular basis is also thought to lower blood pressure high sodium intake from table salt is associated with high blood pressure or hypertension.

'Numerous studies have shown that sodium restriction above does no improve blood pressure control in most people but must also be accompanied by a high potassium intake'

(Mc Keith 2008)

Potassium is important in the diet as it is a diuretic effect on fluid levels in the body and its counteracts the effect of sodium which can cause the body to retain fluid and this potassium sodium balance is very important for those who are retaining fluid around their abdomen or enabled good food sources of potassium include bananas, water cress, cabbage, celery, parsley, courgettes, cauliflower, radishes, mushrooms, molasses and pumpkins.

Olive oil which is a mono unstructured oil is much more resistant to oxidation than oils with high levels of poly unsaturated fats such as com oil, sunflower oil or safflower oil. The substitution of mono unsaturated fats in the diet (a favourite amongst modern cooks) for saturated fats such as butter, lard or dripping, in the diet has shown to decrease total cholesterol, in particular (LDL) bad cholesterol.

You need to follow a few steps if you wish to reduce the risk and help prevent heart disease:

1. Maintain a healthy stable weight. Within your ideal weight range.
2. Lower your blood pressure.
3. Lower level of LDL 'bad' cholesterol
4. Increase level of HDL 'good' cholesterol

Before a myocardial infarction or cardiac arrest occurs the patient can be diagnosed with having angina which is a condition where there is partial blockage of the coronary arteries which feed oxygen and glucose to the heart muscle causing sharp chest pains especially under stress. If you are experiencing sharp chest pains it is best to go to your G.P., or if you are very worried that a heart attack is coming on, ring 999 and go straight to accident and emergency in your local hospital and a "trace" of your heart can be done. In a lot of cases it is not an imminent heart attack but just stress pains.

A stroke can occur because of a blockage in the main artery to the brain, the caratoid artery where part of the brain tissue may die leaving the patient with no feeling down one side of the body. Sometimes this occurs not because of a blockage in the artery in the neck but because the artery ruptures. If a blockage occurs in the legs it can result in severe leg pain which is called a thrombosis in the leg.

Medicine would agree that arteriosclerosis (hardening of the arteries), is a factor which contributes to coronary heart disease. However they may not necessarily agree that taking large doses of Vitamin C can make arteries more supple.

The recently discovered fish oils which constitutes Vitamin F in combination with Vitamin E found mainly in many kinds of nuts such as pistachio nuts, cashew nuts and peanuts are much healthier than foods high in triglycerides such as our typical "Ulster Fry" or "Full English Fry" and/or fish and chips out of the fish and chip shop. If you must go to the fish and chip shop, eat the fish but try not to eat too much of the batter and chips.

Research shows that LDL (low density lipoprotein) is found in large proportions in an individual's cholesterol and it is likely to be deposited in the artery walls. Another lipoprotein called HDL (high density lipoprotein) can transport cholesterol out of the arteries back to the liver. So the higher an individual's HDL compared to their LDL cholesterol, the lower the risk of heart disease.

Taking fish oil supplements, or eating a lot of oily fish is what is understood to protect the Eskimos from having one of the lowest incidences of cardiovascular disease in the world.

In order to lower triglycerides (fats in the blood) avoid fried food as much as possible and reduce the intake of meat and foods high in saturated fat, do not eat more than half a dozen eggs per week although no direct link has been found between eating eggs and high blood cholesterol, or heart disease. Increase foods high in Vitamin F such as salmon, tuna, mackerel, herrings, sunflower oil, saffron oil and olive oil, extra virgin olive oil or rapeseed oil and eat plenty of fresh fruit and vegetables, as well as restricting salt intake which contributes to high blood pressure i.e. hypertension, and take regular exercise to keep your weight under control.

It is highly recommended that as well as dietary changes, odourless garlic capsules prevent the onset of coronary artery diseases. Some nutritionalists also believe that increasing vitamin C intakes can lower blood pressure.

Four steps to achieve a Healthier Heart:

1. Reduce Saturated Fat
2. Reduce Salt
3. Drink five glasses of red wine per week.
4. Increase vitamin C intake. Drink the juice of a lemon or lime daily, or take 1,000mg of vitamin C daily.

EVADING THE OBESITY CRISIS THROUGH EXERCISE

Now that the obesity crisis is literally becoming critical, apart from dieting, there is only one sure way you are going to lose weight and that is to use up excess calories through exercise.

It is easier for children and young people to take regular exercise such as in the gymnasium at physical education lessons at school, basketball, netball, volleyball, swimming lessons, bicycling and playing games with their friends.

Taking part in exercise becomes more difficult for adults, including the mothers of small children. It is easier for young men – they can play football and go running.

Overtraining or vigorous exercise actually can suppress the immune system while the Chinese art of Tai-chi has been shown to increase the T-cells (One of the body's types of immune cells) by 40 percent.

More calming, less stressful forms of exercise are probably best for immunity. This may suppress the immune system. Numerous studies have found that low psychological states of mind such as stress, depression, and grief depress the immune system.

(2000 Holford P.)

In western society, people have lost the art of taking even moderate exercise are in many cases people travel everywhere by cars, buses, trains or in large cities – the tube or metro.

One of the easiest ways of doing moderate exercise is to go for a brisk walk for about twenty minutes at least three times per week which will result in weight loss much quicker than dieting alone. If dieters don't want to go walking, purchasing a treadmill for the home is very beneficial for losing weight and general aerobic exercise.

Aerobic respiration happens when the body produces energy when carbohydrate foods react with oxygen from the air we breathe. Oxygen is the most vital nutrient we take into our bodies, yet most of us breathe in only a third of our lung capacity. By spending 15 minutes a day taking moderate exercise, we can build up stamina, suppleness, strength and a beautiful body, leaving you feeling physically energised. Emotionally balanced, and mentally clear. Too much exercise can elevate levels of the stress hormone. Cortisol is not recommended if you are stressed out.

(2000 Holford P.)

During less strenuous exercise is known as 'aerobic exercise' such as jogging, swimming, walking, cycling, canoeing, skiing or horse riding, carbohydrates yield twice as much energy as fat. During a short burst of 'aerobic' exercise such as sprinting, the body does not use up fat as energy but only carbohydrates.

Athletes eat rice or pasta or other complex carbohydrates a few hours before physical performance, as carbohydrates can be stored as glycogen in the liver and muscles while fat cannot be stored for short term energy release, whilst contrary to popular belief increasing protein intake does not increase physical performance. 62 grams of protein per day is necessary for health.

It is more likely that the leaner you are, the longer you will live. You don't have to suffer malnutrition in order to become slim and fit, or be like an Olympic athlete. Balanced nutrition is about giving the body what it needs and no more. Avoid foods which contain empty calories such as saturated fat, sugar and too much salt as it can increase the blood pressure, and eat nutrient dense foods such as organic vegetables, fruits and nuts, particularly the antioxidant nutrients vitamin A, C, E, selenium and zinc.

Patrick Holford states in his book "The Optimum Nutrition Bible" that if we would only listen to him we could be living to a hundred and twenty years of age.

DESIRED WEIGHT AND MATCHING CALORIE MAINTENANCE CHART.

(based on height: no clothing)

	WOMEN		MEN	
Height	Weight in Pounds	Daily Calories	Weight in Pounds	Daily calories
4'10"	90 – 98	1080 – 1170	95-105	1235 – 1365
4'11"	95 – 102	1115 – 1170	98 – 108	1275 – 1405
5"	95 – 105	1140 – 1260	100 – 111	1300 – 1445
5'1"	97 – 108	1165 – 1295	105 – 117	1365 – 1520
5'2"	100 – 111	1200 – 1335	110 – 123	1430 – 1560
5'3"	105 – 118	1250 – 1415	115 – 128	1495 – 1665
5'4"	110 – 123	1320 – 1475	120 – 133	1560 – 1730
5'5"	112 – 126	1345 – 1515	125 – 138	1625 – 1795
5'6"	117 – 130	1405 – 1560	130 – 143	1690 – 1860
5'7"	120 – 134	1440 – 1610	133 – 148	1730 – 1925
5'8"	125 – 139	1500 – 1670	137 – 153	1780 – 1990
5'9"	130 – 144	1560 – 1730	143 – 159	1860 – 2065
5'10"	135 – 149	1620 – 1790	148 – 164	1925 – 2130
5'11"	140 – 154	1680 – 1850	152 – 168	1975 – 2185
6"	144 – 158	1730 – 1895	155 – 171	2015 – 2225
6'1"	163 – 179	2120 – 2395		
6'2"	167 – 183	2170 – 2380		
6'3"	170 – 188	2210 – 2445		
6'4"	172 – 195	2235 – 2535		
6'5"	178 – 198	2315 – 2575		
6'6"	185 – 206	2405 – 2680		

Write your desired weight goal here _____ pounds

Write your daily calorie allowance here _____ calories

TABLE OF WEIGHTS FOR MALES
(in indoor clothing)

Height (without shoes)	Desirable weight (age 25 and over)			Average weight for age					
	Minimum	Mean	Maximum	20-24	25-29	30 – 39	40 – 49	50 – 59	60 – 69
5'2" 1.58m	8st 3lb 115lb 52kg	9st 1lb 127lb 58kg	10st 4lb 144lb 65kg	9st 2lb 128lb 58kg	9st 8lb 134lb 61kg	9st 11lb 137lb 62kg	10st 0lb 140lb 64kg	10st 2lb 142lb 64kg	9st 13lb 139lb 63kg
5'3" 1.50m	8st 6lb 118lb 54kg	9st 4lb 130lb 59kg	10st 8lb 152lb 59kg	9st 6lb 132lb 60kg	9st 12lb 138lb 63kg	10st 1lb 141lb 64kg	10st 4lb 144lb 65kg	10st 5lb 145lb 66kg	10st 2lb 142lb 64kg
5'4" 1.63m	8st 9lb 121lb 55kg	9st 7lb 133lb 60kg	10st 12lb 152lb 69kg	9st 10lb 136lb 62kg	10st 1lb 141lb 64kg	10st 5lb 145lb 66kg	10st 8lb 148lb 67kg	10st 9lb 149lb 68kg	10st 6lb 146lb 55kg
5'5" 1.85m	8st 12lb 124lb 56kg	9st 11lb 137lb 62kg	11st 2lb 156lb 71kg	9st 13lb 139lb 63kg	10st 4lb 144lb 65kg	10st 9lb 149lb 68kg	10st 12lb 152lb 69kg	10st 13lb 153lb 69kg	10st 10lb 150lb 68kg
5'6" 1.58m	3st 2lb 128lb 58kg	10st 1lb 141lb 64	11st 7lb 161lb 73kg	10st 2lb 142lb 64kg	10st 8lb 148lb 67kg	10st 13lb 153lb 69kg	11st 2lb 156lb 71kg	11st 3lb 157lb 71kg	11st 0lb 154lb 70kg
5'7" 170m	9st 6lb 132lb 60kg	10st 5lb 145lb 66kg	11st 12lb 166lb 75kg	10st 5lb 145lb 66kg	10st 11lb 151lb 68kg	11st 3lb 157lb 71kg	11st 7lb 161lb 73kg	11st 8lb 162lb 73kg	11st 5lb 159lb 72kg
5'8" 1.73m	9st 10lb 136lb 62kg	10st 9lb 149lb 68kg	12st 2lb 170lb 77kg	10st 9lb 149lb 63kg	11st 1lb 155lb 70kg	11st 7lb 161lb 73kg	11st 11lb 165lb 75kg	11st 12lb 166lb 75kg	11st 9lb 159lb 72kg
5'9" 1.76m	10st 0lb 140lb 64kg	10st 13lb 153lb 69kg	12st 6lb 174lb 79kg	10st 13lb 153lb 69kg	11st 5lb 159lb 72kg	11st 11lb 165lb 75kg	12st 1lb 169lb 77kg	12st 2lb 170lb 77kg	12st 0lb 168lb 76kg
5'10" 1.75m	10st 4lb 144lb 65kg	11st 4lb 158lb 72kg	12st 11lb 179lb 81kg	11st 3lb 167lb 71kg	11st 9lb 163lb 74kg	12st 2lb 170lb 77kg	12st 6lb 174lb 79kg	12st 7lb 175lb 79kg	12st 5lb 173lb 78kg
5'11" 1.80m	10st 8lb 148lb 67kg	11st 8lb 162lb 73kg	13st 7lb 184lb 83kg	11st 7lb 161lb 73kg	11st 13lb 167lb 76kg	12st 6lb 174lb 79kg	12st 10lb 178lb 81kg	12st 12lb 180lb 82kg	12st 10lb 178lb 81kg

6'0" 1.83m	10st 12lb 152lb 69kg	11st 13lb 167lb 76kg	13st 7lb 189lb 86kg	11st 12lb 166lb 75kg	12st 4lb 172lb 78kg	12st 11lb 179lb 81kg	13st 1lb 183lb 83kg	13st 3lb 185lb 84kg	13st 1lb 183lb 83kg
6'1" 1.85m	11st 2lb 156lb 71kg	12oz 3lb 171lb 78kg	13st 12lb 194lb 88kg	12st 2lb 170lb 77kg	12st 9lb 177lb 80kg	13st 1lb 183lb 83kg	13st 5lb 187lb 85kg	13st 7lb 189lb 86kg	13st 6lb 188lb 85kg
6'2" 1.88m	11st 6lb 160b 73kg	12st 8lb 176lb 80kg	14st 3lb 199lb 90kg	12st 6lb 174lb 79kg	13st 0lb 182lb 83kg	13st 6lb 188lb 85kg	13st 10lb 192lb 87kg	13st 12lb 194lb 88kg	13st 11lb 192lb 88kg

Table of Weights for Females
(in indoor clothing)

Height (without shoes)	Desirable Weight (Age 25 and over)			Average Weight for Age					
	Minimum	Mean	Maximum	20-24	25-29	30-39	40-49	50-59	60-69
4'10" 1.47M	6st12lb 96lb 44kg	7st9lb 107lb 49kg	8st 13lb 125lb 57kg	7st4lb 102lb 46kg	7st9lb 107lb 49kg	8st3lb 115lb 52kg	8st10lb 122lb 55kg	8st13lb 125lb 57kg	9st1lb 127lb 58kg
4'11" 1.50m	7st 1lb 99lb 45kg	7st12lb 110lb 50kg	9st2lb 128lb 58kg	7st7lb 105lb 48kg	7st12lb 110lb 50kg	8st5lb 117lb 53kg	8st12lb 124lb 56kg	9st 1lb 127lb 58kg	9st 3lb 129lb 59kg
5'0" 1.52m	7st 4lb 102lb 46kg	8st1lb 113lb 51kg	9st 5lb 131lb 59kg	7st10lb 108lb 49kg	8st1lb 113lb 51kg	8st8lb 120lb 54kg	9st1lb 127lb 58kg	9st4lb 130lb 59kg	9st5lb 131lb 59kg
5'1" 1.54m	7st7lb 105lb 48kg	8st4lb 116lb 51kg	9st8lb 134lb 61kg	8st0lb 112lb 51kg	8st4lb 116lb 53kg	8st11lb 123lb 56kg	9st1lb 127lb 58kg	9st4lb 130lb 59kg	9st5lb 131lb 59kg
5'2" 1.58m	7st10lb 108lb 49kg	8st8lb 120lb 54kg	9st12lb 136lb 63kg	8st3lb 115lb 52kg	8st7lb 119lb 53kg	8st11lb 123lb 56kg	9st4lb 130lb 59kg	9st7lb 133lb 60kg	9st8lb 134lb 61kg
5'3" 1.60m	7st13lb 111lb 50kg	8st11lb 123lb 56kg	10st2lb 142lb 69kg	8st6lb 118lb 54kg	8st10lb 122lb 55kg	9st3lb 129lb 59kg	9st10lb 136lb 62kg	10st0lb 140lb 64kg	10st1lb 141lb 64kg
5'4" 1.63m	8st2lb 114lb 52kg	9st2lb 128lb 58kg	10st6lb 146lb 66kg	8st9lb 121lb 55kg	8st13lb 125lb 57kg	9st6lb 132lb 60kg	10st0lb 140lb 64kg	10st4lb 144lb 65kg	10st5lb 145lb 66kg
5'5" 1.65m	8st6lb 118lb 54kg	9st6lb 132lb 60kg	10st10lb 150lb 68kg	8st13lb 125lb 57kg	9st3lb 129lb 50kg	9st9lb 135lb 61kg	10st0lb 143lb 65kg	10st5lb 148lb 67kg	10st9lb 149lb 68kg
5'6" 1.58m	8st10lb 122lb 55kg	9st10lb 136lb 62kg	11st0lb 154lb 70kg	9st3lb 129lb 59kg	9st7lb 133lb 60kg	9st13lb 139lb 63kg	10st7lb 147lb 67kg	10st12lb 152lb 69kg	10st13lb 153lb 69kg
5'7" 1.70m	9st0lb 126lb 57kg	10st0lb 140lb 64kg	11st4lb 158lb 72kg	9st6lb 132lb 60kg	9st10lb 136lb 62kg	10st2lb 142lb 64kg	10st11lb 151lb 68kg	11st2lb 156lb 71kg	11st3lb 157lb 71kg
5'8" 1.73m	9st4lb 130lb 59kg	10st4lb 144lb 65kg	11st9lb 163lb 74kg	9st10lb 136lb 62kg	10st0lb 140lb 64kg	10st6lb 146lb 66kg	11st1lb 155lb 70kg	11st6lb 160lb 73kg	11st7lb 161lb 73kg
5'9" 1.75m	9st8lb 134lb 61kg	10st8lb 148lb 67kg	12st0lb 168lb 70kg	10st0lb 140lb 64kg	10st4lb 144lb 65kg	10st10lb 150lb 68kg	11st5lb 159lb 72kg	11st10lb 164kg 74kg	11st11lb 165lb 75kg
5'10" 1.78m	9st12lb 138lb 63kg	10st12lb 152lb 59kg	12st6lb 174lb 79kg	10st4lb 144lb 65kg	10st8lb 148lb 67kg	11st0lb 154lb 70kg	11st10lb 164lb 74kg	12st1lb 169lb 77kg	-

ROTATIONAL DIET

Most people live on a rotational diet. There could be a dozen or more meals people cook for themselves and their families and friends.

The key to losing weight is to know how to avoid the highest calorie foods and drinks. Spirits are obviously the first drink to avoid if you wish to lose weight.

From this list, people will very quickly work out which foods to avoid and which foods they can eat quite a lot of and still lose weight.

About 2010 I gained weight because of medication for my nervous system. After a couple of years I stopped this medication. Due to my knowledge of the calorific value of foods, I have been a stable weight of between 8st 12lbs and 9 stone for several years, and I am 5' 4" in height.

I know the secret of being able to eat plenty of food and remain slim and some people maintain I am young looking for my age which is 51 years of age. It is a combination of a lower calorie healthy diet, regular exercise, vitamin and mineral supplements and Avon skin products which keep me heathly even if I do smoke cigarettes but I avoid drinking spirits.

As a Nutritional Consultant with a background of Human Nutrition and Dietetics, Health Promotion and Health and Social Care, I wish to help as many people as possible "Crack the Obesity Crisis", as it has become critical.

Miracles don't happen overnight. It can take weeks, even months to lose weight. The key is to have positive mental attitude and general gut determination to achieve results for the rest of your life.

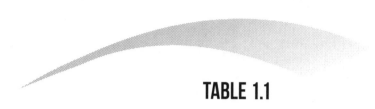

per 100g

TABLE 1.1

Kcal – Kilo calorie
KJ - Kilojoule

Calories in Commonly Eaten Foods

	Kcal	Kj
Tomato Soup, Tinned	51	215
Sweetcorn, Tinned	77	324
Branston Pickle	157	638
Dolmio Bolognese Sauce	44	185
White Dolmio Sauce for Lasagne	98	408
Red Kidney Beans	98	401
Peanut Butter	624	2586
HP Sauce	122	517
Stir Fry Sauce	118	503
Tinned Tomatoes Chopped	22	94
Devon Custard Light	89	378
Honey	334	1417
Greek Style Yogurt	72	304
Dairy Lea Triangles	245	1025
Ski Mousse	127	534
Créme Caramel	110	467

CALORIES IN ALCOHOLIC BEVERAGES PER 100ML

Kcal – Kilo calorie

KJ - Kilojoule

Beers

	Kcal	Kj
Brown Ale, Bottled	28	117
Canned Beer	32	132
Draught Beer	32	132
Lager, Bottled	29	120
Stout, Bottled	37	157
Stout Extra	39	163
Strong Ale	72	301

Cider

	Kcal	Kj
Cider, Dry	36	152
Cider, Sweet	42	176
Cider, Vintage	101	421

Wines

	Kcal	Kj
Red Wine	68	284
Rosé, Medium	71	294
White Wine Dry	66	275
White Wine, Medium	75	311

per 100g

White Wine, Sweet	94	394
White Wine, Sparkling	76	315
Port	157	655
Sherry, Dry	116	481
Sherry, Medium	118	489
Sherry, Sweet	136	568

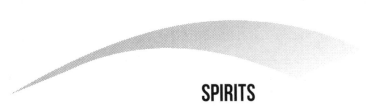

SPIRITS

	Kcal	Kj
70% Proof	222	919

Meats and meat products

	Kcal	Kj
Bacon, lean, raw	147	617
Bacon fat, raw	747	3075
Gammon joint, raw, lean and fat	269	1119
Gammon, lean only	167	703
Gammon rashers, grilled, lean and fat	228	953
Gammon rashers, grilled, lean only	172	726
Rashers, raw, back	428	1766
Rashers, raw, middle	425	1756
Rashers, raw, streaky	414	1710
Rashers, grilled, lean only	292	1218
Rashers, back, lean and fat	405	1681
Rashers, middle, lean and fat	416	1722
Rashers, streaky, lean and fat	422	1749
Beef		
Mince, raw	221	919
Rump steak, raw, lean and fat	197	821
Rump steak, fried, lean and fat	246	1026
Rump steak, lean only	190	797
Rump steak, grilled, lean and fat	218	912
Rump steak, grilled, lean only	168	708
Silverside, salted, boiled, lean and fat	242	1072
Silverside, salted, boiled, lean only	192	806

Sirloin, raw, lean and fat	272	1126
Sirloin, roast, lean and fat	284	1182
Sirloin, lean only	192	806
Stewing steak, raw, lean and fat	176	736
Stewing steak, stewed, lean and fat	223	932
Topside, raw, lean and fat	214	896
Topside, raw, lean only	156	659

Lamb

	Kcal	Kj
Breast raw, lean and fat	378	1564
Breast, roast, lean and fat	410	1697
Breast, roast, lean only	252	1049
Chops loin, lean and fat	377	1558
Chops, grilled, lean and fat	355	1473
Cutlets raw, lean and fat	386	1593
Cutlets, lean only	222	928
Cutlets, lean and fat	122	512
Cutlets, lean only	222	928
Cutlets, lean and fat (weighed with fat and bone)	122	512
Cutlets, raw, lean and fat	386	1593
Cutlets, grilled, lean and fat	370	1534
Leg, raw, lean and fat	240	996
Leg, roast, lean and fat	266	1106
Leg, roast, lean only	191	800
Scrog and neck, raw, lean and fat	316	1309
Stew, lean and fat	292	1216
Stew, lean only	253	1054
Stew, lean only, weighed with fat and bone	128	536
Shoulder, raw, lean and fat	314	1301
Shoulder, roast, lean and fat	316	1311
Shoulder, roast, lean only	196	819

Pork

	Kcal	Kj
Belly rashers, raw, lean and fat	381	1574
Belly rashers, grilled, lean and fat	398	1574
Chops loin, grilled, lean and fat	332	1380
Leg, raw, lean and fat	269	1115
Leg, roast, lean and fat	286	1190
Leg, roast, lean only	185	777

Veal

	Kcal	Kj
Cutlet, fried	215	904
Fillet, raw	109	459
Fillet, roast	230	963

Poultry and game

	Kcal	Kj
Chicken, raw, meat only	121	508
Chicken, raw, meat and skin	230	954
Light meat	116	489
Dark meat	126	528
Chicken, boiled, meat only	183	767
Chicken, boiled, light meat	163	686
Chicken, boiled, dark meat	204	853
Chicken, roast, meat only	148	621
Chicken, roast, meat and skin	216	902
Chicken, roast, light meat	142	589
Chicken, roast, dark meat	155	648
Chicken, wing quarter (weighed with bone)	74	311
Chicken, leg quarter (weighed with bone)	92	388

Duck

	Kcal	Kj
Duck, raw, meat only	122	513
Duck, raw, meat, fat and skin	430	1772
Duck, roast, meat only	189	789
Duck, roast, meat, fat and skin	339	1406
Goose, roast	319	1327
Partridge, roast	212	890
Partridge, roast, weighed with bone	127	533
Pheasant, roast	213	892
Pheasant, roast (weighed with bone)	134	563
Pigeon, roast	230	961
Pigeon, roast (weighed with bone)	101	422
Turkey, raw, meat only	107	454
Turkey, raw, meat and skin	145	606
Turkey, raw, light meat	103	435
Turkey, raw, dark meat	114	478
Turkey, roast, meat only	140	590
Turkey, roast, meat and skin	171	717
Turkey, roast, light meat	132	558
Turkey, roast, dark meat	148	624

Canned meat

	Kcal	Kj
Beef, corned	217	905
Ham	120	512
Ham and pork, chopped	270	1118
Luncheon meat	313	1298
Stewed steak with gravy	176	730

Sausages

	Kcal	Kj
Frankfurters	274	1135
Salami	491	2031
Sausages, beef, raw	299	1242
Sausages, beef, fried	269	1168
Sausages, beef, grilled	265	1104
Sausages, pork, raw	367	1570
Sausages, pork, fried	269	1168
Sausages, pork, grilled	318	1320
Beef burgers, frozen, raw	265	1102
Beef burgers, frozen, fried	264	1099

Meat and Pastry products

	Kcal	Kj
Cornish pastie	332	1388
Pork pie (individual)	376	1564
Sausage roll, flaky pastry	479	1991
Sausage roll, short pastry	463	1929
Steak and Kidney pie (individual)	323	1349

Cooked Dishes

	Kcal	Kj
Beef Steak pudding	223	934
Beef stew	119	498
Bolognaise Sauce	139	579
Canned meat	160	668
Lancashire Hot Pot	114	480
Irish Stew	124	520
Irish Stew (weighed with bones)	114	475
Moussaka	195	811
Shepherds Pie	119	497

Fish and Fish products

	Kcal	Kj
Cod, raw, fresh fillets	76	322
Cod, raw, frozen steaks	68	287
Cod, baked	86	408
Cod, baked, weighed with bones and skin	82	348
Cod, fried in batter	199	834
Cod, grilled	95	402
Cod, poached	94	396
Cod poached (weighed with bones and skin)	82	346
Cod, steamed	83	350
Cod, steamed, weighed with bones and skin	67	283
Cod, smoked, raw	79	333
Haddock fresh, raw	73	308
Haddock fresh, fried	174	729
Haddock fresh, fried (weighed with bones)	160	669
Haddock, steamed (weighed with bones and skin)	75	316
Haddock, smoked, steamed	101	429
Haddock weighed with bones and skin	66	279
Plaice, raw	91	386
Plaice, fried in batter	279	1165
Plaice, fried in crumbs	228	951
Plaice, steamed	93	392
Whiting, fried	191	801
Whiting, steamed	92	389
Whiting, steamed (weighed with bones)	63	265

Fatty Fish

	Kcal	Kj
Black lumpfish caviar	190	360
Eel, raw	168	700
Eel, steamed	201	839
Fillet of anchovies in extra virgin olive oil	185	773
Herring, raw	234	970
Herring, fried	234	975
Herring fried, weighed with bones	206	858
Herring, grilled	199	825
Herring grilled, weighed with bones	135	562
Kipper, baked	205	855
Kipper, baked, weighed with bones	111	464
Kipper Fillets, canned	238	987
Mackerel (raw)	223	926
Mackerel (fried)	188	784
Mackerel, weighed with bones	138	574
Mackerel, in sunflower oil	260	1080
Pilchards canned in tomato sauce	126	531
Salmon, raw	182	757
Salmon, steamed	197	823
Salmon, canned	155	649
Salmon, smoked	142	598
Sardines, canned in olive oil	217	906
Sardines, canned in sunflower oil	230	958
Sardines, canned in tomato sauce	177	760
Sprats, fried	441	1826
Sprats fried, weighed with bones	388	1608
Trout, brown (steamed)	135	566
Trout, steamed, weighed with bones	89	375
Tuna (canned in brine)	105	444
Tuna (canned in oil)	289	1202
Whitebait, fried	525	2174

Cartilaginous fish

	Kcal	Kj
Dog fish fried in batter	265	1103
Dog fish fried (weighed with waste)	244	1016
Skate, fried in batter	199	830
Skate, weighed with waste	163	680

Crustacea

	Kcal	Kj
Crab, boiled	127	534
Crab, boiled, weighed with shell	25	105
Crab, canned	81	341
Crab meat chunks, canned	72	306
Lobster, boiled	119	502
Lobster, boiled, weighed with shell	41	172
Lobster dressed, canned	45	189
Scampi, boiled	316	1321
Shrimps, boiled	117	493
Shrimps, boiled, weighed with shell	39	164
Shrimps, canned	94	398

Molluscs

	Kcal	Kj
Cockles, boiled	48	203
Mussels, raw	66	276
Mussels, boiled	87	336
Mussels, boiled (weighed with shell)	26	111
Mussels, pickled (canned)	97	410
Oysters, raw	51	217
Oysters, raw (weighed with shell)	6	26
Oysters, smoked, in sunflower oil, canned	230	960
Scallops, steamed	105	446
Squid in Olive Oil	66	159
Whelks, boiled	91	385
Whelk, boiled (weighed with shell)	14	59
Winkles, boiled	74	312
Winkle boiled (weighed with shell)	14	60

Fish products and Dishes

	Kcal	Kj
Fish cakes, frozen	178	749
Fish cakes, fried	188	785
Fish fingers, frozen	178	749
Fish fingers, fried	233	975
Fish paste	169	704
Fish pie	128	540
Kedegree	181	633
Roe Cod hard, raw	113	476
Roe, Cod, fried	202	844
Roe, herring, soft, raw	80	337
Roe herring, soft, fried	244	1019

Carbohydrates

	Kcal	Kj
Porridge	44	188
Macaroni raw	357	1515
Macaroni, boiled	117	499
Lasagne Sheets	357	1515
Tagliatelle	357	1515
Conchiglie	357	1515
Medium Egg Noodles	178	748
Rice, polished, raw	361	536
Rice, boiled	123	522
Spaghetti, raw	378	1612
Spaghetti, boiled	117	499
Spaghetti, canned in tomato sauce	59	250

Bread

	Kcal	Kj
Wholemeal	216	918
Brown	223	948
Hovis	228	958
White	233	991
White, toasted	297	1265
Soda	264	1122

Rolls

Brown, crusty	289	1229
White, crusty	290	1231
Chappatis (made with fat)	336	1415
Chappattis (made without fat)	202	860

Breakfast Cereals

	Kcal	Kj
All Bran	273	1156
All Bran Bran Flakes	356	1503
All Bran Sultana Bran	344	1453
All Bran Golden Crunch	405	1701
Cheerios	381	1610
Coco Pops	387	1639
Cornflakes	368	1567
Crunchy Nut Bites	450	1892
Crunchy Nut Clusters	447	1879
Crunchy Nut Cornflakes	402	1701
Crunchy Nut Milk Chocolate Curls	460	1932
Frosties	375	1594
Fruit n Fibre	380	1603
Museli	368	1556
Oats n More, almond	400	1690
Oats n More, honey	374	1581
Oats n More, raisin	367	1555
Quaker Oats	356	1500
Ready Brek	390	1651
Rice Krispies	372	1584
Special K	388	1650
Special K, Creamy Berry crunch	388	1648
Special K, Chocolate & Strawberry	385	1631
Special K, Fruit & Nut	380	1609
Special K, Peach & Apricot	380	1623
Special K, red berries	380	1610
Special K, Strawberry Clusters	389	1648
Special K, Oats & More	379	1604
Special K, Yoghurty	388	1644
Weetabix	340	1444
Weetabix, chocolate	367	1548
Weetabix, crispy minis	375	1585
Weetabix, golden syrup	363	1535

Snack Cereal Bars

	Kcal	Kj
Alpen Snack Bars	419	1767
Caramel and Nut Bars	390	1645
Coco Pops Snack Bar	415	1750
Elevenses Nutrograin	377	1589
Frosties Snack Bar	414	1744
Jordans Fruseli Bar	376	1587
Rice Krispie Snack Bar	413	1742
Special K cereal bars	411	1731
Weetabix Minis, fruit and nut bar	374	1578
Weetabix Oaty Bars	345	1445
Weetos Snack Bar	440	1850

Cheese

	Kcal	Kj
Camembert type	300	1246
Cheddar type	406	1682
Cottage Cheese	439	1807
Cheese Spread	283	1173
Creamy Cheshire	382	1581
Danish Blue type	355	1471
Double Gloucester	404	1675
Edam	304	1262
Emmental	360	1495
French Brie	298	1213
French Roule	293	1231
Goude	362	1501
Low Low Medium White	302	1263
Mozzarella	245	1076
Parmesan	408	1696
Philadelphia, full fat	244	1070
Philadelphia, light		

Philadelphia, chocolate	361	1205
Processed Cheese	311	1291
Red Leicester	390	1619
Swiss Gruyere	413	1714

Eggs

	Kcal	Kj
Whole raw	147	612
White raw	36	153
Yolk	339	1531
Boiled	147	612
Fried	232	961
Poached	155	644
Omelette	190	747
Scrambled	246	1018

Egg and cheese dishes

	Kcal	Kj
Cauliflower cheese	113	471
Cheese soufflé	252	1019
Macaroni Cheese	174	726
Pizza, cheese and tomato	234	982
Scotch Egg	279	1156
Welsh rarebit	365	1523

Yoghurt

	Kcal	Kj
Low fat natural	52	216
Low fat flavoured	81	342
Low fat fruit	95	405
Low fat hazelnut	106	449

Pizza

	Kcal	Kj
Thin & Crispy Pizza, Vegetable	225	944
Thin & Crispy Hawaiian Pizza	233	979
Thin Margarita	298	1251
Thin Pepperoni	295	1238
Deep Loaded Cheese Pizza	295	1238
Deep Loaded Pepperoni	296	1240
Deep Loaded Mozzarella and Cherry Tomato	255	1070
Deep Loaded Vegetable and Goats Cheese Pizza	265	1112
Garlic Bread	358	1500

Cakes, Buns and Pastries

	Kcal	Kj
Chocolate Biscuits, Full Coated	524	2197
Digestive Biscuits, Plain	471	1981
Chocolate Digestive Biscuits	493	2071
Cream Crackers	440	1857
Ginger Nuts	456	1981
Shortbread	531	2242
Fruit Cake, Rich	332	1043
Fruit Cake, Rich, Iced	352	1490
Gingerbread	373	1573
Madeira Cake	393	1573
Sponge Cake, with Fat	464	1941
Sponge Cake, without Fat	301	1280
Doughnuts	349	1467
Eclairs	376	1589
Jam Tarts	384	1616
Mince Pies	435	1826

Sugars & Preserves

Sugars	Kcal	Kj
Glucose Liquid	318	1355
Sugar Demerara	394	1681
Sugar, White	394	1680
Syrup, Golden	298	1269
Treacle, Black	257	1096

Preserves	Kcal	Kj
Cherries Glacé	212	903
Honeycomb	281	2101
Honeycomb in Jars	288	1229
Jam, Fruit with Edible Seeds	261	1116
Jam, Stone Fruit	283	1202
Lemon Curd	283	1202
Marmalade	261	1114
Marzipan Almond Paste	443	1856
Mincemeat	235	1163

Cereals

	Kcal	Kj
Custard Powder	354	1508
Flour, Wholemeal	318	1351
Flour, White Plain	350	1493
Flour, Self Raising	339	1443
Rice, Polished, Raw	361	1536
Pastry, Choux, Raw	214	893
Pastry, Choux, Cooked	330	1379
Pastry, Flakey, Raw	427	1780
Pastry, Flaky, Cooked	565	2356
Pastry, Short Crust, Raw	527	2202
Scones	371	1562

Sauces & Pickles

	Kcal	Kj
Bread Sauce	110	463
Brown Sauce	99	422
Cheese Sauce	198	825
Chutney, Apple	193	824
Chutney, Tomato	154	658
French Dressing	658	2706
Mayonnaise	718	2952
Mayonnaise, Light	265	1092
Onion Sauce	99	413
Piccalilli	33	147
Pickle, Sweet	134	572
Salad Cream	311	1288
Tomato Ketchup	98	420
Tomato Purée	67	286
Tomato Sauce	86	359
White Sauce, Savory	151	630
White Sauce, Sweet	172	722
Salt	0	0

Puddings

	Kcal	Kj
Apple Crumble	208	878
Bread and Butter Pudding	159	159
Cheesecake	421	1747
Christmas Pudding	304	1279
Custard Tart	211	885
Dumplings	211	885
Fruit Pie, with Pastry Top & Bottom	369	1554
Fruit Pie, with Pastry on Top	180	704
Ice Cream, Dairy	167	704
Ice Cream, Non Dairy	165	691

Jelly Packet Cubes	259	1104
Jelly, made with Water	59	251
Jelly, made with Milk	86	363
Lemon Meringue Pie	323	1359
Queen of Puddings	216	910
Triple	160	674
Yorkshire Pudding	215	902

Miscellaneous

	Kcal	Kj
Baking Powder	163	693
Bovril	174	737
Gelatin	338	1435
Ginger, Ground	258	1101
Marmite	179	759
Oxo Cubes	229	969
Mustard, Powder	452	1184
Pepper	308	1312
Vinegar	4	16
Yeast, Bakers	53	226
Yeast, Bread	169	717
Butter	740	3041
Margarine (All Kinds)	730	3000
Chips	253	1065
Crisps	533	2224
Baked Beans	78	329

Confectionary

	Kcal	Kj
Boiled Sweets	327	1397
Chocolate Milk	529	2214
Chocolate Plain	525	2197
Bounty Bar	473	1980

	Kcal	Kjoules
Mars Bar	441	1853
Fruit Gums	172	734
Liquorice Allsorts	313	1333
Pastiles	253	1079
Peppermints	329	1670
Toffees	430	1810

Sugars, preserves and confectionary per 100g

	Kcal	Kjoules
Sugars		
Glucose liquid	318	1355
Sugar Demerara	394	1681
White	394	1680
Syrup, golden	298	1269
Treacle, black	257	1096
Preserves		
Cherries, glace	212	903
Honeycomb	281	1201
In jars	288	1229
Jam fruit with edible seeds	261	1114
Lemon curd (starch based)	283	1201
Homemade	290	1216
Marmalade	261	1114
Marzipan (dried paste)	443	1856
Boiled sweets	327	1397
Chocolate, milk	529	2214
Chocolate, plain	525	2197
Fancy and filled	460	1980
Bounty Bar	441	1853
Mars Bar	441	1853
Fruit Gums	172	734
Liquorice Allsorts	313	1333
Pastilles	253	1079
Peppermints	392	1670
Toffees, mixed	430	1810

Vegetables

	Per 100g	
	Kcal	Kjoules
Asparagus (boiled)	18	75
Aubergines (raw)	14	62
Beans (French boiled)	7	28
Beans (runner raw)	26	114
Beans (runner boiled)	48	206
Beans (butter raw)	273	1162
Beans (butter boiled)	95	405
Beans (haricot raw)	271	1157
Beans (haricot boiled)	93	396
Beans (baked in tomato sauce)	64	270
Beans red kidney (raw)	272	1159
Beans red kidney (canned)	87	369
Beansprouts (canned)	9	40
Beetroot (raw)	28	118
Beetroot (boiled)	44	189
Broccoli (raw)	23	96
Broccoli (boiled)	18	78
Brussels Sprouts (raw)	26	111
Brussels Sprouts (boiled)	18	75
Cabbage, red (raw)	20	85
Cabbage, savoy (raw)	26	109
Cabbage, savoy (boiled)	9	40
Cabbage, spring (boiled)	7	32
Cabbage, white (raw)	22	93
Cabbage, winter (raw)	22	92
Cabbage, winter (boiled)	15	66
Carrots, old (raw)	23	98
Carrots, old (boiled)	19	79
Carrots, young (boiled)	20	87
Carrots, young (canned)	19	82
Cauliflower (raw)	13	56

Cauliflower (boiled)	9	40
Celery (raw)	8	36
Celery (boiled)	5	21
Cucumber (raw)	10	43
Horseradish (raw)	59	253
Leeks (raw)	31	128
Leeks, boiled	24	104
Lentils, raw	304	1293
Lentils, split, boiled	99	420
Lentils, Masur dahl, cooked	90	380
Lettuce, raw	12	51
Marrow, raw	16	69
Marrow, boiled	7	29
Mushrooms, raw	13	53
Mushrooms, fried	210	863
Mustard and Cress, raw	10	47
Okra	17	71
Onions, raw	23	99
Onions, boiled	13	53
Onions, fried	345	1424
Spring, raw	35	151
Parsley, raw	21	88
Parsnips, raw	49	210
Parsnips, boiled	52	238
Peas, fresh, raw	67	283
Peas, boiled	52	223
Peas, frozen raw	53	224
Peas, boiled	41	175
Peas, canned, garden	47	201
Peas, processed	80	339
Peas, dried, raw	286	1215
Peas, dried, boiled	103	438
Peas, split, dried, raw	310	1318
Peas, split, dried, boiled	118	503
Peppers, green, raw	15	65

Peppers, green, boiled	112	518
Peppers, ripe, fresh	267	1126
Potatoes, old raw	87	372
Potatoes, old, boiled	80	343
Potatoes, mashed	119	499
Potatoes, baked	105	448
Potatoes, baked, weighed with skins	85	364
Potatoes, roast	157	662
Chips	253	1065
Old Chips, frozen	109	462
Frozen, fried	291	1214
New, boiled	76	324
Canned	53	226
Instant Powder	318	1356
Made up	70	299
Crisps	533	2224
Doritos	506	2115
Wotsits	547	2290
Pumpkin (raw)	15	65
Radishes	15	62
Spinach (boiled)	30	128
Swedes (boiled)	21	81
Sweetcorn on the cob (raw)	127	538
Sweetcorn on the cob (boiled)	123	520
Canned kernels	76	325
Sweet potatoes (raw)	91	387
Sweet potatoes (boiled)	85	363
Tomatoes (raw)	14	60
Tomatoes (fried)	69	288
Tomatoes (canned)	12	51
Turnips (raw)	20	86
Turnips (boiled)	14	60
Watercress (raw)	14	61
Yam (raw)	131	560
Yam (boiled)	119	508

Fruit per 100g

	Kcal	Kjoules
Apples, eating	46	196
Apples eating (raw)	37	189
Apricots fresh, raw	28	117
Avocado Pears	223	922
Bananas, raw	56	240
Blue lemons raw	29	125
Cherries, eating, raw	47	201
Cranberries, raw	15	63
Currants black, raw	28	121
Dried	243	1039
Damsons, raw	38	162
Dates, dried	248	1056
Figs green, raw	21	174
Figs dried, raw	213	908
Fruit pie filling, canned	95	407
Fruit salad, canned	95	405
Gooseberries green, raw	17	73
Grapes black, raw	61	258
Grapes white, raw	63	268
Grapefruit, raw	22	95
Grapefruit, canned	60	257
Quavas, canned	60	258
Lemons, whole	15	65
Lemon juice, fresh	7	31
Logan berries, raw	17	73
Mandarin Oranges (canned)	56	231
Mangoes, raw	59	253
Manops	77	330
Melons cantaloupe (raw) weighed with skins	15	63
Yellow Honeydew raw weighed with skins	13	56
Watermelon, raw weighed with skins	11	47
Mulberries raw	36	152

Nectarines raw	50	214
Olives in brine	109	422
Oranges raw	35	150
weighed with peel and pips	26	113
Orange juice, fresh	38	161
Passion fruit raw	34	147
Raw weighed with skin	14	60
Dried raw	212	906
Canned	87	373
Pears eating	41	175
Eating (weighed with skin and core)	29	125
Pears, cooking	36	154
Canned	77	327
Pineapple fresh	46	194
Canned	77	327
Plums Victoria dessertraw weighed with stones	36	153
Cooking, raw	26	109
Weighed with stones	20	84
Pomegranate Juice	44	189
Prunes dried raw	161	686
Weighed with stones	134	570
Raisins dried	246	1049
Raspberries raw	25	105
Canned	87	370
Rhubarb raw	6	26
Strawberries raw	26	109
Canned	81	344
Sultanas dried	250	1066
Tangerines raw	34	143
Weighed with peel and pips	23	100

IMPROVING YOUR MENTAL HEALTH

Nutrition isn't the answer to all ailments. But often in conjunction with orthodox medicine it can give patients the strength to pull through many illnesses and surgery.

There are no nutritional answers for many of today's complex illnesses. A few examples are multiple sclerosis, motor neurone disease, autism and learning difficulties.

But orthodox medicine has proved conclusively that drinking alcohol during pregnancy can reduce the intelligent quotient of a baby sometimes to the point of a baby being born with foetal alcohol syndrome. If a mother wishes to have a baby as clever as genetically possible, it is important to avoid alcohol for at least three months before conception and throughout the pregnancy to increase the baby's intelligent quotient. Classic drugs available for depression such as anti-depressants are helpful. Some antipsychotic drugs have dreadful side effects such as weight gain, thirst, drowsiness, lack of appetite and one old fashioned antipsychotic drug first manufactured in the 1950's and still prescribed today reacts with strong sunlight and sunbeds. Chlorpromazine causes itchiness and severe burning in temperatures above 18°C. But there are much cleaner tranquilizers available. A modern tranquilizer with none of these setbacks is a much more expensive drug but it has none of these side effects. It is known as olanzapine. There is a wide range of tranquilizers and sedatives labelled antipsychotic drugs on the market, but one major side effect is they cause weight gain.

Very often psychological problems can be caused as a result of insomnia. But natural remedies are available in health food shops or through the company Avon Cosmetics Ltd. Health food shops sell camomile and lavender oil, and Avon Cosmetics sells a very effective pillow mist containing camomile and lavender spray which is very effective in helping you sleep.

Orthodox medicine often tests psychiatric problems with malfunctioning of parathyroid hormone which they suggest can lead to psychiatric problems, bone pains and constipation but an excess of parathyroid hormone can easily be corrected by surgery to the thyroid gland in the neck.

Conversely calcium insufficiency is also associated with a wide range of psychiatric conditions. The most common symptoms are depression, anxiety, panic attacks, nervous twitches, insomnia and hyperactivity.

So it is advisable to take a calcium supplement, preferably with vitamin D as it is necessary for the absorption of calcium.

The Politics of Health in Britain

Health Promotion

Ethical principles in Health Promotion are simply to do good and avoid harm, or in more academic language the principles of beneficence (doing good) and non-maleficence (not doing harm). Other central ethical principles in health promotion are, respect for autonomy:- that is respect for the rights of people to determine their own lives and justice being fair and equitable, which is about how to respect everyone.

For example, I know I am doing good, avoiding harm, respecting autonomy, and being fair by writing this book which is truthful, none of it imaginative, and it is all from a very good source - University lectures, and from the Open University as well as from Higher Education Colleges.

I would not write anything I am not sure is true like some so called Nutritionists who play with people's health, by advising diets which are not recommended by the Medical Profession. Instead this book is written to be as closely allied to Medicine as possible and Health Promotion itself as an integral part of medicine. In other words I am using the copyright of my Bachelor of Science to help the general public get an insight into looking at their own eating habits and "lifestyle to lead healthier lives; I am also doing something that has never been done before, integrating recipes with theory including, Human Nutrition and Dietetics, Disease, Health Promotion Health Protection, and Health Education.

"The Financial and social costs of acting on advice about moving to a healthier diet might be too great ·for poor families to contemplate. Work pressures might lead to increased use of processed foods, even if these are known to be less nutritious than home cooking. Parents might not be prepared to face the conflict involved in resisting children's demands for junk foods, even if these were recognised to be unhealthy."

(2000 Promotion, Health Knowledge and practice.)

This quotation refers directly to the problems- of especially poor income families achieving a healthy diet. This is one of the problems properly qualified Nutritionists and Dieticians have to cope with. It is difficult to convince families on a low budget that it is as cheap to cook a healthy meal for the family, instead of relying on tinned and processed foods; and feeding their children out of takeaways, and junk food such as fizzy drinks and crisps, sweets etc.

No matter how much orthodox medicine has advanced in the 21st century a major crisis didn't happen regarding AIDs. But luckily not the pandemic feared in the 1980's. As many people are now taking responsibility for their sexual health.

"Disease prevention, health promotion and health education are much public concerns as medical matters. Much of what is involved is a sensible diet, moderate alcohol, more exercise takes place where people live and work in the community - whether in the home, the surgery, pharmacy, consulting room or clinic - are among "key players" in the government's health strategy.

(Jones, Sidell and Douglas 2000)

The message from the Labour Government in the 1990s was basically that various professions allied to medicine including Dietetics; in this case Community Dieticians, Pharmacists and G.P.s need to work together concerning medical matters. There is just one problem and that is that there are not enough Nutritionists or Dieticians employed in the community. More students are needed to be trained for jobs which will help save people's lives. The previous Labour Government gave an indication of this proposed strategy but did not come to fruition.

"There is a real interest in health promotion in general practice, particularly among practise nurses. Health visitors whose remit is to search out a wider health promotion role."

(Caraher and Mac Nab 1996)

Obviously Orthodox Medicine and all branches of medicine wish for a wider health promotion role and more people with specialist roles in diet and nutrition and health promotion itself are needed in the community.

Health promotions have a fairly good understanding of the objectives, aims and goals they are seeking in order to lower the rate of heart disease and cancer in particular.

A lot of books written on the topic of nutrition unfortunately give the profession "a bad name". People are confused. They do not know who to believe. I'm not saying that all other nutritionists say is wrong. Some of it could be correct. But it is often difficult to decipher what is correct and what is incorrect.

Under Tony Blair, the White Paper "Saving Lives - Our Healthier Nation 1999" was not wrong. The Labour Government just did not succeed in implementing all of these changes but there has been a noticeable increase in the number of people who now survive cancer compared to a few years ago.

In England The White Paper Saving Lives Our Healthier Nation, replaced the 27 targets 8) the Health of the Nation with four targets: to reduce heart disease and stroke, accidents, cancer and poor mental health.

Saving Lives: Our Healthier Nation Targets

Under Tony Blair's government - A White Paper stated the aim was to by 2010:

- Reduce the death rate from cancers in people under 75 by at least a fifth – saving 100,000 lives.
- Coronary Heart Disease and stroke - reduce the death rate from coronary heart disease and stroke and related diseases in people under 75 by at least two fifths, saving 200,000 lives.
- Accidents

Reduce the death rate from accidents by at least a fifth and to reduce the rate of serious injury from accidents by at least a tenth - saving 12,000 lives.

Mental Health

Reduce the death rate from suicide and undetermined injury by at least a fifth saving 4,000 lives.

(2000 Katz J, Perberdy A and Douglas J).

The last strategy for anyone going on a diet to try and lose weight is not to follow any diet unless it is approved by a G.P.

There are many complicated models, but a-simplified empowerment model illustrates how people can take control of their own lives.

"The goal here is to encourage personal growth by enhancing self esteem and self-assertiveness. The aim is to teach people the skills to take charge of their own health."

(2000 Katz J, Perberdy A and Douglas J).

"Both men and women in the manual skilled and unskilled socioeconomic groups have poorer health status and lower expectation of life than those in professional groups (McKie 1994, Dreyer and White Health 1997). Not only does health status alter with social class, but so too does health behaviour. Individuals with a lower socio-economic status tend to smoke more and participate less in exercise or any physical activity. In 1984, 36 percent of men in employment were smokers, compared to 61 percent of unemployed men. Men consume more alcohol than women do (Baxter 1990). For all ages, male alcohol consumption also varies between social classes, with those from manual groups drinking more heavily than non-manual workers. Townsend et al (1988) shows that 26 percent of unskilled manual working men were categorised as heavy drinkers where as only 8 percent of professional men were found in the same category. (2000 Katz J, Perberdy and Douglas J)

"Alcohol consumption by semi-skilled manual male workers increased by 30% between 1987 and 1999, whilst consumption by all other male socioeconomic groups fell. (McKie 1994)

"Not surprisingly unemployed men are more likely to drink than those in employment. (Blaxter 1990)"

It is clear that there is a positive correlation between career success, affluence and less alcohol consumption in Britain today. Conversely, there also is a negative correlation between alcohol consumption, social class, lack of success and excessive alcohol consumption.

In today's society, in the U.K., it is no longer Beijing which has more billionaires per square mile in the world. It is London. This may in a round about way make the U.K. a richer country, but these 'fat cats' with their billions do not really help the vulnerable and poor members of society.

Not all the super rich keep their money to themselves. Take for example the singer Madonna. Not only is Madonna such a good single mother – no-body in the world would criticize her as a mother, a few years ago she donated 10 million dollars of her fortune to build a school in Malau, so that some of these poor children would have the chance of an education as she herself did.

The current conservative government does encourage an increase in the private sector in order to make the U.K. a richer country as well as more affluence for those who are ambitious enough to become self made men or women. They encourage as many as possible of us to become self-made millionaires or even billionaires if we wish.

But unfortunately this is not happening in the private sector and in professions allied to medicine. Health professionals are suffering financially but more importantly are suffering low morale as so much pressure is being put on people such as nurses who may only have part-time work. As well as this health professionals who are on sick leave or retire are not being replaced. A huge amount of health professionals are under pressure with heavy workloads and this is resulting in the patient suffering because the pay and conditions are so bad for health professionals including junior doctors. These professionals are not even guaranteed the pensions they thought they were going to receive.

Its similar in the teaching profession. Pay and conditions are so bad in teaching and there are so many social problems with children and young people, very little teaching is being done in lower class areas. It is reducing the morale of teachers too.

A capitalist government has its advantages but a conversely socialist government has its advantages too. But unfortunately there is nobody as inspiring as Mr Tony Blair on the horizon to lead a labour government so the future is uncertain for Britain in the long term. Britain could end up in anarchy.

Britain is overpopulated and under resourced and England itself doesn't have enough agricultural land to justify such a large population which could be around sixty million people.

The obesity crisis itself could bring England to its knees in the future as we have an ageing population and very many sick people who are not fit to do any kind of work and who are a drain on the economy.

During the famine in Ireland in 1845-1847, many Irish people has to travel on ships to the USA to start a new life in the land of the free.

Irish people arrived on what were known as 'Coffin Ships' emaciated and thin from starvation and they had no possessions. At least a million Irish people survived the journey and they prospered to create the modern U.S.A.

Queen Victoria was heavily criticized for being responsible for the deaths of millions in the Great Famine. But it must have been her who provided the ships to transport the starving Irish people to the New World.

In today's society in Britain and the USA especially, people are not dying from starvation. They are dying from eating too much. The wealth of the nation is going down people's throats.

Thousands are dying in hospitals in Britain especially at week-ends with a lack of doctors and nurses on duty – but with clinically and morbidly obese people, surgeons cannot operate on these people because of the amount of fat on their bodies. Even simple operations such as appendectomies, gall stones, an hiatus hernia or more complicated operations such as a coronary artery bypass cannot physically be done by surgeons until people lose the weight and this is why so many obese people are dying in hospital these days.

In ten years time a lot of the obese, clinically obese and morbidly obese people in British and American Society in particular will no longer be with us, they will be dead.

Medicine will not be able to save their lives and in a lot of cases, their heart stops beating with the sheer weight they are carrying around in the form of body fat. There is really only one option – to lose the weight before you become clinically or morbidly obese, or risk dying young.

Because of advances in orthodox medicine and nutrition, it is possible that people will live to a hundred and twenty years of age. Being over fifty will soon no longer be considered to be middle-aged, but still young, for the slim and healthy.

Promoting Health within Local Communities

Health Promotion is an important part of a wide network including those involved in Health Education and Social Care.

Health Promotion includes health education; however, it cannot be denied that it is social and economic factors which determine health status.

From a political perspective under the previous Labour government: white papers included; The Health of the Nation (DoH 1992) and Saving Lives; Our Healthier Nation (DoH 1999), which health professionals operate within as structural groups to promote health.

Collaborative partnerships which are multi professional including medicine, nursing, health visiting, dietetics and other health professionals including social work, community development, work in partnership with each other and within the community they serve.

Establishing these collaborative partnerships requires careful consideration. Constraints within health promotion means that it is necessary for a full understanding of the philosophy which this relatively new profession of Health Promotion is flourishing under within the last few decades.

The most recommended definition of health promotion is:

Health Promotion comprises efforts to enhance positive health and reduce the risk of ill-health, though the overlapping spheres of health education, disease prevention and health protection.

From the aspect of weight control which the previous Labour Government did not address at all Health Promotion is supposed to show "Evidence Based Practice" under The Labour Government, there was a lot of aims, objectives of what they aimed to do. Some of it may have been achieved such as a reduction in deaths from cancer; but the obesity crisis came to the point that it is spirally out of control as this health matter was ignored by the previous Labour Government. We have to rely on the present Conservative Government to get the message through to the general population and show "Evidence Based Practice" that a healthy diet will keep weight within a desirable weight limits. Steps are being taken through T.V. advertisement about the obesity crisis i.e. if your waistline is more than 32 inches for a woman or over 37 inches for a man, you are overweight. This is an easy guide for most people.

One positive step towards improving the health of the Nation and addressing the obesity crisis is when The Chancellor of The Exchequer in his recent budget increased the price of a seemingly harmless but yet very dangerous substance, cane sugar.

The fundamental theory underlying health promotion today is based on the World Health Organisation declaration of 1945 that "health is not merely the absence of disease but a state of complete physical, mental and social well-being.

Health Promotion has a collective approach to promoting health. It aims to involve the inter dependency different but linked aspects of health including medicine, nursing, dietetics and other health professionals to improve their own health and well-being.

Community participation has always been central to the WHO strategy. The Alma Ata declaration 1978 from an international conference on Primary Health Care explicitly stated that "people have a right and a duty to participate individually and collectively in the planning and implementation of their health care (WHO 1978)."

In other words, regarding the obesity crisis, if one is overweight, obese, clinically obese or even morbidly obese, there is no-body who can force someone to lose weight only themselves. It does not mean stopping eating. As illustrated there is wide variety of fruits and vegetables to be eaten which will stop hunger pains and are very tasty and nutritious.

We live in a democracy which gives each and every individual the choice to create autonomy. A sociologist Seedhouse illustrates a distinction between creating autonomy and respecting autonomy which he regards as the central conditions when working for health.

"Creating autonomy is making an effort to improve the quality of a person's autonomy by trying to enhance what the person is able to do. In health promotion work, this is often called empowerment." "1994 Health Promotion Foundations for Practice Naidoo J and Wills J".

The Ottawa Charter 1976 further developed these principals: "Health Promotion works through effective community action in setting priorities, making decisions, planning strategies and implementing them to achieve better health." For example, in today's world with the obesity crisis being a major concern in society; this could involve going on a calorie controlled diet, checking with your GP if you have any contraindications such as diabetes or a bowel disorder such as crohn's disease, diverticulitis, ulcerative colitis or bowel cancer and check your body mass index and a sensible weight loss to aim towards.

"At the heart of this process is the empowerment of individuals and communities to have ownership and control of their own destiny." (WHO 1986),

It is true therefore that the primary health sector with community and self help groups, as well as within general practise is a suitable setting for promoting health.

Inequalities in health however still exist especially between rich and poor. It is more likely that the less affluent members of society are more easily empowered by health promoters than the very wealthy members of society who are generally better informed about aspects of health, especially the well educated. They are able to pay for health care out of their own pockets, but poverty and health indicates that semi-skilled and unskilled groups of society have a lower life expectancy, and experience more ill health than those in the non manual and professional groups.

Many people are either overweight, obese, clinically obese or morbidly obese, particularly in lower socio economic groups of society. Professional groups are less affected as they seem to have more general knowledge about diet and nutrition.

For lower socio economic groups of society, much health education is needed for those people who seem to be empathetic towards their plight, unaware of the health consequence, never mind the physical image. Many people are beyond caring probably because they are in a vicious circle of depression and overeating.

In the past health promoters did not directly approach the problem of obesity. It is an "expanding" problem. There are just too few dieticians qualified in Britain and other countries with the same problem such as the USA to address the problem and consequences of obesity.

A collective approach within communities for overweight people involving self help groups with the help of those qualified in the nutritional field could help reduce the problem of obesity and empower whole communities.

Depression caused by the state of the economy is possibly driving more people to comfort eating and binge eating than ever before.

Self help groups recommended by the past Labour government; in communities with all the information at their fingertips in this book could mean people really could motivate each other to slowly but surely lose weight and develop a whole new relationship with food.

There are slimming groups for women, but they cost money and with money being so scarce it puts people off losing weight.

Men do not normally attend slimming clubs. It would go against most men's macho ideology to attend slimming clubs. But there is no reason why men can't have slimming meetings in each other's houses. This would mean people would be forming collaborative partnerships independently within their own community. The Labour Government indicated self help groups and it is a very good strategy for self motivation and motivating others to lose weight. It could be made sociable and fun, but drinking alcohol is not recommended or it will cancel out the previous weeks dieting as alcohol is so high in calories. Any more than a pint of beer would be too much on a weight reduction diet.

In the field of Health Promotion, The Labour Government had wonderful ideas about Health Action Zones in Northern Ireland as well as in Great Britain.

The Health Action Zone model identifies self-esteem to be a key component in complex issues such as a person's values, drive and self esteem. "Self esteem means the evaluation a person makes of him or herself, a personal judgement in the attitudes a person holds toward themselves.

"1994 Health Promotion Foundations for Practice Nadioo J and Wills J."

This ideology again connects with autonomy but unfortunately in today's society with so many people being obese and having such low self esteem because they are trapped inside fat bodies trying to increase the self esteem of the general public is of little use without firstly reducing the number of obese people in society dramatically.

To prevent a new generation of obese people, it may become considered a form of child abuse if obese parents bring up obese children as it is nobody's fault only the parents.

Obesity is expected to reach 50% of the population of the UK by 2030. But with Health Education, this could be prevented.

The present Conservative Government has achieved very important things including saving Britain from bankruptcy and so far defending our borders from an attack from the Islamic State.

But unfortunately the health service and the department of education are suffering including junior doctors and nurses who are having difficult times regarding pay and conditions.

Health Education

Some definitions of health education suggest that it is concerned with improving the health of the individual as well as the prevention of ill health.

Health Education has been aimed at preventing specific diseases, often through targeting high risk groups who have an increased likelihood of developing the disease. Health education then is seen as disease prevention and interventions are designed to prevent ill health.

For example if a person who has survived a cardiac arrest or myocardial infarction commonly known as a heart attack, the hospital dietician will guide the patient about steps to be taken to prevent a second heart attack. The dietician's advice would include: stopping smoking, lowering saturated fat, salt and sugar in the diet, increasing fibre including fresh fruit and vegetables and Vitamin F including Omega 3, 6 and 9 and taking moderate exercise.

Health Promotions includes a twofold component which gives rise to the following formula:

Health Promotion = Healthy Public Policy x Health Education.

The term "healthy public policy" is borrowed from the Ottawa Charter (1986). The principles of health promotion are developed in the Ottawa Charter which outlines these areas as important for health promotion:

1. Building a healthy public policy,
2. Creating supportive environments,
3. Developing personal skills,
4. Strengthening community action,
5. Reorientation of health services.

The WHO (World Health Organisation) does distinguish between health promotion and prevention; health education is seen as an integral part of health promotion in conjunction with the field of prevention.

The development of health education lies in the nineteenth century when epidemic disease eventually led to pressure for sanitary reform for the overcrowded industrial towns, especially from the time of the cholera epidemics of the early nineteenth century.

Alongside the public health movement emerged the idea of educating the public for the good of its own health. The Medical Officers of Health appointed to each town under the Public Health legislation of 1848 frequently disseminated everyday health advice on safeguards against contracting contagious disease.

Specialist workers who were previously known as Health Education Officers, have frequently changed their title to Health Promotion Officers and recently to Health Promotion Specialists without necessarily changing their professional role.

'The term health promotion and health education are not interchangeable. Health Promotion covers all aspects of these activities which seek to improve the health status of individuals and communities. It therefore includes both health education and all attempts to produce environmental and legislative change conducive to good health. Put another way, health promotion is concerned with making healthier choices, easier choices'.

(Dennis et al 1982)

'Defining and planning health promotion makes a distinction between health education, prevention and health protection'.

(Downie et al 1990)

One of the main domains in which Health Promotion Officers work is in secondary schools advising pupils about important aspects of their life including healthy eating, taking regular exercise, safe sex and hygiene.

The origins of formal health promotion as a modern movement lie in the World Health Organisation declaration of 1946 that "health is not merely the absence of disease, but a state of complete physical, mental and social wellbeing.

In the UK and the Republic of Ireland health services centred around health education, and for many health professionals the focus was around information which would persuade the public to change to healthier habits, for example, giving up smoking.

In the UK a central council for Health Education was first established in 1927, financed by public health departments.

The Health Education Council was created in 1968 in England as a non governmental organisation with an objective to create a climate of opinion generally favourable to health education.

'Similar health education agencies were set up in Scotland, Wales and Northern Ireland and in 1975 the Health Education Bureau was established in the Republic of Ireland'.

(Hensey 1998)

Health Education is a form of communication which aims to give people the knowledge and skills needed to make choices about their health. This might aim to encourage people to change their own behaviour or to change the wider environment. This might include going on a reduction diet if they are risking becoming obese, clinically obese or morbidly obese.

Katherine Weare (1992) maintains that enabling people to be autonomous is a fundamental goal of education.

Regarding the obesity crisis it's entirely up to the individual to make healthy choices. However many "autonomous" people make unhealthy choices. This book is aimed towards helping people make healthy choices, if they wish to be educated about food and nutrition not just to improve the health of the individual but to improve self-esteem and self awareness by taking charge of their own health.

Its another one of Britain's social problems that thousands of parents in the U.K. are not sending their children to school, but claim to be educating them at home. What do these irresponsible parents know academically? Very little. They are just too lazy to get up in the mornings to get their children into uniforms to send them to school, which is unreal in 21st century Britain. It is unfortunately the poor and the vulnerable who are suffering in modern Britain.

WHAT IS GERONTOLOGY?

How to slow down the ageing process

As we enter the twenty first century many scientists and gerontologists seek to prevent the diseases responsible for premature ageing and death. Their aim is to discover what factors determine the maximum possible lifespan.

Optimum nutrition as well as restricting calorie has shown to reduce diseases and cancer meaning that a lifespan in the region of 110 years to 120 years of age is possible in the future.

Research shows that of the 22 million Americans that die each year, 1.8 million die of diet related diseases. By eating less we can live longer. Calorie restriction however is not about malnutrition. It is about giving the body exactly what it needs and no more.

The ageing process currently focuses on the energy factories within the cell, called the mitochondria. The mitochondria are rod like structures inside the cell which are the power house of the cell, and they control the rate of energy production inside the cell.

Damage to the mitochondria can result in damage to the cells. DNA known as deoxyribonucleic acid, and RNA known as ribonucleic acid are the genetic blue print for new cells. If damage to the DNA can be decreased or be repaired, there is a growing consensus amongst gerontologists, and nutritionists in general, that the ageing process can be slowed down or even reversed by repairing the damage done to cells by free radicals.

What are free radicals?

Free radicals are the by-products of energy metabolism. The key to longevity lies in reducing our exposure to free radicals, and increasing the body's protection, against them, by increasing our intake of antioxidants. Free radicals are made in the combustion process including smoking, the exhaust fumes from burning petrol and diesel, radiation, frying, or barbecuing foods, and normal body processes. Eating antioxidant nutrients in the diet especially foods containing Vitamin A, beta-carotene, Vitamin C and E, selenium and zinc are shown to increase longevity.

Well balanced nutrition including generous amounts of Vitamin C and E can contribute to extending the lifespan from the time of prenatal development to old age, even for those who are already middle aged. It is not legal in the Western World to die of old age. A death certificate is required to identify the cause of death. The chance of living to a healthy old age is increased if heart disease and cancer can be prevented and this can be achieved through optimum nutrition.

In the Western World today you have a fifty per cent chance of dying from heart or artery disease. That is the bad news. The good news is that most cases, a cardiac arrest, also known as a myocardial infarction or a cardiovascular accident, commonly known as a stroke is in many cases preventable. There is nothing natural about dying of heart disease. Many cultures do not experience a high incidence of heart attacks or strokes, such as the Eskimos and Japanese. For example, by middle –age British people have nine times more heart disease than the Japanese. This can be connected with the fact that 40% of the total calories is in the form of fat is typical of the British diet, whereas in Japan, Thailand and the Philippines people consume only 15% of their calorie intake in the form of fat. For example Japanese people eat on average 40 grams of fat per day, where British people eat 142grams of fat per day. Most authorities now agree that no more than one third of our total fat intake should be saturated(hard fat).Ideally it should only be 10%.ealthy fats called essential fatty acids, are an important part of a healthy diet. They are found mainly in fish, nuts and seeds. The Eskimos and the Japanese eat a lot of fish sometimes raw fish, a major source of the essential fatty acids, especially omega 3. This is a probable reason why the incidence of cardiovascular disease is lower in these countries than in Britain and the USA

The umbrella term for the essential fatty acids is vitamin F. This includes omega6 the newly discovered omega 7 and omega9. Good dietary sources of omega 3 include specifically oily fish such as salmon, mackerel, herring, tuna and sardines. It plays an important role in controlling high cholesterol levels. Good dietary sources of omega 6 include sunflower oil, corn maize oil, evening primrose oil. It also has cholesterol lowering effect as well as having a blood thinning effect. Good dietary sources of omega 9 include olive oil and rape seed oil which can be produced in Ireland. It again has a cholesterol lowering effect.

A very healthy fish and chip could consist of monounsaturated fat. Fresh or tinned salmon or tuna fish, salad and chips fried in olive oil or rapeseed oil is a healthy meal. But it is important to replace the oil after using more than three times as it is broken down in the frying process from healthy monounsaturated fat into dangerous saturated fat which can cause arterial blockage known as atherosclerosis. A Mediterranean type diet consisting of high levels of olive oil and antioxidant rich fresh fruit and vegetables, shows reduced rates of heart disease and other related diseases such as strokes. A wide variety of citrus fruit is not widely available in Britain and Ireland. Supplements D so vitamin C is recommended for children and adults. Vitamin C has been discovered to increase the elasticity of the arterial walls reducing the chance of arterial blockage. and it also strengthens the collagen and elastin in the epidermis of the skin helping to maintain a youthful appearance.

The National Advisory Council for Nutritional Education, The NACNE Report 1983 states that we need to "lower sugar, salt and saturated fat levels and increase fibre." The same principles apply today.

Northern Ireland and Scotland have the highest rate of Coronary Heart Disease in the world because of our diet which is frightening. But it is the slim, healthy people in future age groups who are likely to work until eighty years of age and live to 120 years of age whereas the prognosis of such a long life is less likely for those suffering from obesity because of medical complications.

Health and Beauty

Many women are under the illusion that it is just what they put on their skin which makes skin look beautiful. It is true we need to moisturise our skin, the skin on our face and body. It is important to remove make up every night with a cleansing wipe or cleanse and tone skin with cotton wool or cotton pad and then apply a night moisturiser. This is important to allow the skin to breathe, instead of allowing it to be clogged with make up, dirt and grime going to bed. In the morning it is also important to apply a light day cream prior to applying make up There is nothing wrong with using skin creams with vitamins added. Using creams with significant amounts of Vitamin A, C and E, the anti-oxidants in creams can penetrate the epidermis, the skins outer layer is important. Avoiding strong sunlight and using high factor sun screen creams or total sunblock.

As well as putting the antioxidant nutrients on your skin it is important to take all round vitamin and mineral supplements plus extra antioxidant ingredients, vitamins A, C and E especially Vitamin C, which is water soluble and needs to be replaced daily in the diet. Taking adequate amounts of the antioxidants can actually slow down the ageing process. Free radicals from environmental pollution, radiation, fried and burnt foods, sunlight and combustion, damage cells including our skin cells, that is, our elastin. It is the dermis consisting largely of collagen which gives the skin its strength and structure. Elastin fibres are woven within the collagen and this gives the skin its elasticity. Collagen makes up to seventy percent of the skin and twenty percent of the entire body.

It is necessary therefore, to take Vitamin C supplements daily, 1000mg of Vitamin C, or the juice of a lemon or lime in water daily for healthy, glowing and beautiful skin.

In heavy smokers especially as they approach middle age, it is noticeable that their skin is often dry and wrinkly. This is because smoking depletes Vitamin C. The collagen structure in the skin is damaged and the flexibility of collagen and elastin fibres is reduced through smoking due to the free radicals produced by smoking.

It is therefore very important for smokers to take Vitamin C supplements daily in the diet to cheat the effects smoking has on the skin. At least 1000mg of Vitamin Cis recommended daily for smokers.

In a normal, balanced diet it should not be necessary to take specific supplements of the other antioxidants Vitamin A and E, a balanced diet and a multivitamin, mineral complex should provide enough of Vitamins A and E. But the health of skin depends on sufficient zinc, which is needed for production of new skin cells. The lack of zinc leads to stretch marks and poor wound healing. Zinc deficiency leads to lowered ability to fight infection. Dermatitis is also primarily caused by skin deficiency and responds exceptionally well to zinc supplementation.

It is possible to buy Vitamin C with zinc in any pharmacy and one chewable tablet or tablet dissolved into water is recommended daily as a dietary supplement for smokers and non smokers, but especially for smokers. The flexibility of collagen and elastin fibres reduces in time because of the damage caused by free radicals. It is possible to slow down the ageing process with the right nutritional approach. However, it can be beyond repair without botox or other types of plastic surgery for those who can afford it.

Selenium is another important antioxidant and a deficiency in selenium can lead to premature ageing.

Keratin is a protein that is waterproof and resistant to friction and helps to resist bacterial infection. The outer layer of skin consists of keratinized tissue. Vitamin A helps to control the rate of keratin accumulation in the skin. A lack of Vitamin A can therefore result in dry, rough skin. The membranes of skin cells are made from essential fatty acids including omega 3,6 and 9. A lack of essential fatty acids results in these cells becoming dry very quickly, resulting in dry skin and an excessive need for moisturisers. It is therefore important to take adequate amounts of these healthy fats in the diet as well as all the vitamins and minerals recommended.

As a user of the antioxidant vitamin and mineral supplements, no matter how much makeup a woman wears, it will not make them look younger if they are not already in good health.

But if you are in good health, even much older people can benefit from a combination of vitamin therapy, and in addition the flattering effect of skin creams and age defying skin products, makeup will make women whose skin is in good condition look and feel younger.

Users of Avon Products including skin products often receive flattering comments about their skin. Avon Products visibly fight the multiple signs of ageing, boost collagen and regenerate surface skin cells. Avon creams contain collagen boosting antioxidant rich pomegranate seeds and chia seeds with added Vitamin E to help target multiple signs of ageing, reducing wrinkles and producing younger looking skin.

In older women with visible deep wrinkles, Avon again provides Pro+ Line Corrector Treatment. However, this is not a lasting permanent means of reversing wrinkles.

It is better to start using skin creams preferably in your 20's to prevent rather than trying to reverse wrinkles in middle age as this may not be very successful without botox or other forms of cosmetic surgery.

Avon Cosmetics Ltd are hugely secretive about the chemical composition of their Anew day and night creams. But users of these products actually visibly are seen to reverse by a number of years the visible signs of ageing.

There are many new and innovative skin products constantly being invented, manufactured and sold by Avon Products Ltd, which helps reduce the onset and also reverse the development of fine lines and wrinkles. These include face masks, facial exfoliators, facial hydrating treatments, multi-line corrector creams, deep recovery creams, youth maximising serums, resurfacing pads and many youth enhancing body products such as dry oil sprays, body lotions; body butters, yoghurt body cleans, yoghurt body scrubs and silky body soufflés, all exclusive to Avon Cosmetics Ltd.

But no matter how youthful your skin is, or how well you know how to apply makeup none of this is flattering if you are overweight or obese.

If you want to take the holistic approach to health and beauty, you need to be within your ideal weight range.

Staying slim, healthy and beautiful it requires a lot of dedication and it costs quite a lot of money. But if you wish to make yourself ten years younger than your age, it is worth spending the money to do so to become truly beautiful.

Avon Cosmetics Ltd products go beyond being a commodity and often more than a necessity but sometimes an addiction.

"The Water of Life"

Approximately 70% of the human body consists of water. Chemically water is known as H20. But water is not simply H20. Natural water provides significant quantities of minerals:-

A typical spring water for instance contains significant amounts of calcium, which is necessary for healthy bones and teeth. The recommended daily intake of water for health is at least one litre per day.

Some health conscious people actually do drink up to one litre of pure water each day. But many people consume water in other ways such as in coffee and tea as well as carbonated minerals such as Coca-Cola and in alcoholic drinks.

Adverse effects of tea and coffee produce "passing of excessive amounts of urine'.

Liquids, which also produce excessive amounts of urine, include alcoholic drinks.

Such liquids are known as a diuretic. Tea and coffee can have some actual beneficial effects however. The stimulant effects of caffeine can have a beneficial effect on 'Asthma'.

Caffeine is chemically similar to the ophyline, a potent medicine used in treating asthma. 'Pain relief caffeine appears to be effective in improving the efficiency of minor painkillers'.

'Nutritional value'. Tea in particular can be a good source of certain minerals especially manganese and fluoride'.

Diuretics however can have adverse effects. 'Poor nutrition and a diuretic effect which results in more zinc being lost in the urine may both contribute to zinc deficiency in alcoholism.

Alcoholics with zinc deficiency can develop a zinc responsive skin rash. Anyone who drinks a lot should be suspected of being zinc deficient. There is a definite relationship between alcohol consumption during pregnancy and foetal abnormalities. There is now considerable evidence for a link between zinc deficiency and alcohol intake in the mothers of these children. It seems likely that zinc deficiency is resulting in the series of congenital abnormalities that are now so well described in the foetal alcohol syndrome'.

Plasma, the clear liquid that 'carries the red blood cells' is 90 percent water. Approximately 55 percent of blood is plasma and the average adult has about five litres of blood inside their body.

Some people are under the illusion that all bottled water is spring water. However not all bottled water is spring water. The carbon molecules in naturally carbonated water actually deplete our minerals.

The carbon molecules in naturally carbonated water are bound to minerals found in the rock bed and deliver them into our bodies, but the carbon in carbonated drinks is unattached and binds to minerals in us, taking them from the body. For this reason people who consume a lot of carbonated drinks tend to have less dense bones that those who do not.

'Water is vital to life'. It is required for all body fluids, e.g. digestive juices, mucus, salvia, blood, lymph, sweat and urine. It is also required in many metabolic reactions. Water keeps linings of mucus membranes, digestive tract and bronchial tubes moist. Some nutrients dissolve in water for proper absorption. Water also lubricates joints and membranes.

Many foods contain water and some such as fruits and vegetables are composed mainly of water.

In addition to the water that is taken in food as liquids, some water is produced during the many metabolic reactions of the body.

'Water should be drunk every day especially in hot weather when much is lost through sweating.

Water is constantly lost in this way through the skin and also from the lungs, kidneys and bowels. Extra water is required.

- During illness where a raised temperature results increased sweating.
- If vomiting or diarrhoea has occurred, both of which can cause dehydration rapidly especially in babies.
- In lactation, when extra water is required for milk production.

Digestion is mainly a chemical process of hydrolysis, which means removal of water.

'Even though it is not' digested, dietary fibre is of great importance as it absorbs a lot of water, and binds other food residues to itself, thus ensuring that the faeces are soft and bulky and pass easily out of the body in the minimum time.

'If the faeces are not removed quickly and regularly', several problems can arise, including:-

Constipation

Many people suffer from constipation. The faeces become very hard and move slowly through the intestine, and a lot of effort is required to remove them. In addition, abdominal discomfort and a general feeling of ill health accompany this condition.

Diverticular disease.

The extra strain put on the muscular walls of the intense through constipation may lead to diverticular disease, which is the development of small blown-out pouches in the walls of the large intestine. If the faeces are small and hard (due to lack of dietary fibre and insufficient water) the muscular walls of the intestine have to work harder to move them along. This causes increased pressure in the intestine pressure in the intestine and leads to pouches of the bowel lining pressure being focused out through the intestine wall. If pouches (called diverticula) become inflamed, this causes discomfort. Part of the treatment for this to put the patient on a high fibre diet.

Tips about Diet Plan

1. Diet of 1200 kcal for women + 1500 kcal for men for weight reduction.
2. Designed for slow steady weight loss along with moderate exercise.
3. Do not go on a crash diet which would bring sudden weight loss – Dangerous as sudden weight loss can easily be regained as soon as previous eating plan is re established.
4. It is important to do 40 minutes exercise 3 times per week on this weight reduction plan. The reason apart from achieving a healthy heart and circulation; moderate exercise as the body decreases, means that loose skin will become toned up gradually as you lose weight to achieve an attractive figure/physique through exercise.
5. Go to the gym, walk briskly, swim, run up and down the stairs. Do floor exercises at home to music, gardening.
6. Eat little but often. Believe it or not snacking will speed up the metabolism as long as it is healthy food like fresh fruit.
7. Look at this diet as a change in eating habits for life.
8. Different people have different metabolic rates. For some people, less food may be needed to achieve weight loss i.e. if weight cannot be lost with this calorific amount try eating less calories by omitting some foods.
9. Don't eat after two hours before you intend to go to bed. The body will be at its Resting Metabolic Rate when you are asleep i.e. just enough energy to keep the functioning of the main arteries heart, lungs, liver etc working. So very few calories will be needed.
10. Some people eat a large meal before they go to bed but this is "comfort eating" unnecessary and it defeats the purpose of being on a diet as all the calories lost during the day when active are regained at night if a large meal is consumed before going to bed and weight will never be lost.

11. Expect to lose 5-7lbs on the first week of this diet plan and approximately 1-2lbs subsequently.

12. For obese people looking for a "quick fix", this diet may not seem appetising, but think about it. You could be losing on the conservative side up to 40lbs to 50lbs per year, i.e. 4 stones to 5 ½ stones per year and change your eating plans for life.

13. Diet and exercise come together. One is not achievable without the other.

14. Set a target for whatever weight you want to be if you are outsize but do not have extremely high aspirations i.e. to be size zero like a model. Aim to be an average size i.e. size 8 to 16. Don't buy many clothes until you reach your target weight.

15. It is important not to break the diet plan by eating out of fast food outlets or Chinese or Indian take-aways until your target weight is reached. An occasional McDonalds, Burger King, Kentucky Fried Chicken, Chinese or Indian take-away or meal will do no harm but not in excess.

16. If you have a weight problem it is practically impossible to eat and drink alcohol as well as alcohol is so high in calories, so cut out the booze and only take an occasional drink when you reach your target weight, to keep your weight stable.

17. If you are on medication for depression, any kind of mental health problem or for any other illness expect losing weight to be more difficult than if you are not on medication. If so consult your GP.

18. If you are on insulin or a non-insulin dependent diabetic consult your GP before starting this diet plan.

19. If going completely without sugar or butter take half sugar and half butter available in most large supermarket chains and the fat should easily melt off you. For Optimum Health.

20. Take a multi-vitamin, multi-mineral capsule daily plus a B-vitamin and Vitamin C supplement daily. The B Complex and Vitamin C are water soluble and must be replaced daily as they are water soluble and cannot be stored in the liver, unlike

the other vitamins A, D, E, F and K which are fat soluble and can be stored in the liver.

21. Of course not everyone is at home every day to eat lunch. If you are on the move, working, shopping etc in large towns and cities, you can replace a meal with a panini, a wrap, a bagel or a sandwich of your choice with fruit juice, bottled water, tea or coffee.

22. When you reach your target weight it is okay to use some of the recipes as they are generally in line with the N.A.C.N.E. recommended at the beginning of the book, i.e. low in fat, sugar, salt and high in fibre, i.e; fruit and vegetable sources. These recipes can be used for a three course meal or a simple lunch. But you cannot eat too many three course meals after you reach your target weight or adipose tissue will start to deposit again i.e. you will start gaining weight again. Three course meals are okay for dinner parties or Sunday lunch, not every day.

23. Don't worry about constantly having to weigh food. After a couple of weeks you will have a good idea what for example 25g of cornflakes is, or 250mls of low fat milk is and you won't have to weigh food.

24. The operative word is moderation. Don't do anything in excess including dieting.

25. When you are being successful and coming within a weight range you are happy with it is okay to cook the recipes at the back of the book to have an occasional dinner party or simple lunch so that losing weight does not become an unhappy chore.

26. In order to commence this diet plan you must have a pair of digital scales. Don't weigh yourself every day, but about once per week. You will need a set of kitchen scales to weigh the food portions and a calculator to count calories. After a few weeks on this diet you will not be depending so much on the kitchen scales or calculator and dieting should become easier.

The method behind giving the reader, not only a flexible calorie controlled reduction diet; is to give the reader the autonomy, in other words the independence and freedom to choose what they want to eat without having to comply rigorously to a calorie controlled diet.

It will be a very big change for people who do not not eat fruit and vegetables, but if they do not they will never lose weight.

As for alcoholism the most overweight type of alcoholic is the type of person who overindulges in alcohol and overindulges in food as well; and if they are a smoker as well, their days are limited.

The operate word is moderation. Unhealthy food, alcohol and smoking will do the human body no harm in moderation. It is okay to go to KFC, Burger King, McDonalds, The Fish and Chip Shop, the pizzeria, the Chinese and the Indian restaurants and take aways occasionally as a treat for yourself or the family, but not on a regular basis.

It does not be advisable to starve for long periods of time eat a huge especially in the evening because the human body "sends out signals". The body will conserve energy from occasional large meals high in fat or meals containing a lot of sugar and turn it to fat in the body. This "conservation mechanism" is natural in the human body and results in a slowing down of the metabolism. The body is storing fat the way a squirrel will store nuts, albeit at a time it will have no food. The safest way to lose weight and stay healthy is to eat little but often.

How to eat yourself into a Healthy and Beautiful Condition

1. Eat a diet low in sugar, salt, saturated fat and high in fruit and vegetables.
2. Eat as much organic food as possible. Buy organic eggs, chicken, beef, milk, fruit and vegetables.
3. Eat three meals per day and snack with fruit or a handful of nuts, seeds or raisins between meals. This can actually boost the metabolism and help you to lose weight.
4. Eat as much fresh food as possible and limit tinned, processed, cook chilled or frozen food.
5. Avoid too many sweet foods.
6. Lower salt levels and use sea salt
7. Limit alcohol to 14 units per week for a woman and 21 units per week for a man.
8. Limit or avoid smoking
9. Drink a litre of water per day,
10. Limit caffeine. Substitute extra cups of tea or coffee for decaffeinated tea or coffee and drink green tea.
11. Try to grill instead of frying food.
12. Boost Omega 3 by eating oily fish such as tuna, salmon, herrings, mackerel or sardines or take a supplement of Omega 3 fish oils.
13. Boost Omega 6 by using plant seed oils e.g. sunflower oil, safflower oil, soya or corn maize oils or take a supplement of Evening Primrose oil.
14. Boost Omega 9 by frying in olive oil.
15. Alternatively, take a supplement containing Omega 3, Omega 6 and Omega 9.
16. Take a good multi vitamin and mineral supplement daily
17. Drink two large glasses of pure fruit juice per day and/or take a supplement of Vitamin C daily of 1000mg.

18. Take a supplement of the B Complex daily
19. Take a supplement of cod liver oil daily to help circulation and joints.
20. Don't go on crash diets. Lose weight slowly and gradually.
21. Don't diet and think that when you reach your target weight that you can go back to your old eating habits. You will put all the weight back on again.
22. Change your eating habits to a healthy eating plan for life.

Conclusion

Dietary Advice

Eat 62g of protein daily

Avoid saturated fat i.e. limit chips and fried foods

Fry occasionally in olive oil (A good source of omega 9), extra virgin olive oil or rapeseed oil (A good source of omega 6)

Lower sugar intake

Lower salt intake

Increase fibre. Eat plenty of fresh fruit and vegetables and roughage.

Eat salmon, tuna, sardines, and mackerel (A good source of omega 3)

Vitamin B complex, brewer's yeast and vitamin C are passed out daily in the urine.

Vitamin A, C, D, E, F and K and all minerals are fat soluble. They are stored in the liver and they need to be replaced no more than a couple of times per week.

Eat plenty of fresh organic food is possible.

Avoid processed and tinned food as much as possible.

Eat free range eggs.

Try to eat organic chicken when available.

Eat nuts. A good source of vitamin E.

Limit smoking.

Limit caffeine.

Limit Alcohol.

CONCLUSION

We have major challenges in the Western World today which would never have been anticipated at the end of World War II when the World Health Organisation was founded. We have problems which only very optimistic people could think there is a solution to. These include the obvious such as Cancer, Heart Disease, The Obesity Crisis and the threat of ISIS.

It's a dark period the Western World is going through especially for the French. But after the First World War, there came a very happy period, the roaring twenties, and after the Second World War, the 1950's were a very happy period in history.

Nuclear bombs are a terrible means of fighting a war, as so many innocent people die, and there is long term effects on those who even experience nuclear fallout, such as cancer.

The nuclear bombs had to be dropped on Hiroshima and Nagasaki in 1945 by the American President Mr Harry Truman as the war was over but the Japanese would not surrender They wanted to continue fighting.

We just have to be optimistic and hope that whatever happens, it is in the best interest for Christians especially. Good always wins over evil.

MENU PLANNING

SOUPS & STARTERS

Avocado Prawn Cocktail

For 4 servings:
- 2 ripe avocados
- 3 tbsp mayonnaise
- 2 tbsp tomato puree
- 1 small onion, finely chopped
- 1 tbsp chopped fresh dill
- salt and pepper
- 175g (6oz) frozen prawns, thawed.

Garnish
- 4 slices cucumber
- 4 slices lemon
- 4 sprigs fresh dill.

Preparation
1. Mix together mayonnaise, tomato puree, chopped onion, dill and seasoning. Drain prawns, reserve 4 for garnish and add remainder to mayonnaise. Stir gently to coat.
2. Cut avocados in half lengthways and remove stone. Squeeze lemon juice onto cut surfaces of avocados.
3. Put each half onto a small serving plate and divide prawn mixture between avocados.
4. To garnish, put cucumber slice onto lemon slice and cut from centre to edge. Twist edges away from each other and place on prawns. Add reserved prawns and dill and serve.

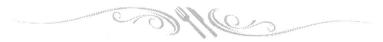

Carrot and Coriander Soup

Healthy Option
Origin: England

For 4 servings
- 2 tbsp extra virgin olive oil
- 5 large carrots sliced
- 2 large onions chopped
- 25g (1oz) lentils
- 1 tsp powdered coriander
- 1 chicken stock cube
- 125mls (¼ pint) single cream

Timing
5 minutes

Cooking:
20 minutes

Preparation
1. Fry carrots and onion in extra virgin olive oil with lentils for 5 minutes. Add chicken stock and simmer for 20 minutes. Add coriander.
2. Cool and add cream, liquidise in a food processor or liquidise and reheat but do not boil and serve.

Nutritional Information		
Calories	Fat	Fibre
2000 (serves 4)		
500 calories per serving		
Good source of Vitamin A and Omega 9.		

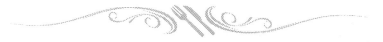

Chili & Tomato Soup with Roasted Peppers

(Serves 4)

Ingredients:
- 1 onion, chopped finely
- 3 cloves garlic, chopped finely
- 2 or 3 red, yellow or orange peppers, deseeded and chopped into chunks
- 2 cartons of Chopped Tomatoes with chili
- 1 red chili, deseeded and chopped finely
- Drizzle of oil
- 1 pint of chicken stock

Method:

(1) Prepare all vegetables as described.
(2) Fry off the onions, garlic, peppers and chili until softened.
(3) Add the chopped tomatoes and stock.
(4) Bring to the boil, and then simmer for a further 20-25 minutes.
(5) When simmered, blend until smooth.
(6) Serve with crusty or wheaten bread and ENJOY!!

Classic Minestrone

Healthy option
Origin: Italy

For 4 servings
- 1 large leek, finely chopped
- 2 carrots, chopped
- 1 courgette, thinly sliced
- 115g (4oz) whole green beans, halved
- 2 celery sticks, thinly sliced
- 45ml (3tbsp) olive oil
- 1.5 litres (2 ½ pints) (6 ½ cups) stock or water
- 400g (14oz) can tomatoes
- 15ml (1 tbsp) chopped fresh basil
- 5ml (1 tbsp) chopped fresh thyme or 2.5ml (½ tsp) dried salt and black pepper
- 400g (14oz) can cannelloni or kidney beans
- 50g (2oz) small pasta shapes or macaroni
- Finely grated Parmesan cheese, to garnish (optional)
- Fresh parsley, chopped, to garnish

Preparation:
1. Put all the fresh vegetables into a large saucepan with the olive oil. Heat until sizzling then cover, lower the heat and sweat the vegetables for 15 mins, shaking the pan occasionally.
2. Add the stock or water, tomatoes, herbs and seasoning. Bring to the boil, replace the lid and simmer gently for about 30 minutes.
3. Add the canned beans and their liquor together with the pasta and simmer for a further 10 minutes. Check the seasoning

and serve hot, sprinkled with the Parmesan cheese, if using, and chopped fresh parsley.

Nutritional Information		
Calories	Fat	Fibre
1331 total (serves 4) 332 per serving	Low	High

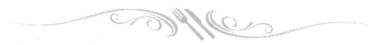

Creamy Courgette Soup

Healthy Option
Origin: Ireland

For 4 servings
- 500g (116oz) courgettes
- 1 large tub of Philadelphia light 300g
- 150mls (1½) pints of chicken stock
- 1 tbsp medium curry powder

Preparation
1. Cut courgettes, minus top and tail, into slices about 2cm in diameter and boil with the stock in a large saucepan for 20 minutes.
2. Remove from heat, add soft cheese.
3. Put in a blender, mix until the whole mixture is smooth.
4. Return to heat. Heat through but do not boil. Serve as a healthy nutritious starter.

Nutritional Information		
Calories	Fat	Fibre
300 cals (serves 4) 75 calories per serving	Medium	High
Generous Vitamin C content		

Creamy Fish Chowder

Origin - Ireland

For 4 servings:
- 2 tbsp olive oil
- 125g (8oz) potato, finely diced
- 1 onion, sliced
- 2 celery sticks sliced
- 25g (1oz) flour
- 500ml (1pt) fish stock
- 225g (8oz) unfried cod fillet
- 225g (8oz) haddock fillet, skinned
- 150g (5oz) peeled prawns
- 200g (7oz) can sweet corn, drained
- 30ml (½ pt) single cream
- Salt and pepper
- 3 tbsp freshly chopped parsley
- Parsley to garnish (optional)
- Croutons to serve (optional)
- 1 diced potato (large)
- 1 large onion diced
- 2 sticks of celery sliced

Timing
Preparation:
5 mins

Cooking:
35mins

Preparation
1. Melt butter in a large saucepan. Add potatoes, onion, celery and sauté for 5 mins.

2. Stir in flour and cook for 1 min. Pour in stock, stir and bring to boil. Reduce heat to a simmer and cook for 20 mins or until potatoes are cooked.
3. Cut cod and haddock into cubes and add to pan with the prawns, sweetcorn and cream. Season and stir in parsley.
4. Heat gently for 10 mins, stirring. Garnish with parsley if using, top with croutons and serve.

Nutritional Information		
Calories	Fat	Fibre
1921 500 per serving	Low	Medium

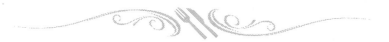

Fruity Prawn Cocktail

Origin: England

For 4 servings:
- 275g (10oz) peeled prawns
- 225g (8oz) can pineapple pieces in fruit juice
- ½ lollo rosso or small lettuce
- ¼ cucumber
- Paprika to garnish
- Whole prawns to garnish (optional)

Sauce:
- 200ml (7fl oz) thick mayonnaise
- 1 tbsp tomato ketchup
- 2 tsp lemon juice
- dash Tabasco sauce
- salt and pepper.

Timing
Preparation: 25mins

Preparation:
1. To make sauce, mix together mayonnaise, tomato ketchup, lemon juice, Tabasco and seasoning
2. Add the prawns to the sauce. Drain pineapple and add to sauce, stirring gently to coat.
3. Arrange lollo rosso leaves on four individual plates. Peel cucumber skin in narrow strips to give striped effect. Slice cucumber and arrange on top of lettuce. Top with prawn cocktail.
4. Dash with paprika and serve garnished with whole prawns if using.

Nutritional Information		
Calories	Fat	Fibre
1300 total (serves 4) 325 per serving	Low	Low

Home Made Coleslaw

200g white cabbage
100g onion peeled
100g carrot
25g low fat (light) mayonnaise

Slice cabbage, onion and carrot or a grater. Mix with mayonnaise and serve.

Italian Tomato Soup

Healthy Option
Origin: Italy

For 4 servings
- 1 tbsp olive oil
- 1 onion, chopped
- 1 clove garlic, chopped
- 25g (1oz) wholemeal or plain flour
- 600ml (1pt) vegetable stock
- 675g (1 ½ lb) ripe tomatoes peeled
- 2 tbsp tomato puree
- 2 bay leaves
- 2 tsp fresh chopped basil
- Salt and pepper
- 50ml (2fl oz) double cream
- Chopped parsley, to serve.

Timing
Preparation:
25mins

Cooking:
45mins

Preparation:
1. Heat oil in a large saucepan, add the onion and garlic and fry gently for 5mins. Stir in flour.
2. Remove from heat and gradually stir in stock. Bring to boil, stirring continuously until thickened.
3. Chop tomatoes, removing seeds, if wished. Add to pan with tomato puree, bay leaves, and seasoning. Cover and simmer for 30 mins.

4. Remove bay leaves. Stir in cream, basil and parsley. Heat gently to warm through.

Nutritional Information		
Calories	Fat	Fibre
640 total (serves 4) 160 per serving	Low	Med
Good source of Vitamin C, folic acid, phosphorus, potassium		

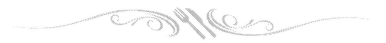

Leek and Potato Soup

Healthy Option
Origin: Wales

For 4 servings:
- 350g (12oz) potatoes
- 3 leeks
- 25g (1oz) butter
- 1 onion, chopped
- 850ml (1½ pt) vegetable stock
- 150ml (¼ pt) single cream
- Snipped chives, to garnish

Timing
Preparation:
10mins

Cooking:
20mins

Preparation:
1. Cut potatoes into thick slices. Trim and slice leeks.
2. Melt butter in a saucepan, add leeks and onion and cook gently for 5 mins without browning. Add potatoes and cook for 3 minutes.
3. Add stock, bring to boil, cover and simmer gently for 20-30 mins. Leave to cool.
4. Puree or push through a sieve until smooth. Return to a cleaned pan.
5. Reheat gently, stir in the cream and seasoning. Top with chives and serve.

Nutritional Information		
Calories	Fat	Fibre
955 total (serves 4) 240 per serving	Low	Med
Good source of Vitamin C		

Potato and Onion Soup

Healthy Option
Ireland

For 4 servings
- 2tbsp olive oil
- 3 onions chopped
- 375g (12oz) diced potatoes
- 900ml (1 ½) pints of vegetable stock
- 1 tbsp chopped parsley
- 1 tsp chopped thyme
- Sprinkle of salt and pepper
- 150ml (¼ pint) single cream
- ½ red pepper, seeded and thinly sliced
- .Grated red Leicester cheese
- Chopped parsley to serve

Timing
Preparation:
10mins

Cooking:
20-25mins

Preparation
1. Melt butter in a large saucepan, add the onions and sauté for 4 – 5 mins.
2. Add potatoes and stock and bring to the boil.
3. Cover and cook for 10 – 15 mins or until potatoes are soft.
4. Put in a blender or food processor with parsley, thyme and seasoning and puree until smooth.

5. Return to cleaned pan, add cream and red pepper. Gently re-heat.
6. Serve in individual bowls, sprinkled with cheese and parsley.

Nutritional Information		
Calories	Fat	Fibre
1370 (serves 4) 343 per serving	Low	Medium
Good source of Omega 9		

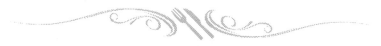

Prawn Cocktail

- Lettuce (3 slices, chopped)
- 100g prawns
- 25g low calorie mayonnaise
- 25g tomato ketchup
- Dash lemon juice
- Dash Worchester Sauce
- Slice of lemon
- 1 King Prawn in shell
- Dash of paprika

Chop lettuce and put in bottom of a large wine glass. Put prawns on top of lettuce. Mix light mayonnaise, tomato ketchup, dash of lemon juice and dash of Worchester sauce together and blend into a creamy mixture.

Place on top of prawns. Add a sprinkling of paprika on top, with a slice of lemon and/or King Prawn in shell to decorate.

148 kcal per small serving.

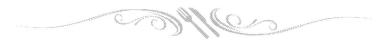

Special Egg Mayonnaise

Origin: England

For 4 servings
- 4 eggs
- 25g (1oz) butter
- 1 clove garlic crushed
- 1 tbsp fresh chopped parsley
- 4 slices French Bread
- 4 tbsp mayonnaise
- 2 tbsp soured cream
- 1 tsp lemon juice
- 2 tsp horseradish sauce
- salt and pepper
- mustard and cress and salad leaves to garnish (optional)

Preparation
1. Put eggs in a saucepan and cover with cold water. Bring to boil and simmer for five minutes. Plunge eggs into cold water to prevent them from cooking further and leave to cool.
2. Mix together butter, garlic, and parsley. Brush half butter onto bread. Put under a preheated grill and cook for 3 minutes, until golden. Turn and repeat with second side. Leave to cool.
3. Shell eggs and arrange on slices of bread.
4. Mix together mayonnaise, soured cream, lemon juice and horseradish. Season to taste. Spoon over eggs coating completely. Garnish with mustard and cress and salad and serve.

Nutritional Information		
Calories	Fat	Fibre
1200 total (serves 4) 300 per serving	High	Low

Spring Rolls

Origin: China

For 8 rolls:
- 100g (4oz) plain flour
- Pinch salt
- 1 egg
- 30ml (½ pt) milk
- Oil for frying

Filling:
- 1 tbsp vegetable oil
- 100g (4oz) button mushrooms, chopped
- 1 stick celery, finely chopped
- 3 spring onions, chopped
- 100g (4oz) cooked pork, finely chopped
- 100g (4oz) beansprouts
- 1 tsp cornflour
- 2 tbsp dry sherry
- 1 tbsp soy sauce
- 1 beaten egg
- soy sauce to serve.

Timing
Preparation:
30mns

Cooking:
40mins

Preparation
1. Sift together flour and salt. Add egg and half the milk and beat until smooth. Gradually beat in remaining milk.

2. Heat a little oil in a large frying pan until hot. Drain off any surplus oil. Pour in just enough batter to thinly coat base of pan.
3. Cook for 1-2 minutes until a light golden colour, turn and cook other side. Repeat with remaining mix to make 7 more pancakes.
4. Heat vegetable oil in a frying pan. Add mushrooms, celery, and spring onions and sauté for 2-3 minutes. Add pork and beansprouts and sauté for 2 minutes. Blend cornflour with 1 tablespoon of water. Add sherry and soy sauce. Stir into pan and cook for 2 minutes.
5. Spoon equal portions of filling into centre of each pancake. Brush edges with beaten egg and roll, folding edges in so that the filling is completely enclosed.
6. Heat oil to 180C/350F and fry rolls in batches until golden.

Nutritional Information		
Calories	Fat	Fibre
1282 total (makes 8) 160 per roll	Low	Medium

Spring Vegetable Soup

Healthy Option
Origin: England

For 4 servings
- 2 leeks, finely sliced
- 1 potato, grated
- 2 carrots, grated
- 1 swede, grated
- 1 chicken breast
- 2 sticks celery, finely sliced
- 6 sprigs parsley, chopped
- 25g (1oz) butter
- Pepper
- 1 chicken stock cube

Timing
Preparation:
10mins

Cooking:
30mins

Preparation:
1. Put chicken breast in a saucepan and add 600ml (1pt) cold water. Bring to boil and simmer for 30 mins. Remove from stock and leave to cool, reserving stock for the soup. Shred chicken finely.
2. Melt butter in a saucepan and add vegetables. Sauté until they are totally coated with butter.
3. Measure chicken stock and add sufficient water to make up 1 litre (2pt). Add to vegetables with stock cube.

4. Bring to boil and simmer for 5 mins before adding shredded chicken. Simmer for another 15 minutes until vegetables are tender. Season with pepper and serve.

Nutritional Information.		
Calories	Fat	Fibre
345 total (serving 4) 86 per serving	Med	High

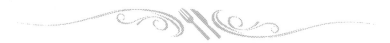

Stir Fried Mange Touts

For 4 servings
- 25g (1oz) sesame seeds
- 1 tbsp vegetable oil
- 1 tsp salt
- 1 clove garlic crushed
- 200g (8oz) mange touts, topped and tailed
- 2 tbsp water

Timing
Preparation:
10 mins

Cooking:
6 minutes

Preparation
1. Heat a heavy frying pan or wok. Add sesame seeds and shake over heat until seeds turn golden brown. Set aside.
2. Heat oil in wok and add garlic and salt. Sizzle over high heat for a few seconds and add mange touts. Stir fry over high heat for 2-3 minutes.
3. Add water, cover with a lid and cook for another 3 minutes or until water has evaporated. Add sesame seeds, toss and serve.

Nutritional Information		
Calories	Fat	Fibre
260 total (serves 4) 65 per serving	Med	High

Strawberry And Banana Smoothie

Ingredients

- 2 punnets of fresh strawberries
- 2 large bananas
- 1 medium glass of pure orange juice
- 1 tub of Low fat Onken yoghurt
- Other fruits can be used including:
- Raspberries
- Mango
- Blueberries
- Melon
- Passion Fruit
- Kiwi Fruit
- Nectarines
- Pears
- Blackberries
- Or frozen fruit can be used.

Method.

Chop fruit into small pieces, add orange juice and yoghurt, and blend in a liquidiser until smooth. Serve in a tall glass and drink through a straw.

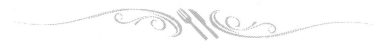

Tuna Stuffed Tomatoes

Healthy Option
Origin: Italy

For 4 servings:
- 8 tomatoes
- salt and pepper
- 198g (7oz) can tuna in oil, drained
- 5 tbsp mayonnaise
- 1 tbsp stuffed olives, chopped
- 2-3 drops Tabasco
- 2 tsp lemon juice
- 8 sprigs parsley
- lettuce leaves to serve.

Timing
Preparation:
10mins

Preparation:
1. Cut the tops of the tomatoes and set aside. Scoop out the seeds from the tomatoes and discard. Season insides of cases with salt and pepper.
2. Mix together tuna, mayonnaise, olives, Tabasco and lemon juice.
3. Divide tuna mixture between the tomato cases, filling each one generously.
4. Place tomato lids on top of stuffing, pressing down gently to secure. Garnish with parsley and serve on a bed of lettuce leaves.

Nutritional Information		
Calories	Fat	Fibre
597 total (serves 4) 149 per serving		
Good source of Omega 3.		

MAIN COURSES

BEEF

Beef and Pineapple Curry

Healthy Option
Origin: China

For 4 servings
- 1 tbsp seasoned flour
- 675g (1 ½ lb) braising steak
- 2 tbsp rapeseed oil
- 225g (8oz) button mushrooms
- 1 tbsp madras curry powder
- 1 clove garlic, crushed
- 100g (4oz) creamed coconut, dissolved in 150ml (½ pt) warm water.
- 1 tbsp soy sauce
- Salt and pepper
- 200g (7oz) can pineapple chunks in natural juice
- 1 apple, peeled, cored and chopped.

Timing
Preparation:
10 mins

Cooking:
1 hour.

Preparation
1. Toss beef in seasoned flour until evenly coated. Heat oil in a flameproof casserole and fry beef for 8 mins, until browned on all sides. Add onions and cook for 2 mins. Stir in curry powder and cook for a further two mins.
2. Stir in the garlic, coconut mixture, soy sauce and seasoning. Bring to boil, cover and simmer for 30 mins.

3. Add pineapple and apple pieces and simmer for a further 15 mins, until beef is tender. Adjust seasoning and serve.

Nutritional Information		
Calories	Fat	Fibre
1320 total (serves 4) 330 per serving	Med	Med
Good source of protein, iron and omega 6.		

Beef and Tomato Stroganoff

Healthy Option
Origin: Germany

For 4 servings:
- 700g (1½ lb) rump or fillet steak, cut into thin strips
- 2 tbsp seasoned flour
- 25g (1oz) butter
- 1 tbsp rapeseed oil
- 1 onion, chopped
- 175g (6oz) button mushrooms, wiped and sliced
- 1 tsp paprika
- Salt
- 225g (8oz) can chopped tomatoes
- 1 tbsp chopped parsley
- 200ml (7fl oz) soured cream

Preparation
1. Cut steak into thin strips about 2.5cm (1in) long. Coat with seasoned flour.
2. Heat butter and oil in a frying pan, add steak and onion and fry for 3-4 mins, until meat is browned on all sides.
3. Add mushrooms and fry for 2-3 mins. Stir in paprika and salt and fry for one min.
4. Add the chopped tomatoes and the parsley. Cook for 4-5 mins.
5. Lower heat, add soured cream and heat through. Serve.

Nutritional Information		
Calories	Fat	Fibre
1656 total (serves 4) 414 per serving	Low	Low
Good source of iron and omega 6		

Beef with Grapes

Healthy Option
Origin: Italy

For 6 servings:
- 2 tbsp vegetable oil
- 2 onions, sliced
- 2 cloves garlic, crushed
- 900g (2lb) top rump or chuck steak, cut into 12 large pieces
- 2 tbsp plain flour
- 600ml (1pt) beef stock
- salt and pepper
- 100g (4oz) seedless white grapes, halved
- 1 tbsp chopped fresh rosemary
- 1 tbsp chopped fresh parsley

Timing
Preparation:
25mins

Cooking:
2 ¾ hours

Preparation:
1. Preheat oven. Heat oil in a large ovenproof casserole dish. Add onions and garlic and fry until softened. Remove from pan with slotted spoon and set aside.
2. Add meat and cook until browned. Remove from pan.
3. Add flour to casserole and blend with juices. Lower heat and gradually add stock, stirring continuously. Bring to boil, stirring, until thickened.

4. Return meat and onions to casserole, season, cover and cook over a very low heat for 2½ hours.

5. Gently stir in grapes, top with herbs and serve.

Nutritional Information		
Calories	Fat	Fibre
1770 total (serves 6) 295 per serving		
Good source of iron		

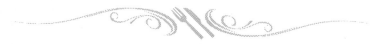

Beef with Soured Cream

Origin: France

For 4 servings
- 350g (12oz) cold roast topside of beef, sliced
- 6 tbsp soured cream
- 4 tbsp crème fraiche
- 2 tbsp horseradish sauce
- 3 tbsp chopped parsley
- Few drops Tabasco sauce
- Salt and pepper
- 4 pimento stuffed green olives, quartered
- Chopped fresh parsley, to garnish

Timing
Preparation
20mins

Preparation
1. Cut the beef slices into strips approximately 2.5cm (1in) wide.
2. Mix together the soured cream, crème fraiche and horseradish.
3. Stir in the chopped parsley, Tabasco sauce and olives. Season with salt and pepper.
4. Arrange the beef on a serving platter and spoon the sauce over the top. Garnish and serve on a green salad.

Nutritional Information		
Calories	Fat	Fibre
1106 total (serves 4) 277 per serving		
Good source of protein and iron.		

Brown Stew

- 1lb stewing steak
- 2 onions peeled
- 3 carrots
- 1 pint beef stock
- 1 tbsp bisto
- 1 tsp extra virgin olive oil

Cut stewing steak into cubes, chop onion into small pieces, slice carrots, brown meat on all sides in olive oil. Add carrots and onions. Add beef stock.

Cook in a moderate oven 180°C, gas mark 5 for two hours

Test meat. When meat is tender remove from oven and thicken with bisto.

Serve with mashed potatoes.

Carbonade of Beef

(Origin: France)

For 4 servings:
- 1½ lb chuck steak
- 1oz. butter
- 2 tablespoons salad oil
- 2 medium onions, chopped
- 1 level tablespoon flour
- ½ pint light ale
- ¼ pint water
- pinch dried thyme
- bay leaf
- 1 level teaspoon sugar
- Salt and pepper.

Preparation:
1. Cut beef into strips, 1-inch-wide, 2 inches long and about 1/2 inch thick. Melt butter in a pan with oil and brown meat quickly on all sides.
2. Remove meat from pan; add onions to fat and fry until golden brown. Blend in flour and cook for 1 minute. Blend in light ale and water, then bring to boiling point and simmer until thickened.
3. Add meat, thyme, bay leaf, sugar and seasoning. Cover pan and simmer over a very low heat for 2 hours or until meat is tender.

Chilli Con Carne

Healthy Option
(Origin: Mexico)

For 4 servings

Ingredients
- 1 tbsp extra virgin olive oil
- 25g (1oz) butter
- 2 medium onions, finely chopped
- 2 cloves garlic, crushed
- 100g (4oz) streaky bacon, chopped
- 675g (1 ½ lb) stewing steak
- 60g (2 ¼ oz) tomato puree
- ¾ pint beef stock
- 2 tsp chilli powder
- 400g (16oz) canned red kidney beans
- 1 tbsp corn flour
- 4 tsp cumin

Preparation
1. Heat oil in a pan, add butter and fry onion and garlic until soft and pale golden brown. Remove from pan and put to one side on kitchen roll to soak up excess fat.
2. Cut streaky bacon into 1cm (½ inch) pieces and stewing steak into 2cm (1 ½ inch) pieces. Add to pan and fry until pale golden brown.
3. Replace onion and garlic to pan, add tomato puree, cumin, stock, salt and pepper and chilli powder. Bring to boil, cover and simmer for 3 hours.
4. Add Kidney beans and simmer for a further 10 minutes. Thicken with corn flour, dissolved in a little water. Serve on a bed of rice.

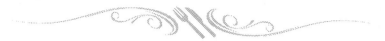

Fillet Steak Royale

Origin: England

For 4 servings
- 4 fillet steaks, about 175g (6oz) each.
- 4 tbsp olive oil
- 1 onion, finely chopped
- 175g (6oz) button mushrooms, sliced
- 200ml (7 fl oz) white wine.
- 150ml (5fl oz) double cream.
- 2 tsp French Mustard
- 2 tbsp chopped fresh tarragon
- 1 clove garlic, crushed
- salt and pepper
- Tarragon sprigs, to garnish (optional).

Preparation
1. Flatten steaks with your fist or a meat mallet. Heat 2 tbsp oil in a frying pan and fry steaks, turning regularly, according to taste. For a rare steak, fry for 2 minutes, for a medium, 6 minutes, and for a well done steak, fry for 8 minutes
2. Meanwhile, heat oil in another frying pan and sauté onion for 3 mins under a gentle heat.
3. Add mushrooms and cook for a further 2 mins. Add wine and simmer for 5 mins.
4. Stir in cream, mustard, tarragon, garlic and seasoning and heat gently to warm through.
5. Serve steaks on a bed of mushroom sauce, garnished with tarragon sprigs, if liked.

Nutritional Information		
Calories	Fat	Fibre
3360 total (serves 4) 840 per serving	High	Low
Good source of Omega 3.		

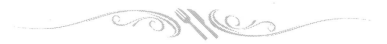

Greek Style Beef

Healthy Option
Country of Origin: Greece

For 4 servings:
- 1 tbsp olive oil
- 175g (6oz) button onions, peeled
- 2 garlic cloves, crushed
- 675g (1½ lb) braising steak, trimmed and cubed
- 25g (1oz) flour
- 2 tbsp tomato puree
- 350g (12oz) tomatoes, peeled and halved
- 300ml (½ pt) red wine
- 300ml (½ pt) beef stock
- 100g (4oz) button mushrooms, wiped and halved
- 3 tbsp freshly chopped coriander
- salt and black pepper
- coriander sprigs, to garnish (optional)

Preparation
1. Preheat oven. Heat oil in a frying pan, add onions and garlic and sauté for 5 mins.
2. Add meat and cook for 5 mins, or until sealed, stirring.
3. Stir in flour and cook for 1 min. Add the tomato puree, tomatoes, wine and stock.
4. Bring to boil, stirring. Add mushrooms and coriander. Season well.
5. Transfer to a flame- proof casserole dish. Cover and cook for 1¼ hours or until meat is tender. Garnish if wished, and serve with rice.

Nutritional Information		
Calories	Fat	Fibre
1122 total (serves 4) 280 per serving	Med	Low
Good source of protein, iron and omega 3.		

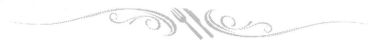

Horseradish Roast Beef

Healthy Option
Origin: England

For 6 servings
- 700-900g (1½ - 2lb) fillet or sirloin of beef
- 3 tbsp hot horseradish sauce
- 1 clove garlic, crushed
- 1 tbsp fresh chopped parsley
- Salt and pepper
- 100g (4oz) streaky bacon, rinded

Timing
Preparation:
15 mins

Cooking:
50-60mins

Cooking temperature
180C/350F/gas 4.

Preparation
1. Mix together horseradish sauce, garlic, parsley and seasoning. Remove string, if any, from beef.
2. Spread horseradish mixture over top and sides of beef
3. Stretch bacon rashers with the back of a knife. Wrap around beef joint and secure with cocktail sticks
4. Put on a roasting rack in a roasting tin and cook for 18-24 minutes per 450g (1lb) depending on how well done you like your beef, plus 20 minutes.

5. Remove from oven, cover with foil and allow to stand for 5 minutes before carving.

Nutritional Information		
Calories	Fat	Fibre
3041 (serves 6) 507 per serving	Med	Low
Good source of protein and iron.		

Mexican Beef Stew

Healthy Option
Mexico

For 4 servings

- 2 tbsp olive oil
- 450g (1lb) stewing steak
- 2 onions, sliced
- 2 cloves garlic, crushed
- 1 tbsp tomato puree
- 215g (8oz) can tomatoes
- ¼ tsp salt
- 1 tsp ground cumin
- ¼ tsp coriander
- 1 tsp chilli powder
- 1 tsp brown sugar
- 1 tsp vinegar
- ½ tsp Tabasco sauce
- 200 ml (7 fl oz) beef stock
- 1 red and 1 green pepper, seeded and cut into rings
- 435 g (1 lb) can red kidney beans, drained

Timing
Preparation
10minutes

Cooking
3 hours 10 minutes

Oven setting
150C/300F/Gas Mark 2

Preparation

1. Preheat oven, cube meat or use diced stewing steak. Heat oil in a wok and brown the beef. Remove with a slotted spoon.
2. Add onions and garlic and gently fry for 5 mins.
3. Put tomato puree, tomatoes, cumin, salt, chilli powder, coriander, brown sugar, vinegar and Tabasco in a blender and process until smooth.
4. Mix meat, onions and garlic with stock and put in a casserole.
5. Cover tightly and cook in oven for 2 hours. Add peppers and kidney beans. Cover again and cook for 1 hour.

Calories	Fat	Salt	Sugar	Fibre
2000 total, serves 4	Medium	Low	Low	High
500 calories per serving				

TIPS

For a real Mexican flavour serve this stew with saffron rice and taco shells.

SAFFRON RICE

Add equal amounts of long grain white rice and water with a pinch of salt and a ½ tsp of tumeric. Boil until water is saturated and serve Mexican Beef Stew on a bed of Saffron Rice.

Porc a La Crème

Origin: France

4 servings
- 750g (1½ lb) pork fillet or boned loin of pork
- 2 tbsp extra virgin olive oil
- 1oz butter
- 1 onion, peeled and chopped
- 1 level tbsp paprika pepper
- 1 level tbsp flour
- 500ml (½ pt) water
- 1 beef stock cube
- 5 tbsp sherry
- 1 level tbsp tomato puree
- salt and pepper
- 6oz button mushrooms
- 1 level tbsp corn flour
- 125g (5oz) carton double cream

Preparation
1. Cut pork into 1½ inch (3cm) pieces. Heat oil in a pan, add butter. Then fry pork pieces until they are just beginning to turn brown. Remove from pan and drain on kitchen paper.
2. Fry onion and paprika for 2 minutes. Blend in flour and cook for a further minute. Remove from heat and blend in stock. Add sherry and tomato puree, return to heat and simmer until thick. Season with salt and pepper then add the meat. Cover and simmer for 30-40 minutes or until the pork is tender.
3. At the end of cooking time, add mushrooms to pan. Blend 2 tbsp of corn flour to a smooth paste with 2 tbsp of cold water and add to pan. Re-boil and just before serving blend

in cream. This can be decorated with triangles of fried bread and sprigs of parsley.

Nutritional Information		
Calories	Fat	Fibre
2400 total (serves 4) 600 per serving	Low	Low
Good source of protein and omega 3.		

Shepherd's Pie (Vegetarian)

Serves 4

- 6oz (175g) brown/green lentils
- 4oz (100g) split peas green or yellow
- 1 pint (500mls) hot water
- 1 medium onion, peeled and chopped
- ½ green pepper, chopped
- 2 carrots, chopped
- 2 sticks celery, chopped
- 1 clove garlic, crushed
- ½ teaspoon dried mixed herbs
- 2 pinches ground mace
- ¼ teaspoon cayenne pepper
- 25g low fat margarine
- Sprinkle of flaxseed

For the topping

- ½ 1lb tomatoes (200g) peeled and sliced
- 1 ½ lbs cooked potatoes (700g)
- 3oz (75g) cheddar cheese, grated
- 1 small onion, chopped
- 2oz low fat margarine (50g)
- 2 tablespoons milk
- Salt and freshly milled black pepper.

Wash the lentils and split peas then put them in a saucepan with hot water and simmer gently covered for approximately 45 – 60 minutes, or until the peas and lentils have absorbed the water and are soft. Pre heat the oven to gas mark 5, 375°F (190°C).

Meantime melt some low fat margarine in a frying pan, add the celery, onion, carrots and chopped pepper, and cook gently until softened. Then mash lentil mixture and add to the vegetables. Add seasoning and a pinch of salt. Then spoon the mixture into a large pie dish (3 pint or 1.75 litre) and arrange the sliced tomatoes on top.

Next prepare the topping by softening the onion in low fat margarine in a small pan, then mash the potatoes, add the cooked onion, margarine, milk and grated cheese and mix thoroughly. Season well then spread on top of the ingredients in the pie dish. Bake for about 20 minutes or until the top is lightly browned. Sprinkle with a tsp flaxseed.

As an alternative to a low fat margarine instead of butter, you can compromise and use half butter, half margarine available in most supermarkets.

For a meat shepherd's pie just replace lentils and split peas with 1lb minced steak.

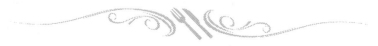

Simple Beef Wellington

Origin: England

For 4 servings:
- 900g (2lb) piece beef fillet
- salt and pepper
- 1 tbsp rapeseed oil
- 40g (1½ oz) butter
- 225g (8oz) button mushrooms, sliced
- 3 tbsp horseradish sauce
- 175g (6oz) full fat soft cheese
- 4 tbsp double cream
- 350g (12oz) puff pastry
- beaten egg, to glaze

Timing
Preparation:
40mins

Cooking:
1 hour

Cooking temperature
200C/425F/gas 7

Preparation:
1. Trim excess fat from beef fillet and tie at intervals to keep in shape. Season.
2. Heat oil and half the butter in a large frying pan. Add the beef and fry for 10 mins until browned on all sides.
3. Remove from heat and put to one side to cool.
4. Add remaining butter to frying pan, add mushrooms and fry for 5 mins. Leave to cool.

5. Preheat oven. Mix together the horseradish sauce, cheese, cream, seasoning and mushrooms.

6. On a lightly floured surface roll out pastry to a rectangle 25x35cm (10x14in).

7. Remove string from beef and cut meat into thick slices.

8. Arrange the slices along the centre of pastry, sandwiching together with mushroom sauce. Reserve any left over sauce.

9. Brush edges of pastry with a little beaten egg. Fold pastry lengthways over beef, making sure edges are well sealed. Fold ends over and put on a lightly greased baking tray. Brush with beaten egg.

10. Bake for 45 mins, reducing oven temp to 190/375F/gas 5 after 20 mins. Cover loosely with foil if pastry starts to brown too quickly. Serve with extra mushroom sauce at side.

Nutritional Information		
Calories	Fat	Fibre
2280 total (serves 4) 570 per serving	Med	Low
Good source of protein, iron and omega 6.		

Steak and Kidney Pie

For 6 servings:
- 675g (1½ lb) stewing steak, cubed
- 225g (8oz) ox kidney, cut into small even-sized pieces
- 2 tbsp flour
- salt and pepper
- 25g (1oz) butter
- 2 tbsp oil
- 2 onions, chopped
- 100g (4oz) mushrooms, sliced
- 200ml (7fl oz) dry red wine
- 200ml (7fl oz) beef stock
- 1 bay leaf
- 350g (12oz) shortcrust pastry
- 1 egg, beaten, to glaze

Preparation
1. Mix the flour with seasoning.
2. Coat the steak and kidney in seasoned flour
3. Put butter and oil in a large pan, add onion and fry for 5 mins until soft.
4. Add meat and sauté for 5 mins until browned.
5. Stir in mushrooms. Add stock, wine and bay leaf, and bring to the boil. Cover and simmer for 1½ - 2 hours or until meat is tender stirring occasionally. Leave to cool.
6. Preheat oven. Add meat mixture to pie dish. Roll out pastry 2.5cm (1in) larger than the top of the dish. Cut off 1cm (½ in) strip from outer edge to line dampened rim of dish.
7. Dampen pastry rim and cover with pastry lid. Trim and seal edge. Make small slashes in lid to allow steam to escape during cooking. Decorate with pastry leaves, brush with beaten egg and bake for 20 minutes. Reduce heat to 180C/350F/gas 4 and bake for a further 20 mins or until crust is golden.

Steak and Kidney Pudding

(Origin: England)

For 4 servings:

For the filling:
- 1lb skirt beef stewing steak
- 4oz ox kidney
- 1oz seasoned flour
- 1 onion, peeled and chopped

For the pastry
- 8oz self raising flour
- ½ level teaspoon salt
- 4oz. shredded suet
- 8 tablespoons cold water

Preparation:
1. Cut steak in 1-inch cubes. Remove skin, core and fat from kidney then cut into ½ inch pieces. Coat the steak with seasoned flour.
2. Sieve flour and salt for pastry into a bowl. Stir in suet, then add enough water to make a fairly soft dough. Roll out two-thirds of pastry to a circle large enough to line a greased 2-pint pudding basin. Roll out the remaining pastry to a circle the size of the top of the basin.
3. Put steak, kidney, and onion in alternate layers in basin, then add sufficient water to come within 1-inch of the top of the basin. Moisten edges of pastry "lid" and press firmly on top. Cover with lid of greaseproof paper, then cover with a lid of foil; both pleated to allow for expansion. Steam or boil the pudding for 4 ½ hours, topping up with boiling water as necessary.

Steak with Blue Cheese

For 4 servings:
- 4 fillet steaks
- 175g (6oz) Gorgonzola cheese
- salt and pepper
- 25g (1oz) butter
- 50ml (2 fl oz) dry sherry
- 300ml (½ pt) single cream

Preparation:
1. Cut a horizontal slit into the side of each steak. Halve the cheese. Cut one half into four and put a square inside each steak.
2. Season steaks with salt and pepper. Melt butter in a frying pan, add steaks and fry for 4-5 mins, according to taste.
3. Transfer steaks to a warmed serving plate. Add sherry to pan juices and stir in cream. Crumble remaining cheese and add to pan.
4. Heat gently until the cheese melts. Season sauce and serve separately.

Steaks with Onion Sauce

Healthy Option
Origin: England

For 4 servings:
- 675g (1 ½ lb) rump steak, trimmed
- 2 small onions
- 50g (2oz) butter
- 2 tbsp light soy sauce
- white pepper
- 1 tsp mustard powder
- salt
- flat leaved parsley, to garnish (optional).

Timing
Preparation:
7mins

Cooking:
25mins

Preparation:
1. Put steaks on board and tenderize with a meat mallet until 1.25cm (½ in) thick. Slice onions.
2. Melt 25g (1oz) butter in a frying pan and sauté onions for 5 mins. Add soy sauce. Remove onions from pan with a slotted spoon and keep warm.
3. Melt remaining butter in pan and add steaks. Fry for 5 mins each side. Add pepper, mustard powder and salt.
4. Return onions to pan and cook, stirring for 5 mins. Serve, garnished with parsley, if using.

Nutritional Information		
Calories	Fat	Fibre
1503 total (serves 4) 376 per serving	Low	Low
Good source of protein and iron		

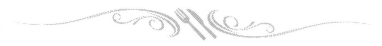

Stir fried Beef

For 4 servings:
- 450g (1lb) rump or sirloin steak, cut into thin strips
- 3 tbsp soy sauce
- 1 leek
- 1 carrot, peeled
- 100g (4oz) cup mushrooms
- 1 red pepper
- 2.5cm (1in) piece root ginger, peeled
- 3 tbsp sesame oil OR vegetable oil
- 75g (3oz) bean sprouts

Preparation:
1. Put beef in a shallow bowl and add soy sauce, coating the meat well. Leave to marinate for at least 30 mins.
2. Cut leeks and carrots into matchstick sized strips. Slice mushrooms, chop pepper and cut ginger into thin strips.
3. Heat oil in a wok or frying pan. Drain beef and add to wok reserving marinade. Stir fry for 2-3 mins. Remove with a slotted spoon and keep warm.
4. Add vegetables and stir fry for 3-4 mins, then add beef, marinade and bean sprouts. Cook for 2-3 mins until vegetables are cooked but still crisp. Season and serve.

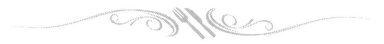

Stuffed Rib of Beef

Healthy Option
Origin: England

For 6 servings:
- 1kg (2¼ lb) fore rib of beef, boned and rolled
- 1 tbsp rapeseed oil
- 2 sticks celery, trimmed and finely sliced
- 4 spring onions, trimmed and sliced
- 25g (1oz) canned sweetcorn, drained
- 50g (2oz) fresh white breadcrumbs
- 1 tbsp chopped fresh thyme
- salt and pepper
- 3 tbsp horseradish sauce
- 1 egg, beaten
- 10-12 sprigs thyme

Preparation:
1. Preheat oven. Untie beef and unroll. Wipe with dampened kitchen paper.
2. Heat oil in a frying pan and fry celery and onions for 3 mins.
3. Add sweetcorn, breadcrumbs, herbs, and seasoning.
4. Remove pan from heat and stir in horseradish sauce and beaten egg. Work mixture together to form a soft stuffing.
5. Spread stuffing over beef. Re-roll and tie.
6. Make slits in meat and slot in thyme sprigs. Cook for 1½ hours or until juices run clear.

Nutritional Information		
Calories	Fat	Fibre
2143 total (serves 6) 357 per serving	Med	Low
Good source of protein, iron and omega 6.		

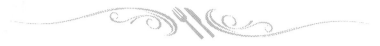

Swiss Steak

(Origin: Switzerland)

For 4 servings:
- 4 slices topside of beef, each weighing about 6 oz.
- 1½ oz flour
- 1 level teaspoon salt
- ¼ level teaspoon pepper
- 2 tbsps extra virgin olive oil
- 2 onions, finely sliced
- 2 sticks celery, chopped
- 8oz can tomatoes
- 2 level teaspoons tomato puree
- ½ teaspoon Worcestershire sauce
- ¼ pint water.

Preparation:
1. Cut steak in 8 pieces. Mix together flour, salt and pepper. Toss meat in flour mixture, pressing it in so that all the flour is used. Heat olive oil in a pan and fry meat quickly on all sides until it is brown. Transfer meat to an ovenproof casserole.
2. Add onion and celery to fat remaining in pan. Fry until pale golden brown, then add to meat with the tomatoes, tomato puree, Worcestershire sauce and water.
3. Cover casserole and cook in a very moderate oven for 2 ½ hours or until meat is tender.

Winter Beef Casserole

For 4 servings:
- 25g (1oz) butter or 2 tbsp vegetable oil
- 1 onion, chopped
- 700g (1½ lb) lean braising steak, cubed
- 25g (1oz) plain flour
- salt and pepper
- 600ml (1 pt) beef stock
- 2 bay leaves
- 2 carrots, thickly sliced

Preparation:
1. Heat the butter or oil in a flameproof casserole. Add the onion and fry for 3-4 mins.
2. Add the meat and fry until lightly browned, stirring occasionally.
3. Stir in the flour and salt and pepper. Cook, stirring for 1 min. Gradually add the stock, stirring continuously and scraping any sediment from the bottom of the casserole. Add bay leaves, bring to the boil, cover and cook over a very low heat for 1 ½ hours. If preferred, cook in oven at 170C/325F/gas 3.
4. Add the carrots to casserole stir well and cook for 1 hour.

Yoghurt-Marinated Beef

For 4 servings:
- 575g (1¼ lb) lean beef topside, cubed
- 150ml (¼ pt) natural yoghurt
- 1 tbsp fresh root ginger, grated
- ½ tsp grated nutmeg
- salt and pepper
- 15g (½ oz) butter
- 1 tbsp vegetable oil
- 50ml (2 fl oz) milk
- 1 tbsp soy sauce
- 3 tbsp crème fraiche

Preparation
1. Put meat in a bowl; add yoghurt, ginger, nutmeg, salt and pepper and mix. Cover, chill and marinate overnight.
2. Heat butter and oil in a frying pan
3. Add beef and fry for 4-5 mins, to brown. Add milk and soy sauce. Bring to boil.
4. Cover and simmer for 30 mins. Stir in crème fraiche. Simmer for 3-4 mins to heat through and serve.

POULTRY

Barbeque Chicken

For 4 servings
- 4 chicken portions or 8 drumsticks
- 1 tsp salt
- 2 tbsp soy sauce
- 2 cloves garlic, crushed
- 2-3 drops Tabasco
- 2 tsp vegetable oil

Sauce
- 2.5cm (1in) piece fresh root ginger
- 1 tbsp rapeseed oil
- 300ml (½ pt) tomato juice
- 2 tsp cornflour
- 3 tbsp red wine vinegar
- 1 tsp brown sugar

Preparation
1. Preheat oven. Rub chicken with salt. Mix together soy sauce, garlic, Tabasco and oil and brush over chicken. Put chicken pieces in a shallow ovenproof dish and bake for 30 – 50 mins.
2. Meanwhile, make sauce. Peel ginger and grate or chop finely.
3. Heat oil for sauce, add ginger and cook for 2-3 mins. Blend a little of the tomato juice with cornflour, then stir in remainder of juice. Add to pan.
4. Bring to boil, stirring continuously until thickened. Stir in vinegar and sugar.
5. Serve chicken portions with sauce poured over and accompanied by boiled rice.

Nutritional Information		
Calories	Fat	Fibre
2140 total (serves 4) 535 per serving	Low	Low
Good source of protein and omega 6.		

Bombay chicken

For 4 servings:
- 8 chicken pieces approx 100g 4oz) each
- 2 onions
- 1 large cooking apple
- 50g (2oz) butter
- 4 cloves garlic, crushed
- 1 tbsp mild curry powder
- 1 ½ tbsp salt
- black pepper
- 1 tbsp tomato purée
- 50g (2oz) desiccated coconut
- 300ml (1/2 pt) chicken stock

Preparation
1. Peel onions and apple and chop roughly.
2. Heat butter in a heavy casserole dish. Add onions and sauté for 5 mins, stirring occasionally to prevent burning.
3. Add garlic, apple, curry powder and seasoning and stir well.
4. Add chicken, tomato to puree, coconut and stock. Mix together and cover tightly. Cook over a medium heat for 30 mins. To see if chicken is cooked, pierce with a skewer and if blood runs, cook for a little longer, until juices run clear.
5. Remove chicken from casserole and keep warm. Boil sauce rapidly to reduce it by half. Return chicken to sauce and serve with pilau rice and a choice of accompaniments such as mango chutney, roasted peanuts and a yoghurt and mint sauce.

Caribbean Chicken

Origin: Caribbean

For 6 servings
- 6 chicken portions
- 1 tbsp plain flour
- 2 tsp salt
- 2 tsp mild curry powder
- 25g (1oz) butter

Sauce
- 2 onions, chopped
- 175g (6oz) streaky bacon, chopped
- 2 tbsp vegetable oil
- 2 apples, peeled and diced
- 2 tsp mild curry powder
- 2 tbsp plain flour
- 2 tbsp tomato puree
- 400ml (12fl oz) chicken stock
- 225g (8oz) can pineapple pieces in natural juice.

Preparation
1. Preheat oven. To make sauce, heat oil in a saucepan, add onion and bacon and fry for 3-4 minutes. Add apple and curry powder and cook, stirring for 1 minute.
2. Stir in tomato puree and flour. Gradually blend in the stock and bring to boil, stirring continuously.
3. Add pineapple pieces, reserving a few for garnish, together with juice. Cover and simmer for 10 minutes.
4. Meanwhile, mix together flour, salt and curry powder. Add chicken and toss to coat.

5. Heat butter in an ovenproof casserole dish, add chicken pieces and fry on both sides to brown.
6. Pour over sauce, cover and cook in oven for 30 minutes or until chicken is tender. Serve garnished with pineapple pieces.

Nutritional Information		
Calories	Fat	Fibre
3884 total (serves 6) 647 per serving	Med	Low
Good source of protein.		

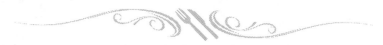

Cheesy Chicken with Mustard

For 4 servings
- 4 boneless chicken breasts
- 100g (4oz) blue cheese OR cream cheese with chives
- 200ml (7fl oz) double cream
- 1 tbsp French mustard
- 25g (1oz) butter
- Salt and pepper
- 1 tsp chopped fresh tarragon OR thyme
- Freshly ground pink peppercorns, to serve.

Preparation
1. Preheat oven. Make a deep slit in the side of each chicken breast to form a pocket. Put a piece of cheese into each pocket.
2. Put chicken into a shallow, ovenproof dish. Mix together the cream and half the mustard. Pour around base of chicken.
3. Melt butter and add seasoning, herbs and remaining mustard. Brush onto exposed chicken.
4. Bake for 40 minutes until golden. Serve, topped with pink peppercorns.

Nutritional Information		
Calories	Fat	Fibre
2400 total – serves 4 600 per serving	High	Low
Good source of protein and calcium.		

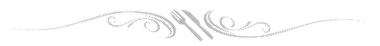

Chicken a la King

Origin: France

For 4 servings
- 1 tbsp extra virgin olive oil
- 450g (1lb) cooked chicken breast
- 1 medium onion, diced
- ½ red pepper, thinly sliced
- ½ green pepper, thinly sliced
- 100g mushrooms, sliced
- 1 packet of white sauce
- ½ pint semi-skimmed milk
- 1 glass cheap white wine
- 125mls (4fl oz) double cream
- 200g long grain white rice
- 400mls water
- salt and pepper to taste
- sprig of parsley

Preparation
1. Slice chicken into 2cm strips. Add diced onion and fry for 5 minutes.
2. Add mushrooms and peppers and fry for another 5 minutes.
3. Mix packet white sauce with semi-skimmed milk and add to mixture.
4. Add cream and wine and heat through
5. Meanwhile cook rice in water and a pinch of salt until rice has absorbed all the water.
6. Serve chicken dish on a bed of rice, topped with a sprig of parsley.

Nutritional Information		
Calories	Fat	Fibre
1633 total (serves 4) 408 per serving	Med	Low
Good source of protein and omega 3.		

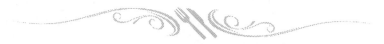

Chicken Cordon Bleu

For 4 servings
- 4 small chicken breasts, skinned and boned
- Salt and pepper
- 4 slices Mozzarella Cheese
- 4 small slices ham
- 1 egg, lightly beaten
- 6 tbsp dried wholemeal breadcrumbs
- 25g (1oz) butter
- 1 tbsp vegetable oil.

Preparation
1. Put chicken breasts between two sheets of greaseproof paper and flatten with mallet or rolling pin. Season.
2. Put a piece of cheese and a piece of ham on top of each piece of chicken, then fold chicken over to enclose filling.
3. Coat pieces first with egg then with breadcrumbs.
4. Heat butter and oil in large frying pan and fry for 5 minutes on each side or until the juices run clear and the breadcrumbs are golden.
5. Drain on absorbent paper and serve.

Nutritional Information		
Calories	Fat	Fibre
1340 total (serves 4) 335 per serving	Med	Med
Good source of calcium and omega 6.		

Chicken Curry

For 4 servings
- 1 tbsp vegetable oil
- 8 small or 4 large chicken pieces
- 25g (1oz) butter
- 1 onion, chopped
- 3 – 4 tsp mild curry powder
- 25g (1oz) plain flour
- 450ml (1/2 pint) chicken stock
- 2 tbsp chopped parsley.

Preparation
1. Heat oil in a frying pan, add the chicken pieces and fry for 4 – 5 mins each side until brown. Remove with a slotted spoon and set aside.
2. Add butter and onion to pan and fry for 5 mins, until softened. Stir in curry powder. Return chicken to pan and stir in flour.
3. Gradually add stock and bring to boil, stirring continuously. Cover and simmer for 30 mins, until chicken is tender and juices run clear. Serve garnished with parsley.

Chicken Satay

For 4 servings
- 450g (1lb) skinless chicken breast fillets, cubed.
- 2 tbsp vegetable oil
- 3 tbsp soy sauce
- 3 tbsp sherry.

Sauce
- 2 red peppers, halved, seeded and sliced.
- 300ml (1/2 pt) vegetable stock.
- 2 tbsp soy sauce
- 2 tbsp dry sherry
- 2 tbsp sugar
- 100g (4oz) peanut butter
- 25g (1oz) creamed coconut
- 1 tsp chilli powder
- 1 clove garlic, crushed
- ½ tsp cornflour, blended with 1 tbsp cold water.

Preparation
1. Thread chicken onto skewers. Mix together oil, soy sauce and sherry and brush over chicken. Cover and leave to marinate for 1 hr.
2. Put peppers and stock in a saucepan. Add soy sauce, sherry and sugar and bring to boil. Simmer for 5 mins.
3. Add peanut butter, creamed coconut, chilli and garlic. Stir in cornflour, bring to boil and simmer gently for 10 mins.
4. Meanwhile, put the chicken under a preheated grill and cook for 10 mins or until juices run clear, turning occasionally and basting with remaining marinade. Serve with peanut sauce.

Nutritional Information		
Calories	Fat	Fibre
1769 total (serves 4) 442 per serving	Med	Med
Good source of vitamins A, C, E, and omega 6.		

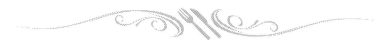

Duckling a L'Orange

Healthy Option
Origin: France

For 4 servings
- 1 oven ready duckling – 2 kilos – 1600g-2000g (L-5lbs)
- Salt and pepper to taste
- 1 large onion, peeled
- 2 oranges
- 1 level tbsp bisto
- 1 tbsp chopped parsley
- 1 small packet potato crisps
- 4 bunches of watercress.

Preparation
1. Sprinkle the duckling with salt and pepper. Cut the onion in half and put inside bird.
2. Place bird on a trivet in a roasting tin and roast in a pre heated moderately hot oven for 20 minutes per pound plus 20 minutes over.
3. Halfway through cooking time taste duckling and spoon surplus fat from roasting tin.
4. Meanwhile grate rind from the one orange, peel and cut into slices, squeeze juice from other orange.
5. Place cooked duckling on a warm serving dish, pour off rest of surplus fat.
6. Blend bisto with orange juice, stir into pan, add grated orange rind and sufficient stock from giblets to make a smooth pouring sauce.
7. Decorate with orange slices dipped in parsley, potato crisps and watercress.

Nutritional Information		
Calories	Fat	Fibre
961 total serves 4 240 per serving	High	Low

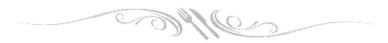

Festive Stuffed Turkey

For 8 servings
- 3kg (7lb) oven ready turkey
- 50g (2oz) butter

Stuffing
- 50g (2oz) butter
- 1 onion, finely chopped
- 175g (6oz) breadcrumbs
- 100g (4oz) "no need to soak" dried apricots, finely chopped
- 50g (2oz) walnuts, chopped
- 1 tbsp chopped fresh parsley
- Salt and pepper
- 1 tsp grated nutmeg
- 1 egg, lightly beaten

Preparation
1. Preheat oven. Remove giblets from turkey. Wash turkey and dry thoroughly.
2. To make stuffing, melt butter in a frying pan, add onion and fry for 3-4 minutes until soft. In a bowl, mix together onions, breadcrumbs, apricots, walnuts, parsley, salt and pepper, and nutmeg. Stir in egg and leave until cold.
3. Fill neck end of turkey with stuffing. Fold skin over and secure on the underside of turkey with wooden cocktail sticks.
4. Put turkey in roasting tin, melt butter and brush over turkey. Cover with greased foil and roast for 3 hours, basting occasionally. Remove foil for last 15 minutes to brown the skin.

Nutritional Information.		
Calories	Fat	Fibre
3000 total (serves 8) 375 per serving	Low	Med
Good source of protein.		

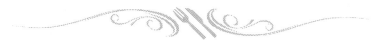

St David's Chicken

Healthy Option
Origin: Wales

For 4 servings
- 4 boneless chicken breasts, approx 100g (4oz) each.
- 100g (4oz) smoked back bacon, rinded.
- 1 large leek, trimmed
- 50g (2oz) butter.
- 2 tbsp clear honey
- 150ml (½ pint) chicken stock.
- salt and pepper
- 1 tbsp chopped fresh parsley.

Preparation
1. Wash chicken and pat dry. Dice bacon and slice leek.
2. Melt butter in a large frying pan or wok. Add chicken and bacon and fry for 10 mins, turning frequently.
3. Add leeks. Stir in honey and stock and season to taste. Reduce heat and simmer for 20 mins, or until chicken is cooked.
4. Adjust seasoning and stir in parsley.
5. Remove chicken from pan with a slotted spoon. Cut each piece diagonally into four and fan out on a serving plate. Spoon over sauce and serve.

Nutritional Information		
Calories	Fat	Fibre
1371 total (serves 4) 343 per serving	Med	Low
Good source of protein.		

Stir Fried Cabbage

For 4 Servings
- 450 (lb) green cabbage
- 1 tbsp vegetable oil
- 2 tsp salt
- 1 tbsp grated fresh root ginger
- 1 clove garlic, crushed
- 125ml (4 fl oz) chicken stock

Timing
Preparation:
5mins

Cooking:
10mins

Preparation
1. Cut cabbage into 2.5cm (1in) strips.
2. Heat vegetable oil into a large saucepan or wok and add salt, ginger and garlic.
3. Add cabbage and stir fry over a high heat for 2 mins
4. Add chicken stock, cover and cook for 5 minutes. Stir and cook for a further 3 minutes. Serve immediately.

Nutritional Information		
Calories	Fat	Fibre
231 total (serves 4) 58 per serving	Low	High

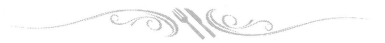

Tandoori Chicken

Origin: India

For 4 servings
- 4 chicken joints
- 1 tbsp lemon juice
- 2 tbsp tandoori mix
- 200ml (7fl oz) low fat natural yoghurt
- 2 tbsp rapeseed oil
- 225g (8oz) long grain rice
- 1 red pepper, seeded and diced
- 100g (4oz) French beans, topped and tailed
- 25g (1oz) butter

Preparation
1. Mix together lemon juice, tandoori mix, yoghurt and oil.
2. Make cuts in the chicken, almost to the bone. Coat with marinade, cover and chill for at least 2 hours.
3. Preheat oven. Put chicken in a shallow baking tin and cook for 30-40 minutes
4. Meanwhile, boil rice for 10-12 minutes. Add peppers and cook for further 5 minutes.
5. Cook beans until tender. Melt butter in a frying pan and sauté beans for 2-3 minutes. Serve chicken and beans on bed of rice.

Nutritional Information		
Calories	Fat	Fibre
23000 total (serves 4) 575 per serving	Low	Low
Good source of Omega 6.		

PORK

Apple and Sage Roast Pork

Origin: England

For 6 servings
- 2kg (4 ½ lb) pork loin, boned
- 300ml (½ pt) cider
- salt, for sprinkling

Stuffing
- 25g (1oz) butter
- 1 onion, chopped
- 1 Bramley apple, peeled, cored and diced
- 50g (2oz) Wensleydale cheese, grated
- 50g (2oz) fresh breadcrumbs
- 1 tbsp fresh chopped sage
- finely grated rind of ½ orange
- salt and pepper
- 1 egg, beaten

Preparation
1. Melt butter in a frying pan and fry onion and apple for 10 minutes, until softened. Remove from heat.
2. Stir in cheese, breadcrumbs, sage, orange rind, seasoning and egg. Mix until well blended.
3. Preheat oven. Unroll meat and spread with stuffing. Re-roll and secure with string
4. Put meat rind side down in a casserole dish. Pour over the cider and roast, uncovered, for 15 minutes.
5. Turn joint over so that rind is on top. Sprinkle with plenty of salt. Roast for a further 30 minutes. Reduce oven temperature to 180C/350F/gas 4 and continue cooking for 2 hours.

6. Transfer meat to a serving plate and keep warm. Bring meat juices to the boil and boil rapidly until reduced by half. Pour into gravy boat and serve with meat.

Nutritional Information		
Calories	Fat	Fibre
4710 total (serves 6) 785 per serving	Med	Low
Good source of protein.		

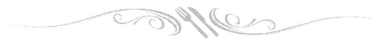

Baked gammon with cloves

Origin: England

For 10 servings
- 3.5kg (8lb) gammon joint
- 2 tbsp French mustard
- 3 tbsp Demarara sugar
- about 24 cloves

Preparation
1. Soak the gammon overnight in cold water. Drain and pat dry with kitchen paper.
2. Wrap joint in a large sheet of kitchen foil, making sure join is on top. Put in a roasting tin and bake for 2½ hours.
3. Increase oven temperature to 220°C/425F/gas 7. Open up foil, taking care not to let the meat juices escape. With a sharp knife, cut rind from joint, leaving behind a layer of fat.
4. Score the fat in a criss-cross pattern. Spread mustard onto the fat, making sure it is evenly coated.
5. Sprinkle sugar over gammon and press down firmly. Push in cloves.
6. Return gammon to oven, uncovered, and cook for a further 15-20 minutes, until golden. Remove joint from oven, leave in foil and allow to cool.

Nutritional Information		
Calories	Fat	Fibre
8479 total (serves 10) 848 per serving	Med	Low
Good source of protein.		

Bavarian Pork chops

Origin: Germany

For 4 servings
- 2 tbsp rapeseed oil
- 1 large onion, chopped
- 100g (4oz) button mushrooms, sliced
- 1 clove garlic, crushed
- 4 tomatoes, chopped
- 2 tbsp fresh parsley
- 150ml (¼ pt) white wine
- 1 tsp dried basil
- 1 tbsp fresh chopped coriander
- 1 tsp cornflour, blended with 1 tsp water
- salt and pepper
- 4 boneless pork chops, trimmed
- sprigs of parsley to garnish (optional)

Preparation
1. Heat half the oil in a saucepan and sauté onion for 5 minutes. Add mushrooms and garlic and sauté for 5 minutes. Stir in tomatoes and parsley and cook for 1 minute.
2. Add wine, basil, coriander, cornflour and seasoning. Bring to boil, stirring. Cover and simmer for 15 minutes.
3. Meanwhile heat remaining oil in a frying pan and fry pork chops on both sides for 15 minutes, until tender. Using a slotted spoon, transfer chops to serving plate. Spoon over sauce and garnish with sprigs of parsley.

Nutritional Information		
Calories	Fat	Fibre
2027 total (serves 4) 506 per serving	Med	Low
Good source of omega 6.		

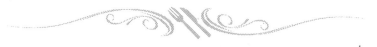

Celebration Pork

(Origin: England)

For 4-6 servings:
- 4 ½ lb, loin of pork with skin
- cooking oil
- salt
- 8 eating apples
- 6oz, granulated sugar
- 1 pint water
- pink food colouring
- few sprigs parsley

Oven setting
350°F/Gas mark 4

Preparation:
1. Have the loin of pork chinned and the skin scored. Put the joint in a roasting tin with the skin side upwards. Brush and sprinkle with salt. Roast in a moderate oven for approximately 2 hours.
2. Meanwhile prepare the sugared apples for decoration. Peel and core the apples. Dissolve the sugar in the water over a gentle heat, and then bring to boil. Add 1 teaspoon pink food colouring. Poach apples gently in the syrup until tender and well coloured (about 20 minutes). Remove on to a plate.
3. Boil syrup rapidly to reduce, and pour over the apples. Serve joint surrounded with sugared apples and decorate with parsley.

Citrus Pork Chops

For 4 servings:
- 4 pork chops
- 1 tomato, chopped
- 1 orange, peeled and diced
- 1 spring onion, finely chopped
- 3 tbsp chopped parsley
- salt and pepper
- 1 tbsp lime juice

Marinade:
- 2 tbsp olive
- 2 tbsp lime juice
- grated rind ½ lime
- ½ tsp cayenne pepper

Preparation
1. Combine marinade ingredients. Put pork chops in a shallow dish and coat with marinade. Cover and leave overnight to marinate.
2. Heat a heavy-based frying pan, add pork chops and marinade. Cook over medium heat for 20-25 mins, turning often
3. Remove chops with a slotted spoon and keep warm. Meanwhile, mix together remaining ingredients.
4. Add 2 tbsp of water to pan, scraping any residue from base and stirring into liquid.
5. Add orange mixture and bring to boil. Simmer for a few mins to heat through and serve spooned over pork chops.

Country Pork Casserole

For 4 servings:
- 450g (1lb) pork fillet
- 1 onion
- 2 carrots
- 50g (2oz) butter
- 1 clove garlic, chopped
- 2 tbsp tomato puree
- 300ml (½ pt) vegetable stock
- 100g (4oz) button mushrooms
- salt and pepper
- 1 tbsp fresh chopped dill
- 125ml (¼ pt) whipping cream

Preparation
1. Cut pork into cubes, chop onion and turnip and slice carrots.
2. Melt butter in a large flameproof casserole. Add onion, turnip and carrot and sauté for 4-5 mins. Add meat and sauté until brown.
3. Add garlic, tomato purée, stock and mushrooms. Bring to boil, cover and simmer for 30 mins.
4. Season to taste. Stir in dill and cream and gently heat through before serving.

Crispy Roast Pork

For 4 servings:
- 700g (1½ lb) belly pork
- 1 tsp salt
- 1 tbsp freshly ground black pepper
- 3 tbsp soy sauce
- 1 tbsp grated fresh root ginger
- 1 tbsp chopped fresh rosemary
- 200ml (7fl oz) water

Preparation
1. Preheat oven. Remove skin from pork and score fat. Rub with salt and pepper, and then brush with soy sauce.
2. Sprinkle with ginger and rosemary. Put in an ovenproof dish and pour water into base.
3. Cook for 1 ¼ hours or until juices run clear.
4. Leave to stand for 10 mins, loosely covered with aluminium foil. Slice and serve.

Crispy-coated Pork with Onions

For 4 servings:
- 4 large boneless pork chops
- 60g (2½ oz) dried wholemeal breadcrumbs
- salt and pepper
- 2 tbsp ground cumin
- 1 tbsp paprika
- 1 egg, lightly beaten
- 2 tbsp vegetable oil

Sauce
- 25g (1oz) butter
- 2 onions, chopped
- 3 cloves garlic, crushed
- 1 tbsp plain flour
- 150ml (¼ pt) milk
- 150ml (¼ pt) single cream
- 2 tbsp grated Parmesan cheese

Preparation
1. Trim chops to remove any excess fat. Mix together bread-crumbs, seasoning, cumin and paprika and put in a shallow dish.
2. Coat chops first in beaten egg and then in crumb mix.
3. Heat oil in a frying pan and fry chops for 5-6 mins per side, or until juices run clear and breadcrumbs are golden. Keep warm.
4. Meanwhile, make sauce. Heat butter in saucepan, add onions and garlic and cook for 5 mins until softened.
5. Add flour to onions and stir well. Gradually add milk and cream and bring to boil, stirring continuously until thick. Stir in cheese. Serve chops on a bed of onion sauce.

Crunchy Stuffed Pork

(Origin: England)

For 4 – 6 servings:
- 3lb joint belly pork with skin
- 4oz soft white breadcrumbs
- 1 onion, peeled and grated
- 1 lemon rind, grated
- 1 stick celery, washed and chopped
- ½ teaspoon nutmeg
- 1oz walnuts, chopped
- 2oz seedless raisins
- 1 egg
- 1oz butter, melted
- salt and pepper
- olive oil

Preparation
1. Score the pork skin and remove the bones from the joint.
2. To make the stuffing, mix together remaining ingredients except olive oil and season to taste. Flatten the meat, skin side down and spread with the stuffing. Roll and secure with a little olive oil and sprinkle liberally with salt. Roast for 30 minutes to the pound and 30 minutes over in a moderately hot oven.
3. Serve with apple sauce, buttered carrots and sprouts.

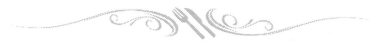

Curried Pork with Pineapple

Origin: China

For 4 servings
- 450g (1lb) pork tenderloin, trimmed of fat
- 1 large leek, trimmed and sliced
- 25g (1oz) butter
- 1½ tbsp flour
- 1½ tbsp curry powder
- 300ml (½ pint) vegetable stock
- 220g (8oz) can pineapple rings

Preparation
1. Cut pork into thin strips approximately 5cm (2in) long. Melt butter in a saucepan and add pork and leeks. Stir-fry for 10 minutes, until pork is browned.
2. Stir in flour and curry powder. Cook, stirring for 1 minute. Stir in stock. Cover and cook for 20 minutes, or until pork is cooked.
3. Drain pineapple rings and reserve juice. Cut pineapple into chunks and add to pan with 3 tbsp juice. Heat gently to warm through.

Nutritional Information		
Calories	Fat	Fibre
945 total (serves 4) 236 per serving	Low	Low
Good source of protein.		

Harvest Home Casserole

For servings
- 2 onions
- 2 tbsp extra virgin oil
- 1 lb baby marrows
- 3 mushrooms, peeled and sliced
- 1 lb belly pork, diced
- garlic salt
- salt and pepper to taste
- 1 tbsp tomato puree
- ½ pint chicken stock, made up with ½ chicken stock cube

Preparation (Time 5 mins):
1. Peel and slice the onions
2. Melt the lard and fry them in a saucepan for 5 mins
3. Keep the saucepan covered so onions remain soft
4. Remove stalks and seeds from the peppers and chop
5. Wash and cut up unskinned marrow into small pieces and add these with the mushrooms and pork to the saucepan
6. Stir well and season to taste
7. Mix the tomato puree with the stock and add to the saucepan
8. Cover the lid and simmer gently for 1 hour
9. This dish can be cooked slowly in the oven

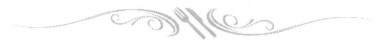

Italian Pork chops

Origin: Italy
Healthy Option

For 4 servings
- 4 pork chops
- Salt and pepper
- 1 tsp dried oregano
- 1 tsp dried marjoram
- 25g (1oz) butter
- 400g (14oz) can tomatoes
- 1 tbsp tomato puree
- Grated rind and juice 1 lemon
- 1 clove garlic, crushed
- Chopped parsley to garnish

Preparation
1. Sprinkle both sides of chops with salt, pepper, oregano and marjoram. Melt butter in a frying pan, add the chops and cook for 4-5 minutes each side, to brown.
2. Add the tomatoes, tomato puree, lemon juice and garlic
3. Bring to boil, cover and simmer for 10-15 mins.
4. Serve topped with lemon rind and parsley.

Nutritional Information		
Calories	Fat	Fibre
1232 total (serves 4) 308 per serving	Low	Low
Good source of protein, and potassium.		

March Pork Casserole

(Origin: England)

For 4 servings:
- 1 small sweet green pepper
- 2 oz bacon dripping
- 1 onion, peeled and chopped
- 1 leek, washed and chopped
- 2oz button mushrooms
- 1 teaspoon curry powder
- ½ teaspoon salt
- ½ teaspoon pepper
- 1oz flour
- 1 ½ lb hand or shoulder pork, diced
- 1 8oz can tomatoes
- Pinch mixed sweet herbs.

Oven setting
335°F/gas mark 3

Preparation:
1. Remove stalk and seeds from the pepper and chop it. Melt the fat and fry the onion, leek, pepper and mushrooms for 3 minutes. Transfer to a casserole.
2. Add the curry powder, salt and pepper to the flour, and then toss the pork in this mixture. Fry the coated pork for 5 minutes, stirring well, then put into the casserole with the vegetables, tomatoes and herbs.
3. Cover tightly and cook for 1 ¾ hours in a very moderate oven. Serve with jacket potatoes.

Mustard Baked Pork

Origin: France

For 4 servings:
- 675g (1 1/2lb) piece of cooked pork loin roast
- 40g (1 1/2oz) butter
- 40g (1½ oz) flour
- 300ml (½pt) milk
- 2 tbsp Dijon mustard
- salt and pepper
- 75g (3oz) dried wholemeal breadcrumbs
- 1 ½ tbsp soft light brown sugar

Red wine sauce:
- 25g (1oz) butter
- 75ml (3fl oz) vegetable stock
- 2 tbsp soft light brown sugar
- 200ml (7fl oz) red wine

Preparation
1. Preheat oven. Slice pork and put in shallow ovenproof dish.
2. Melt butter in a saucepan; add flour and cook, stirring for 1 minute. Remove from heat and stir in milk and mustard. Return to heat and bring to boil.
3. Mix together breadcrumbs and brown sugar and sprinkle on top of sauce. Bake for 30 minutes.
4. To make the red wine sauce, melt butter in a saucepan, add stock, sugar and red wine and bring to boil. Serve separately.

Nutritional Information		
Calories	Fat	Fibre
2169 total (serves 4) 542 per serving	Med	Low
Good source of protein.		

Old English Pork Casserole

(Origin: England)

For 4 servings
- 6oz leeks
- ¼ pt olive oil
- 1¼ lb shoulder of pork
- 2 oz seasoned flour
- ½ pt brown ale
- dash Tabasco Sauce
- piece lemon peel
- 3oz button mushrooms
- bouquet garni
- salt and pepper to taste

Preparation
1. Clean and chop the leeks. Heat the olive oil in a flameproof casserole. Fry the leeks for a few minutes.
2. Meanwhile, cut the pork into 1 inch squares and toss in the seasoned flour. Add this to the leeks and cook for 5 minutes. Add the ale, Tabasco sauce, lemon peel, mushrooms and bouquet garni. Bring to the boil. Put lid on and reduce heat. Simmer for 1 ¼ hours. Remove bouquet garni.
3. Season to taste. Serve with mashed potatoes and buttered carrots.

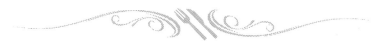

Orchard Pork Casserole

Origin: England

For 4 servings
- 450g (1lb) lean pork
- 350g (12oz) potatoes
- 1 tbsp rapeseed oil
- 1 clove garlic, crushed
- 1 onion, chopped
- 25g (1oz) flour
- 300ml (½ pt) cider
- 2 tbsp chopped fresh parsley
- salt and pepper
- 50g (2oz) no-need-to-soak dried apricots, sliced
- 2 dessert apples, peeled, cored and sliced

Preparation
1. Preheat oven. Cut pork into 2.5cm (1in) cubes. Peel potatoes and cut into small dice. Heat oil in frying pan, add pork, potatoes, garlic and onion and sauté for 7 minutes.
2. Stir in the flour. Add cider, parsley and seasoning. Cook, stirring until thickened.
3. Layer pork mixture and apricots in four individual ovenproof dishes or one large ovenproof dish.
4. Arrange the apple slices on top. Cover and cook for 1 ½ hours. Remove covering and cook for a further 15 minutes, until apples are golden. Serve.

Nutritional Information		
Calories	Fat	Fibre
1412 total (serves 4) 353 per serving	Low	Med
Good source of protein, omega 6.		

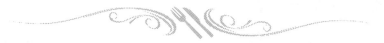

Oriental Honeyed Pork

Healthy Option
Origin: China

4 serving:
- 300g (¾ lb) pork fillet
- 2 level tsp seasoned corn flour
- 6 tbsp extra virgin oil
- 1 clove garlic, crushed
- 1 medium sweet green pepper
- 200g (8oz) canned pineapple chunks
- 3 mushrooms; peeled and sliced
- 2 ripe tomatoes, quartered

For the sauce
- 1 tsp soy sauce
- 1 chicken stock cube
- 2 tbsp honey

Preparation
1. Cut the pork in 1 inch (2cm) cubes and toss in the seasoned cornflour. Remove stalk and seeds from pepper and chop. Drain pineapple chunks, reserving juice.
2. Heat garlic in the oil, fry pork cubes briskly until brown on all sides. Lower heat, add chopped pepper and cook over a gentle heat for 10 minutes, adding pineapple chunks, mushrooms and tomatoes for last 4 minutes. Transfer to a warm serving dish.
3. Meanwhile, make sauce by dissolving chicken stock cube in a ¼ pint boiling water, mix with honey and soy sauce.
4. Blend rest of corn flour with a little pineapple juice, add to mixture. Bring to boil, cook for 3 minutes, stirring all the

time. Pour over the meat in the serving dish and serve with boiled rice.

Nutritional Information		
Calories	Fat	Fibre
2,000 total (serves 4) 500 per serving	Med	Low
Good source of protein, Omega 3.		

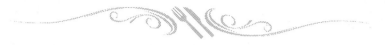

Pan Fried Pork

(Origin: England)

For 4 servings:
- 1lb shoulder or belly pork, thinly sliced
- 1 egg, beaten and seasoned with salt and pepper
- 1 packet sage and onion stuffing or 4oz medium oatmeal
- ½ pt olive oil
- ¾ lb potatoes, boiled
- 1 large onion
- 1 heaped tablespoon chopped parsley.

Preparation:
1. Flatten the slices of pork with a rolling pin and cut into portions. Dip each slice into the seasoned beaten egg and toss in the dry stuffing or oatmeal. Fry in a little hot olive oil on both sides until brown and tender (about 15 minutes). Place in a hot serving dish.
2. Meanwhile, cut the potatoes into ½– inch dice. Peel and chop the onion finely. Pour in rest of olive oil and cook onions gently until just brown but not crisp. Stir in potatoes, increase heat and cook, stirring occasionally, until potatoes are brown. Sprinkle over the meat.
3. Decorate with parsley and serve with a green vegetable.

Pork and Tomato Casserole

Origin: Italy

For 4 servings
- 2 tbsp rapeseed oil
- 675g (1 ½ lb) lean pork, cubed
- 12 button onions
- salt and pepper
- 1 tbsp paprika
- 150ml (½ pint) passata OR sieved tomatoes
- 150ml (¼ pint) dry white wine
- 1 clove garlic, crushed
- 6 tomatoes, skinned
- 75g (3oz) blanched almonds

Preparation
1. Heat oil in a saucepan and sauté pork and onions for 10 minutes, until browned on all sides. Stir in seasoning and paprika and cook, stirring for 2 minutes.
2. Gradually stir in sieved tomatoes, wine and garlic. Bring to boil, cover and simmer for 30 minutes.
3. Meanwhile heat a non-stick frying pan and dry fry almonds for 5 minutes, until browned on both sides. Stir into casserole with whole tomatoes and cook for a further 10 minutes. Remove from heat and serve.

Nutritional Information		
Calories	Fat	Fibre
1693 total (serves 4) 423 per serving	Low	Low
Good source of protein, omega 6.		

Pork Barbeque Style

For 4 servings:
- 4 pork chops
- ½ level teaspoon each salt and pepper
- ½ level teaspoon castor sugar
- ½ level teaspoon ground ginger
- 1oz butter.

For the barbeque sauce:
- ½ - 1 tablespoon chilli sauce
- 1 tablespoon mushroom ketchup
- I tablespoon Worcestershire sauce
- 2 level teaspoons castor sugar
- 2 tablespoons vinegar
- 2 tablespoons tomato ketchup
- 1 teaspoon soy sauce
- 2 cloves garlic, crushed
- 2 bay leaves

Preparation
1. Trim pork chops carefully. Mix together salt, pepper, sugar and ginger and rub over chops. Heat the butter in a heavy meat tin and add the chops. Brown in a moderately hot oven, turning chops once to brown on both sides.
2. Meanwhile, mix together thoroughly all the ingredients for the barbeque sauce.
3. When chops are brown pour off all the fat from baking tin, pour sauce over and cover with a lid of foil. Bake for 20 to 30 minutes, basting occasionally, until tender. Then arrange on a serving dish and spoon sauce over. Decorate with parsley.

Pork Chops with Cider

(Origin: England)

You will need
- 4 pork loin chops
- 1 oz. butter
- 1 large onion, chopped
- 1 large cooking apple, peeled, cored and chopped
- ½ pint cider
- salt and pepper
- ¼ pint double dairy cream

For the garnish:
- parsley sprigs

Preparation
1. Fry chops in butter on both sides for 5 minutes. Remove and place in a casserole.
2. Fry onion and apple together for 5 minutes and add to chops. Pour over cider and season with salt and pepper. Cover and bake in a moderate oven for 45 minutes or until the chops are tender.
3. Spoon over the cream and garnish with parsley sprigs.

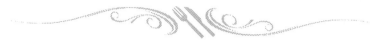

Pork in a Blanket

(Origin: England)

For 4 servings:
- ¾ lb pork fillet, cut in ½ inch slices
- 2 red-skinned eating apples
- 1 large onion, peeled
- 2 oz. butter or margarine
- 1 oz flour
- 1 chicken stock cube
- ¼ pint milk
- salt and pepper to taste
- 1 packet instant potato (serves 4)

Preparation
1. Peel, core and chop one apple. Chop the onion finely. Melt the butter in a frying pan, place sliced pork in the centre and chopped onion round the edge. Cook very gently, covered, for 5 minutes. Turn pork slices, stir onions and add chopped apple. Cover and cook for another 5 minutes. Remove pork to warm serving dish.
2. Stir flour into pan, cook for 2 minutes. Dissolve chicken stock cube in ¼ pint boiling water, add to pan with the milk. Cook until smooth and thick, stirring gently. Taste and correct seasoning. Pour sauce over pork.
3. Make up mashed potato, according to directions on packet. Pipe or spread round serving dish, slide under grill for 2 minutes to brown. Meanwhile core and slice remaining apple. Use to decorate.

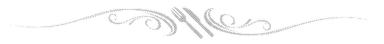

Pork in Mushroom Sauce

(Origin: England)

For 4 servings:
- 4 pieces pork fillet
- 1 oz flour
- salt and pepper
- 2 oz butter
- 4 oz button mushrooms thinly sliced
- 1x16oz can carrots
- ¼ pint double dairy cream
- 1 tablespoon chopped olives

Preparation
1. Bat out pork fillet until thin and coat in flour, seasoned with salt and pepper. Fry in butter for about 5 minutes on each side or until cooked. Place on serving dish and keep warm.
2. Add mushrooms to butter in pan and fry for 3-4 minutes or until cooked. Stir in any remaining flour and cook for a minute. Drain carrots and diced.
3. Remove from heat and stir in cream and a third of the carrots. Reheat very gently until piping hot. *Do not allow to boil.* Season to taste and pour over pork. Garnish with piles of remaining heated carrots, sprinkled with chives.

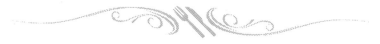

Pork Parcels

(Origin: England)

For 4 servings:
- 4oz long-grain rice
- 1 5oz packet frozen sweetcorn
- 1 5oz packet frozen peas
- 4 spring onions
- salt and pepper to taste
- 4 pork chops
- 1 tablespoon soy sauce
- 4 tablespoons cider

Oven setting
350°F/Gas mark 4

Preparation:
1. Cook the rice, put into a basin. Meanwhile cook the sweetcorn and peas in boiling salted water for 2 minutes. Clean and chop the onions, add to the rice and mix well together. Season to taste.
2. Cut 4 large squares of aluminium foil and put a chop on to each piece. Sprinkle well with soy sauce. Put one quarter of the mixture on top of each chop. Add a spoonful of cider.
3. Wrap into a parcel and place on a tin. Bake in a moderate oven for about 40 minutes. Serve direct from the foil on the serving plate.

Pork Tandoori

(Origin: India)

For 4 servings:
- 4 pork chops
- 8oz Patna rice
- ¼ teaspoon powdered saffron

For the marinade:
- 2 5oz.cartons natural yoghurt
- ½ teaspoons ground ginger
- ¾ teaspoon paprika pepper
- ¼ teaspoon garlic powder or 1 clove garlic, finely crushed
- 4 bay leaves
- 6 peppercorns
- 1 tablespoon tomato puree
- grated zest of 1 lemon
- 1 teaspoon salt

Preparation:
1. Prick pork chops well with a fork or skewer and place in a casserole dish. Place ingredients for marinade in a bowl or jug and mix well. Pour over pork chops making sure that they are all covered with the marinade.
2. Cover dish with foil or lid and leave for 6-8 hours. At the end of the time remove bay leaves and peppercorns. Remove lid from casserole dish and baste pork. Re-cover and bake in a moderate oven for about 1 ½ hours, basting occasionally until all the marinade is used. 15-20 minutes before the end of cooking time, cook rice in boiling salted water with the saffron.
3. Drain rice and place on a round serving dish. Top with the chops and serve. Peas can be added to the rice if liked.

Pork with Almonds

For 4 servings:
- 675g (1½ lb) lean pork
- 1 tbsp seasoned flour
- 2 onions
- 4 sticks celery
- 2 tbsp vegetable oil
- 2.5cm (1 in) piece fresh root ginger, grated
- 2 tbsp soy sauce
- salt and pepper
- 300ml (½ pint) vegetable stock
- 25g (1oz) butter
- 100g (4oz) whole blanched almonds

Preparation
1. Cut pork into even-sized cubes and toss in the seasoned flour.
2. Slice onion and celery.
3. Heat the oil in a flame-proof casserole, add the pork and fry until browned.
4. Add the onion, celery and ginger and cook for 4-5 mins. Stir in the soy sauce, seasoning and vegetable stock.
5. Bring to the boil, cover and simmer for 20 mins.
6. Meanwhile, melt the butter in a frying pan, add the almonds and fry until golden. Serve pork topped with almonds.

Pork with Mushroom Sauce

For 4 servings
- 575g (1 ¼ lb) pork fillet
- 2 tbsp Parmesan Cheese
- Salt and pepper
- 40g (1 ½ oz) dried breadcrumbs
- 1 egg, lightly beaten
- 25g (1oz) butter
- 1 tbsp oil

Sauce
- 25g (1oz) butter
- 200g (7oz) button mushrooms, sliced
- 125ml (4 fl oz) dry white wine
- 1 egg yolk
- Salt and pepper to taste
- 150ml (5fl oz) double cream

Preparation
1. Cut pork fillet into 8 slices. Mix together cheese, seasoning and breadcrumbs.
2. Dip pieces of pork in beaten egg and then coat with breadcrumb mix.
3. Melt butter and oil in a large frying pan. Add pork slices and fry for 5-6 mins per side until meat is cooked and breadcrumbs golden. Put to one side and keep warm.
4. To make sauce, melt butter in a saucepan, add mushrooms and sauté for 2-3 mins. Add wine and simmer for 5 mins.

5. Mix egg yolk, seasoning and cream together. Stir into sauce and heat gently, stirring until slightly thickened. Do not boil.
6. Serve two pieces of pork per person with a little of the mushroom sauce at the side.

Nutritional Information		
Calories	Fat	Fibre
2108 (serves 4) 527 per serving	High	Low

Provencal Roast Pork

For 4 servings:
- 1kg (2lb) pork loin roast
- 50g (2oz) butter
- 1 small onion, finely chopped
- 1 clove garlic, crushed
- 1 tbsp chopped fresh parsley
- 1 tbsp chopped fresh sage
- salt and pepper

Preparation
1. Using a sharp knife, cut between the meat and fat to remove the hard rind and leave a thin layer of fat. Put joint in a roasting tin and score fat in a criss-cross pattern.
2. Soften the butter and add onion, garlic, parsley, sage and salt and pepper. Mix well to combine.
3. Spread herb butter over scored surface.
4. Roast for 1½ hours, basting occasionally to keep meat moist. Allow to stand for 10 mins before carving.

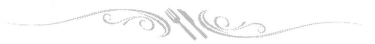

Spare Rib Chops with Almonds

(Origin: England)

For 4 servings:
- 1 tablespoon mustard
- 1 tablespoon brown sugar
- 4 spare rib pork chops
- 1 oz. almonds, shredded
- salt and pepper
- 1 12oz packet frozen chips
- cooking oil for frying

Preparation
1. Mix the mustard and sugar together and rub over the chops. Grill on both sides until tender, about 12 minutes altogether. Sprinkle almonds over the chops and season with salt and pepper.
2. Return the chops to the grill to brown the almonds. Meanwhile, fry the frozen chips in the cooking oil.
3. When cooked, let the chips drain on crumpled kitchen paper. Place the chops on a serving dish surrounded by the chips and serve with a green vegetable.

Suffolk Roast Pork

For 4 servings:
- 900g (2lb) boneless rolled loin of pork

Stuffing
- 1 small onion, finely chopped
- 15g (½ oz) butter OR margarine
- 50g (2oz) fresh white breadcrumbs
- finely grated rind and chopped flesh of 1 large orange
- 25g (1oz) raisins
- 1 tbsp chopped fresh sage
- salt and pepper
- 1 egg, beaten

Preparation
1. Preheat oven. To prepare stuffing, fry onion in butter for 5-6 mins. Stir in breadcrumbs, orange rind and flesh, raisins, sage and seasoning.
2. Add enough beaten egg to blind the mixture.
3. Spread onto pork and tie joint with string.
4. Roast joint for 1 ½ hrs until tender.
5. Remove string and carve.

Thai Pork

For 4 servings:
- 1 tbsp vegetable oil
- 675g (1½ lb) belly pork slices, cut into chunks
- 2 onions, chopped
- 2 tbsp soy sauce
- 4 tbsp hoisin sauce
- salt and pepper
- 2 tbsp ground cinnamon
- 1 tbsp anchovy essence
- 2 tbsp cornflour
- 1 leek, cut into matchstick sized strips

Preparation
1. Heat oil in a frying pan and fry the pork for 4-5 mins to brown.
2. Add the onions, soy sauce, hoisin sauce, seasoning, cinnamon, anchovy essence and 300ml (½ pt) water.
3. Bring to boil, cover and simmer for 1 hr or until pork is tender.
4. Mix the cornflour with 2 tbsp water and stir into the pan.
5. Add the leeks and simmer for 2-3 mins.
6. Adjust seasoning and serve.

LAMB

Curried Lamb

(Origin: India)

For 4 servings:
- 1½lb lamb, cooked
- 1 tablespoon oil
- 1 onion
- 1 apple
- 2 tablespoons coconut, sweetened
- 1 dessertspoon curry powder
- 1 tablespoon flour
- ½ lb tomatoes
- salt and pepper to taste
- 8oz rice.

Preparation:
1. Peel onion and chop. Peel core and chop apple. Skin, seed and chop tomatoes. Chop lamb in small dice and fry quickly in heated oil. Remove from pan. Fry onion and apple until softened; stir in curry powder and flour, mixing well. Cook for several minutes.
2. Meanwhile pour ½ pint boiling water over coconut and stir well. Strain liquid onto onion and apple mixture gradually, stirring until blended. Return meat to pan with tomatoes and seasoning, cover and simmer for 25 minutes. Sprinkle the rice into a saucepan of fast boiling water- ½ teaspoon salt and ½ pint water to each ounce of rice. After 12 minutes test a grain and when tender strain and put on a serving dish in the oven to dry out.
3. Serve curry on the rice on one dish or in individual portions. Fried poppadums or chapattis may be served as an accompaniment.

Fricassee of Lamb

(Origin: France)

For 4 servings:
- 1½ lamb (leg or shoulder), diced
- 1oz seasoned flour
- 1oz butter
- 1 large carrot, peeled and sliced
- 1 large onion, peeled and sliced
- 1 4¾ can button mushrooms
- salt and pepper to taste
- 1 bay leaf
- good pinch rosemary
- 1 tablespoon cream
- 1 tablespoon chopped parsley

Preparation:
1. Coat diced meat with seasoned flour. Fry onion and carrot gently in the butter for two minutes without allowing to brown. Add the meat; turn in the hot fat to seal. Sprinkle in rest of flour, stir well, turn into an ovenproof casserole and add sufficient water to cover. Add the bay leaf and rosemary. Cover.
2. Cook in a moderate oven for 1½ hours, adding mushrooms for the last 15 minutes of cooking time. Taste and correct seasoning if necessary.
3. Remove lid, stir in cream, sprinkle with parsley and serve at once.

Oven setting:
350°F/Gas Mark 4

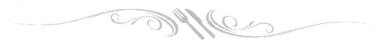

Honey Glazed Lamb

(Origin: England)

For 4-6 servings:
- 1 small leg or shoulder of lamb
- sprig of rosemary or bay leaf
- pinch ground cinnamon
- seasoned flour
- 1 carrot, peeled and sliced
- 1 onion, peeled and chopped
- 1 stick celery, washed and chopped
- 1 tablespoon thick honey
- 4 fresh pears
- 2 oz glace cherries
- few sprigs watercress

Oven setting
350°F/Gas Mark 4

Preparation:
1. Rub the meat all over with a mixture of cinnamon and seasoned flour. Place the prepared vegetables in the bottom of a roasting tin, with the rosemary or bay leaf. Place the meat on top. Bake in a moderate oven allowing 25 minutes per pound plus 25 minutes over. After one hour, turn the joint and baste well.
2. Half an hour before serving, lift out the meat and drain all fat from roasting tin. Replace meat, best side up, and spread with honey, add peeled and cored pear halves. Return to the oven and continue cooking, basting meat and pears once or twice.
3. Serve meat, surrounded with pears and watercress. Place 2 cherries in each pear half.

Honey Roast Lamb

Origin: England

For 6 servings
- 2kg (4.5lb) lean leg of lamb
- 1 large clove garlic crushed
- 4 tbsp liquid honey
- 1½ tsp dry mustard
- Salt and pepper
- 10-12 small sprigs fresh rosemary

Preparation
1. Preheat oven. If preferred trim lamb of excess fat.
2. Mix together garlic, honey and dry mustard. Spread half over lamb with a spatula or palette knife. Season.
3. With a sharp pointed knife or pair of small scissors, make 10-12 cuts into the joint. Push a sprig of rosemary into each slit.
4. Put in roasting tin and roast for 30 minutes.
5. Spread lamb with remaining honey mixture and roast for a further 30 minutes.
6. Cover joint with a piece of tinfoil and continue roasting for a further 50-80 minutes, depending on whether meat is to be served medium or well done.
7. Leave to rest for ten minutes before serving.

Nutritional Information		
Calories	Fat	Fibre
3800 total (serves 6) 633 per serving		
Good source of protein.		

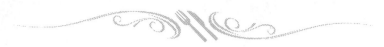

Hungarian lamb

(Origin: Hungary)

For 4 servings:
- 1 oz extra virgin olive oil;
- 2lb middle neck of lamb, cut into joints
- 1 onion, chopped
- 1 clove garlic, crushed
- 2 level tablespoons paprika pepper
- 15 oz can tomatoes
- bay leaf
- salt and pepper
- ½ level teaspoon sugar
- 1lb potatoes
- 1 tablespoon chopped parsley.

Oven setting:
335°F/Gas Mark 3

Preparation:
1. Heat the olive oil in a pan and brown pieces of lamb on both sides for about 5 minutes. Remove meat from the pan and put in an ovenproof casserole. Fry onion in fat remaining in the pan, until soft, add garlic, paprika and continue to cook for a further minute. Add tomatoes and juice, bay leaf, salt, pepper and sugar. Bring the mixture to the boil, and pour over the meat.
2. Cover casserole and cook for 1 hour in a very moderate oven, then remove from the oven. Allow the fat to settle, then skim it off.
3. Peel the potatoes and cut in ¾ inch cubes; place on top of contents of the casserole, put on the lid and cook for a further four, removing lid for the last half hour. Scatter chopped parsley over potatoes.

Irish Stew

Serves 4.

Ingredients
- 1lb potatoes
- 3 large carrots sliced
- 2 onions chopped
- ½ pint water
- ½ pint Guinness
- 1 lamb stock cube
- 1lb neck of lamb
- 1 tbsp extra virgin olive oil

Method
1. Dice lamb into 1cm cubes
2. Slice carrots and chop onions
3. Peel and slice potatoes
4. Fry lamb in a large pot for 2 minutes on all sides.
5. Add onions, carrots and potatoes
6. Half fill with a pint of lamb stock and Guinness
7. Simmer for 1 ½ - 2 hours stirring occasionally until vegetables are softened and meat is tender and serve.

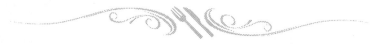

Lamb and Leek Casserole

(Origin: Wales)

For 4 servings:
- 8 lamb cutlets
- 2 tbsps extra virgin olive oil
- 2 leeks, washed and sliced
- 1 onion, peeled and sliced
- 1 turnip, peeled and diced
- ½ lb new carrots, scraped
- 1 pint stock or water
- salt and pepper to taste
- 2 sprigs mint
- 4oz shelled peas or 1 4 oz packet frozen peas.

Oven setting
350°F/Gas mark 4

Preparation:
1. Prepare and trim the cutlets, fry in the fat for 5 minutes to brown. Drain, and place in a casserole.
2. Add lamb, leeks, turnip, onion and carrots to the casserole with the stock or water. Season with salt and pepper and add the mint. Cover the casserole and place in a moderate oven for about 1 ½ hours.
3. If fresh peas are used cook them separately and stir into the casserole just before serving. If frozen peas are used stir them into the casserole about 15 minutes before serving.

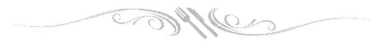

Lamb and Mushroom Pie

(Origin: England)

For 4 servings:
- 1 Spanish onion
- 4oz mushrooms
- 1 oz butter
- 1lb lamb
- ½ pint lamb stock
- salt and pepper
- pinch mace
- 4oz frozen puff pastry
- 1 egg, beaten

Oven setting:
350°F/Gas Mark 4

Preparation:
1. Peel and chop onion. Wash and roughly chop mushrooms. Fry both gently in butter until soft.
2. Cut meat into 1-inch pieces and add to pan. Cook for 10 minutes. Add stock and seasoning. Cover and simmer for 20 minutes.
3. Place mixture in pie dish, cover with pastry, trim edges and flute. Brush with beaten egg and bake in centre of oven for 30 minutes. Reduce temperature to 350°F; Gas mark 4 after 15 minutes.

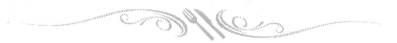

Lamb and Tomato Casserole

Origin: France
Healthy Option

For 4 servings
- 2 tbsp rapeseed oil
- 700g (1½ lb) lamb, cubed
- 225 (8oz) shallots, peeled
- 1 tbsp plain flour
- 150ml (¼pt) lamb stock
- 150ml (¼pt) white wine
- 1 tbsp tomato puree
- 1 clove garlic, crushed
- salt and pepper
- 4 tbsp crème fraiche
- 4 tomatoes, skinned, seeded and diced
- 2 tbsp chopped fresh parsley.

Preparation
1. Heat oil in a large flameproof casserole and sauté lamb for 5 mins until brown. Remove from pan with a slotted spoon.
2. Add shallots to casserole and fry for 5 minutes, until brown. Return lamb to casserole; add flour and cook, stirring for 2 mins. Gradually add in stock, wine and tomato puree and bring to boil. Cover and simmer for 40 minutes.
3. Add garlic, seasoning and crème fraiche and cook for further 20 minutes.
4. Add tomatoes and parsley and cook for a further 10 minutes. Serve.

Nutritional Information		
Calories	Fat	Fibre
704 total (serves 4) 176 per serving	Med	Low
Good source of protein.		

Lamb Chops with Ratatouille

(Origin: Italy)

For 4 servings:
- 2oz butter
- 1 tablespoon olive oil
- 4 loin chops
- ½ level teaspoon mixed herbs

For the ratatouille:
- 2 large green peppers
- 2 medium onions, quartered
- 2oz butter
- 2 small aubergines
- 8oz tomatoes
- salt and pepper
- mustard and cress

Oven setting:
400°F/Gas Mark 6.

Preparation:
1. Melt 2oz butter with oil in a meat tin. Add chops, sprinkle with dried herbs and cook in a hot oven for 15 minutes or until tender.
2. Meanwhile prepare ratatouille. Cut peppers in half, remove seeds and cut in ½ inch wide strips. Shred onions coarsely. Melt butter in a pan and fry peppers and onions for about 5 minutes or until they are soft and onion is pale golden brown. Remove stalks from aubergines and cut them in ¼ inch thick slices. Plunge tomatoes in boiling water for 10 seconds then drain and remove skins. Quarter then and remove seeds. Add aubergines and tomatoes to pan and cook for a further 5 minutes.
3. Season the ratatouille with salt and pepper. Turn it on to a serving dish and arrange chops on top. Decorate with mustard and cress.

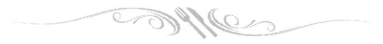

Lamb Chops with Spinach

(Origin: England)

For 4 servings:
- 3lb spinach
- salt and pepper
- ¼ teaspoon grated nutmeg
- ¼ pint double dairy cream
- 8 lamb chops
- 4 tomatoes, halved
- 2 oz butter

Preparation:
1. Wash spinach in several changes of water. Discard any discoloured leaves and tough stalks. Put into a large pan without water and sprinkle in 1 teaspoon salt. Heat gently, pushing leaves down very well in the pan. When liquid is running from spinach, cover and bring to the boil. Simmer gently for about 10 minutes or until tender.
2. Sieve spinach or put into a blender. Season with salt and pepper and stir in nutmeg and cream. Reheat very gently stirring. Turn on to serving dish. Meanwhile cook chops.
3. Dot lamb chops and tomatoes with butter and season with salt and pepper. Grill chops for 10 minutes or until tender, turning once and grill tomatoes until soft. Arrange chops on the bed of spinach with the tomatoes.

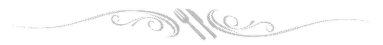

Lamb Pilaff

(Origin: Greece)

For 4 servings:
- 1 small sweet red or green pepper
- ½ oz cornflour
- salt and pepper to taste
- 1lb stewing lamb, boned and diced
- 3 tablespoons olive oil or corn oil
- 3 onions peeled and sliced
- 3 tomatoes, peeled and sliced
- 1 chicken stock cube
- 1oz seedless raisins
- 1 tablespoon lemon juice
- 6oz long grain rice

Oven setting
350°F/Gas Mark 4.

Preparation:
1. Remove stalk and seeds from pepper and chop finely. Season the cornflour and toss the diced lamb in it. Heat the oil and lightly brown the meat on all sides. Remove and keep warm.
2. Lightly fry the onions and chopped pepper in the remaining oil, add the tomatoes, stock cube, raisins, lemon juice and ¾ pint boiling water. Stir in the rice, transfer to an ovenproof casserole. Season to taste.
3. Place meat on top of the rice, cover and cook in a moderate oven for 30-40 minutes or until rice has absorbed all the liquid. Turn on to a warm plate and serve immediately.

Lancashire Hot Pot

Origin: England

For 4 servings
- 3 tbsp vegetable oil
- 450g (1lb) lean boneless lamb, diced
- 1 onion, sliced
- 25g (1oz) plain flour
- 450ml (¾ pint) lamb stock using lamb stock cubes
- 3 carrots
- 2 leeks
- 2 parsnips
- 2 tsp chopped fresh mint
- salt and pepper
- 900g (2lb) potatoes thinly sliced
- mint sprig to garnish

Preparation
1. Preheat oven. Cut carrots, parsnips and leeks into thick slices. Heat 2 tbsp oil in a frying pan, add the lamb and onion and fry until browned.
2. Stir in the flour then gradually add stock. Bring to the boil stirring continuously.
3. Add vegetables, meat and seasoning.
4. Line base of a casserole dish with half the potatoes. Add meat and vegetables.
5. Arrange remaining potato slices on top overlapping one another. Brush with remaining oil.
6. Cover and cook for 1 ¾ hours. Increase oven to 200C/400F/ gas 6.

7. Remove lid and cook for 30 minutes or until potatoes are golden. Garnish with mint sprigs and serve.
8. Sprigs of thyme, rosemary or bay leaves may be used to flavour this casserole.

Nutritional Information.		
Calories	Fat	Fibre
2300 total (serves 4) 575 per serving	Low	High
Good source of iron, protein, vitamin A+C.		

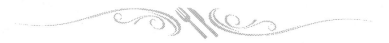

Layered Lamb Casserole

(Origin: England)

For 4 servings:
- 2lb middle neck of lamb, chined
- 1 small white cabbage (about 1 ½ lb)
- 1 heaped teaspoon caraway seeds
- salt and pepper to taste
- 1lb potatoes, peeled
- ½ lb small tomatoes, halved
- 1oz butter or margarine

Preparation:
1. Cut the lamb into chops and trim off excess fat; place in bottom of a large strong saucepan or flameproof casserole. Shred the cabbage, discarding hard core. Wash well, drain, and put half on top of the fat trimmings. Arrange the chops on this bed of cabbage, sprinkle with caraway seeds and season. Top with potatoes and the rest of the cabbage, and dot with butter.
2. Cover pan and bring to the boil, then simmer for 1 ¼ hours. (No water need be added).
3. Half an hour before the dish is ready, add tomato halves. A little water can be added at this stage if the pan seems dry. Cover and finish cooking.

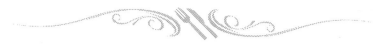

Monday Pie

(Origin: England)

For 4 servings:
- 1 small onion, peeled and chopped
- 2oz mushrooms, sliced
- 2 tbsps extra virgin olive oil
- 1lb cooked lamb, minced
- ½ teaspoon Worcestershire sauce
- salt and pepper to taste
- ½ pint gravy
- 1 lb potatoes, boiled and mashed
- 1 egg, lightly beaten

Oven setting
400°F/Gas Mark 4

Preparation:
1. Fry the onion and mushrooms for a few minutes in the olive oil. Reserve a few mushroom slices for decoration. Add the lamb, Worcestershire sauce, salt, pepper and gravy. Mix well and place in an ovenproof dish.
2. Pile the mashed potato on top and rough up with a fork or pipe it on with a large forcing bag or tube. Brush the top with beaten egg.
3. Cook in a moderately hot oven for about 40 minutes until golden brown. Decorate with mushroom slices and return to the oven to reheat for a few minutes.

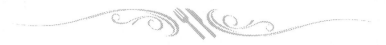

Moussaka

Origin: Greece

For 4 servings
- 3 tbsp olive oil
- 1 small onion, finely chopped.
- 400g (1lb) cooked lamb mince
- 200g (12oz) canned tomato puree
- Pinch salt and pepper
- ½ lb raw potato, sliced
- 1 large aubergine, sliced
- 1 clove garlic, crushed
- ½ tomato, peeled and sliced
- ½ pint cheese sauce
- 50g (2oz) cheese, grated
- 1 egg yolk
- Sprig of parsley

Preparation
1. Heat a third of the oil in a frying pan. Add onion and allow to colour, then add the meat and shake over a brisk heat for a few minutes. Remove from heat. Add tomato puree and season lightly. Put in an ovenproof dish and keep warm.
2. Heat the remaining oil in the frying pan; put in the potatoes and fry gently until brown. Then take out and arrange on top of the meat.
3. Add the aubergine to the frying pan and cook for 5-7 minutes. Then add the garlic and sliced tomatoes. Continue cooking for another 5 minutes and then pour over the potatoes. Meanwhile prepare the cheese sauce, stir in the egg yolk and pour over the dish.

4. Sprinkle top with grated cheese and bake in a moderate oven for 15-20 minutes until well browned. Decorate with parsley.

Nutritional Information		
Calories	Fat	Fibre
2160 total (serves 4) 540 per serving	Med	Med
Good source of calcium, protein and omega 3.		

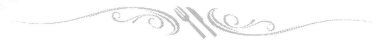

Pork and Lamb Casserole

Origin: England

For 4 servings:
- 350g (12oz) pork fillet
- 225g (8oz) lean leg lamb
- 1 tbsp seasoned flour
- 1 small cabbage
- 6 baby carrots
- 450g (1lb) small new potatoes
- 200g (7oz) French beans
- 450ml (3/4pt) dry cider
- salt and pepper
- 2 tbsp chopped parsley

Preparation
1. Cut meat into thin strips, removing any fat. Toss in seasoned flour.
2. Cut the cabbage into thin wedges. Remove outer leaves and cut out most of the tough stalk, leaving just enough to hold the leaves together. Scrub carrots and potatoes, peel onions and top and tail beans.
3. Put vegetables and meat into a flame- proof casserole. Add cider, seasoning and parsley
4. Bring to the boil, cover and simmer for 25-30 mins, stirring occasionally, until the vegetables are tender.

Nutritional Information		
Calories	Fat	Fibre
1684 total (serves 4) 421 per serving		
Good source of protein.		

Roast Lamb Lyonnaise

(Origin: France)

For 4-6 servings:
- 1½ lb potatoes, peeled
- 8oz onions, sliced
- 2tbsps extra virgin olive oil
- 3lb leg of lamb
- salt and pepper
- 1 or 2 cloves garlic

Oven setting:
350°F/Gas Mark 4

Preparation:
1. Cut potatoes into ½ inch thick slices. Arrange onions in a heavy ovenproof dish. Put potato slices, overlapping slightly, on top.
2. Spread olive oil over lamb and season with salt and pepper. Cut garlic in small pieces and insert pieces in fat of lamb. Place joint on top of potatoes in dish.
3. Roast in a moderate oven, allowing 30 minutes to the pound plus 30 minutes over. Baste from time to time. Remove the joint and place on a serving dish. Surround with potatoes and onions.

Skewered Lamb with Beetroot

(Origin: England)

For 4 servings:
- 1lb lean lamb, diced
- 3 tablespoons oil
- 3 tablespoons vinegar
- pinch thyme
- 4 rashers bacon
- 1 4oz can pineapple cubes
- 1 small beetroot, cooked and peeled
- salt and pepper to taste
- clove of garlic (optional)
- few strips sweet green pepper
- 12oz rice, cooked and buttered.

Preparation:
1. Make a marinade with the oil, vinegar, thyme and seasoning. Pour over the lamb and leave for at least one hour. Trim rind from bacon rashers, cut in half and form into bacon rolls. Dice cooked beetroot. Cut diamond shapes from green pepper.
2. Rub 4 skewers with the garlic clove. Thread on to the skewers the lamb alternately with pineapple, bacon rolls and beetroot, beginning and finishing with green pepper. Brush over with the marinade. Grill slowly turning the skewers several times for about 10 minutes.
3. Place skewers on a bed of buttered rice to serve.

Spring Lamb Noisettes

Origin: England
Healthy Option.

For 6 servings
- 6 large or 12 small lamb noisettes
- 3 lemons
- 120ml (4 fl oz) olive oil
- 2 tbsp chopped fresh mint
- salt and pepper
- 200g (7oz) Greek yoghurt
- mint sprigs and lemon twists, to garnish

Preparation
1. Put noisettes in a shallow dish. Mix together rind and juice of 2 lemons, olive oil, 1 tbsp mint and seasoning.
2. Pour liquid over noisettes. Cover, refrigerate and leave to marinate for 3-4 hours, turning occasionally. Mix together the remaining lemon rind and juice, mint and yoghurt. Put in a small bowl for serving.
3. Put noisettes on a grill rack and cook under a low grill for 15-20 minutes, turning occasionally and basting frequently with marinade.
4. Garnish with mint sprigs and lemon twists and serve with creamy mint sauce.

Nutritional Information		
Calories	Fat	Fibre
2904 total (serves 6) 488 per serving	Med	Low
Good source of Omega 3.		

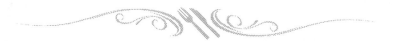

Stir Fried Lamb

Origin: England
Healthy option

For 4 servings
- 750g (2lb) boned leg of lamb
- 2 tbsp soy sauce
- 2 tsp sugar
- 2 tsp cornflour
- 2 tbsp vegetable oil
- 2.5cm (1in) piece fresh root ginger, grated
- 2 cloves garlic, crushed
- 2 leeks, sliced into 2.5cm (1in) strips
- 150ml (¼ pt) sherry.

Preparation
1. Cut lamb into thin strips about 5cm (2in) long. Put into a bowl, add soy sauce, sugar and cornflour and mix well.
2. Heat 1 tbsp oil in a heavy frying pan and add ginger and garlic. Sizzle for 1 minute.
3. Add lamb and stir fry over high heat for 8 minutes, until meat has browned. Remove with a slotted spoon and keep warm.
4. Wipe frying pan and heat remaining oil. Add leeks and stir fry for 3 minutes.
5. Return lamb to pan. Add sherry and bring to boil. Cook, stirring until the sauce thickens. Serve.

Nutritional Information		
Calories	Fat	Fibre
2515 total (serves 4) 644 per serving	Med	Med
Good source of protein,		

Stuffed Aubergines

For 4 servings:
- 2 aubergines
- ½ tsp salt
- 3 tsp olive oil
- 1 onion, chopped
- 275g (10oz) minced beef
- 225g (8oz) can tomatoes, drained
- 1 tsp thyme
- 1 tbsp chopped parsley
- 3 tbsp dried breadcrumbs
- 1 clove garlic
- 1 tbsp tomato puree
- 2 large tomatoes, sliced
- 50g (2oz) grated cheddar or Gruyere Cheese

Timing
Preparation
10mins

Cook time
1 hour

Cooking temperature
180C/350F/gas 4

Preparation
1. Preheat. Cut aubergines in half lengthways.
2. Sprinkle flesh with salt and spoon over 2 tbsp olive oil. Bake for 25-30 minutes, or until just soft at 200C/400F/gas 6.

3. Heat the remaining oil in a saucepan; add the onion and sauté for 4-5 minutes to soften. Add the minced beef and sauté until browned.
4. Scoop the flesh out of the aubergines, being careful to leave the skin intact.
5. Add tomatoes and aubergine to mince and cook for 2-3 minutes. Add thyme, parsley, breadcrumbs, garlic and tomato puree. Mix well and pour into aubergine skins.
6. Top aubergines with tomato slices and cheese and bake for 15 minutes or until cheese has melted. Serve.

Nutritional Information		
Calories	Fat	Fibre
1517 total (serves 4) 379 per serving		
Good source of Omega 3		

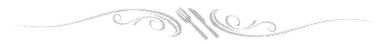

Tasty Lamb Kebabs

Origin: Greece

For 4 servings
- 700g (1½ lb) boneless leg lamb, fat removed
- 2 onions, cut into eighths
- 4 tomatoes, quartered.

Marinade
- 75ml (3fl oz) dry white wine
- 4 tbsp olive oil
- 1 bay leaf
- 2 cloves garlic, crushed
- 1 small stick celery, finely chopped
- 2 tbsp chopped basil (optional).

Preparation
1. Cut lamb into cubes and put into a shallow dish.
2. Mix together wine, olive oil, bay leaf, garlic, celery and basil, if using.
3. Pour marinade over meat and stir to coat. Cover, chill and leave to marinate for 1-2 hours.
4. Preheat grill. Arrange meat, onions and tomatoes on 8 skewers. Grill for 10-15 minutes, basting with marinade from time to time. Turn over halfway through cooking time.

Nutritional Information		
Calories	Fat	Fibre
1552 total (serves 4) 388 per serving	Med	Low
Good source of protein and co-enzyme Q10.		

SEAFOOD

Baked trout fillets

Origin: France

For 4 servings:
- 25g (1oz) butter
- 1 carrot, peeled and cut into thin strips
- 4 spring onions, finely shredded
- 2 sticks celery, finely sliced
- salt and pepper
- 4 medium trout, filleted
- 8 sprigs coriander
- 150ml (¼ pt) white wine
- 300ml (½ pt) double cream

Preparation
1. Melt butter in a small saucepan. Add the vegetables and sauté for 5 mins. Season.
2. Preheat oven. Put each trout fillet on a sheet of foil. Divide the filling between the fillets. Add a sprig of coriander and fold fillet over.
3. Fold up edges of foil and pour wine over each piece of fish. Wrap fish in foil, making sure parcels are tightly sealed. Put on a baking tray and bake for 25 mins.
4. Open parcels and pour juice into a small saucepan. Bring to boil and simmer until only 2 tbsp liquid remains. Add double cream and bring back to boil. Taste and season.
5. Serve trout still in its foil, if liked, with sauce separately.

Nutritional Information		
Calories	Fat	Fibre
1717 total (serves 4) 429 per serving	High	Low
Good source of Omega 3.		

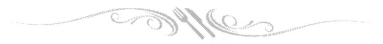

Cheesy Prawn Bake

Origin: England

For 4 servings:
- 4 hard boiled eggs
- 25g (1oz) butter or margarine
- 25g (1oz) plain flour
- 300ml (½ pint) milk
- 3 tbsp chopped fresh dill (optional)
- Salt and pepper
- ¼ tsp dry mustard
- 300g (10oz) peeled prawns
- 3 tbsp grated Emmanthal or cheddar cheese

Preparation:
1. Preheat oven. Shell and slice the hard boiled eggs
2. Melt butter or margarine in a saucepan and stir in flour. Cook, stirring, for one minute. Remove from heat and gradually add milk. Bring to the boil, stirring until thickened.
3. Stir in salt, pepper, mustard, parsley and dill if using.
4. Arrange prawns and eggs in an ovenproof dish. Pour over sauce and sprinkle top with grated cheese.
5. Bake for 15-20 minutes until top is golden and bubbling.

Nutritional Information		
Calories	Fat	Fibre
1308 total (serves 4) 372 per serving	Med	Low
Good source of Vitamin B, Vitamin A, iron and calcium.		

Creamy Fish Chowder

Origin - Ireland

For 4 servings:
- 2 tbsp olive oil
- 125g (8oz) potato, finely diced
- 1 onion, sliced
- 2 celery sticks sliced
- 25g (1oz) flour
- 500ml (1pt) fish stock
- 225g (8oz) unfried cod fillet
- 225g (8oz) haddock fillet, skinned
- 150g (5oz) peeled prawns
- 200g (7oz) can sweet corn, drained
- 30ml (½ pt) single cream
- Salt and pepper
- 3 tbsp freshly chopped parsley
- Parsley to garnish (optional)
- Croutons to serve (optional)
- 1 diced potato (large)
- 1 large onion diced
- 2 sticks of celery sliced

Timing
Preparation:
5 mins

Cooking:
35mins

Preparation
1. Melt butter in a large saucepan. Add potatoes, onion, celery and sauté for 5 mins.

2. Stir in flour and cook for 1 min. Pour in stock, stir and bring to boil. Reduce heat to a simmer and cook for 20 mins or until potatoes are cooked.
3. Cut cod and haddock into cubes and add to pan with the prawns, sweetcorn and cream. Season and stir in parsley.
4. Heat gently for 10 mins, stirring. Garnish with parsley if using, top with croutons and serve.

Nutritional Information		
Calories	Fat	Fibre
1921 500 per serving	Low	Medium

Crunchy Topped Fish Bake

(England)

You will need
- 4 plaice fillets
- 1x10oz tin condensed mushroom soup
- 4oz grated cheese
- 2oz butter
- 1 teaspoon grated onion
- Dash Worcester sauce
- Dash garlic salt
- 1 small bag crisps
- Few anchovies

Preparation time
10 minutes

Cooking time
35 minutes

Oven Setting
350°F/Gas Mark 4

Preparation
1. Put fillets in greased ovenproof dish. Spread with soup and top with cheese
2. Melt butter, add onion, Worcester Sauce and garlic salt. Mix well. Add crushed potato crisps and mix again.
3. Spread mixture over fillets and bake in centre of oven for 35 minutes. Garnish with criss-cross of anchovies and serve with tomato salad.

Serves 4

Cucumber Crunchy Herrings

(England)

You will need
- 4-6 small herrings
- salt and pepper
- pinch mustard
- approx. 1 oz. medium oatmeal
- ½ cucumber
- 1 small carton soured cream
- grated rind and juice of 1 orange
- orange segments

Preparation time
20 minutes

Cooking time
15 minutes

Preparation:
1. Clean and bone fish by removing head, entrails, gills and fins.
2. Wash fish well under cold, running water. Make a slit from belly to tail and place slit down on board. Press backbone firmly with knuckles, turn over and remove backbone. Season well with salt, pepper and mustard. Roll each in oatmeal. Fry or grill for 20 minutes, turning frequently.
3. Peel cucumber and dice. Put into bowl with ½ tea spoons salt. Toss and leave for 15 minutes. Mix cream with orange rind and juice. Rinse and drain cucumber. Add cream and mix well.
4. Arrange herrings on serving platter. Garnish with orange segments. Serve cucumber mixture separately from a bowl.

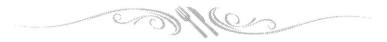

Curried King Prawns

Origin: China

For 4 servings
- 25g (1oz) butter
- 1 red pepper, cut into thin strips.
- 1 leek, cut into matchstick-sized strips
- 16-20 King Prawns peeled.
- 1 tsp curry powder
- ½ tsp paprika
- 2 tbsp brandy
- 2 – 3 drops Tabasco sauce
- ½ tsp mild chilli powder
- 300ml (½ pint) double cream.
- Salt.

Preparation
1. Melt butter in a large frying pan; add red pepper and sauté for 3–4 mins. Add leeks and sauté for 2 mins.
2. Add prawns to frying pan. Stir in curry powder and paprika and cook for 2 mins.
3. Stir in brandy and cook for 1 min.
4. Add Tabasco, chilli powder and cream. Season with salt and cook gently to heat through.
5. Serve on a bed of boiled rice.

Nutritional Information		
Calories	Fat	Fibre
1950 total (serves 4) 487 per serving	High	Low

Devilled Lobster

(England)

You will need
- 1 small lobster, boiled
- 2oz butter, melted
- 2oz white breadcrumbs
- 2 tablespoons thick cream
- 1 teaspoon cayenne pepper
- 2 lemons
- 1oz cheese, grated
- few stuffed olives, sliced
- Few sprigs parsley.

Preparation time
10 minutes

Cooking time
20 minutes

Oven setting
350°F/Gas Mark 4

Preparation:
1. Remove claws from lobster and pick out meat. Cut shell in half lengthwise, remove intestinal cord and sac (the grey-greenish matter from head end). Carefully remove white meat and chop finely with claw meat. Wash and dry hands.
2. Mix the meat, butter, 1½ oz breadcrumbs, cream and cayenne pepper together. Pile mixture back into shells and sprinkle with remaining breadcrumbs, juice of 1 lemon and cheese.
3. Bake in centre of preheated oven for 20 minutes. Serve hot, garnished with lemon slices, olives and parsley.

Serves 4

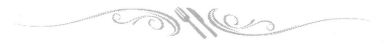

Fish Curry

Origin: India

You will need
- 2lb cod
- salt and pepper
- juice of ½ lemon
- 1 onion
- 2 oz. butter
- 2 oz. plain flour
- 1 tablespoon curry powder
- 1 pint stock or water
- 1 small cauliflower
- 1 teaspoon chopped parsley

Preparation time
15 minutes

Cooking time
25 minutes

Preparation:
1. Cut fish into small pieces. Season well. Sprinkle with lemon juice. Peel and grate or chop the onion. Fry in butter until transparent. Add fish and fry gently for 5 minutes.
2. Remove fish and keep to one side.
3. Add flour and curry powder to butter, mix well and cook for 5 minutes, stirring frequently. Remove pan from heat and gradually add stock or water. Return to heat and bring to the boil, stirring until thickened. Cook for 5 minutes. Add fish to sauce and cook for further 10 minutes.
4. Cook cauliflower sprigs in salted, boiling water. Drain and arrange around edge of dish. Pour fish and sauce into centre.
5. Garnish with parsley.

Fish in Spinach Sauce

(Denmark)

You will need
- 2 large plaice, filleted
- 4 oz. fresh or frozen prawns
- salt and pepper to taste
- 1 packet instant potato (for 4)
- ½ lb. fresh or 5½ oz. packet frozen spinach
- 1 oz. flour
- ¼ pint milk
- 2 tablespoons cream

Preparation time
15 minutes

Cooking time
10 minutes

Oven setting
375°F; Gas Mark 5

Preparation:
1. Roll the fillets skin side inwards, and place on end close together in an ovenproof dish.
2. Fill centres with peeled prawns, reserving a few for decoration. Melt the butter, and pour half of it over them. Sprinkle well with salt and pepper. Cover with foil and bake in a moderately hot oven for 10 minutes. Place on a warm serving dish.
3. Meanwhile, make up the mashed potato and keep hot. Cook the spinach in as little water as possible; when tender, press through a sieve.

4. Blend the flour with the rest of the butter, stir in the milk, then the spinach puree. Season with salt and pepper. Cook, stirring, for 3 minutes, then withdraw from heat and add cream. Taste and correct seasoning. Pour over the plaice rolls. Top each with a prawn and pipe or fork mashed potato round the sides of the serving dish.

Greek-Style Baked Cod

For 4 servings:
- 450g (1lb) cod filet, skinned
- 2 tbsp olive oil
- 2 tbsp lemon juice
- 1 garlic clove, crushed
- 2 tbsp chopped fresh parsley
- 4 tbsp Retsina OR dry white wine
- 3 tomatoes, chopped
- 25g (1oz) fresh white breadcrumbs

Preparation
1. Preheat oven. Put fish in a shadow ovenproof dish and brush with a little olive oil.
2. Mix together lemon juice, remaining oil, garlic, ½ tbsp parsley and Retsina.
3. Arrange tomatoes on top of fish. Pour wine mixture over fish.
4. Sprinkle with the remaining parsley and top with breadcrumbs.
5. Cook for 20 mins or until fish is cooked through. For a crispier topping, put the dish under a medium grill for 5–10 mins before serving.

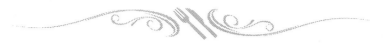

Grilled Salmon Steaks

Origin: England

For 4 servings
- 4 salmon steaks
- salt
- 1 tbsp olive oil
- 1 tbsp grated lemon rind
- lemon slices and dill sprigs, to serve

Potato Salad
- 675g (1½ lb) new potatoes, cooked
- 100g (4oz) radishes, sliced.
- 1 tbsp capers, optional
- mixed salad leaves e.g. iceberg
- 2 tbsp chopped fresh parsley
- salt and pepper
- 3 tbsp olive oil
- 1 tbsp white wine vinegar.
- 2 courgettes

Preparation
1. Scrub potatoes and cook in lightly salted boiling water until just tender. Leave to cool.
2. Slice radishes and potatoes and put into bowl. Add capers, if using.
3. To make dressing, whisk together oil and seasoning, add vinegar and beat well. Pour over potato salad.
4. Wash salad leaves and finely shred. Put in serving dish and arrange potato on top. Sprinkle with parsley.
5. Preheat grill. Sprinkle the salmon steaks with a little salt, brush with oil and top with lemon rind.

6. Cook under a medium grill for 7 – 10 mins on each side, occasionally brushing with a little oil.
7. Serve the salmon with lightly cooked sliced courgettes and garnished with lemon and dill. Serve potato salad separately.

Nutritional Information		
Calories	Fat	Fibre
1950 total (serves 4) 487 per serving	Low	Low
Good source of Vitamin C, protein and Omega 3.		

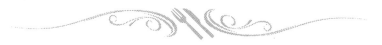

Herrings with Mustard Sauce

Origin: England

For 4 servings
- 4 large herrings
- salt and pepper
- 1 oz. butter
- 1 oz. plain flour
- 2 teaspoons mustard
- pinch curry powder
- ½ pint fish stock or water
- 1 lemon, cut into wedges
- few sprigs parsley

Preparation time
15 minutes

Cooking time
15 minutes

Preparation:
1. Remove heads and entrails from fish. Wash well. Remove scales, cut off fins and gills. Season well. Make 2 slits on each side of fish and grill for 10 minutes.
2. To make sauce, melt butter, add flour, mustard and curry powder. Mix well and cook for 2-3 minutes. Remove pan from heat and add stock or water, stirring all the time. Return to heat and bring to the boil, stirring until thickened. Correct seasoning.

3. Arrange fish on large platter. Garnish with lemon wedges or slices and parsley sprigs. Pour sauce into a decorative line over fish.

Nutritional Information		
Calories	Fat	Fibre
1095 total (serves 4) 279 per serving	Low	Low
Good source of omega 3.		

Mackerel en Papillotes

(France)

You will need
- 4 mackerel
- salt and pepper
- 2oz butter
- grated rind and juice of 1 orange
- dash garlic salt
- 1 small onion
- 1 orange, cut in wedges
- 4 sprigs parsley

Preparation time
10 minutes

Cooking time
30 minutes

Oven setting
375°F/Gas Mark 5

Preparation
1. Remove head, entrails, fins and gills. Clean fish under cold, running water. Season well.
2. Beat butter until soft. Add orange rind and juice, beating until smooth. Add garlic salt. Peel and grate or chop onion, add to butter and beat well. Divide between the mackerel and spread inside each fish. Place each on square of greased foil making a double fold along the top and at each end. Place on baking tin and bake for 30 minutes in preheated oven.
3. Carefully fold back the foil, crimping the edges decoratively. Garnish each fish with orange wedges and parsley. Serve hot or cold.

Serves 4

Oriental Prawns

For 4 servings
- 2 tbsp vegetable oil
- 1 Onion, finely chopped
- 2 sticks celery, cut into thin sticks
- 2 carrots, cut into thin sticks
- 450g (1lb) large prawns
- 227g (8oz) can water chestnuts, drained

Sauce
- 227g (8oz) can pineapple pieces in natural juice
- 2 tbsp tomato ketchup
- 3 tbsp soy sauce
- 3 tbsp white wine vinegar
- 1 tbsp brown sugar
- 1 tbsp cornflour
- salt and pepper

Preparation
1. To make sauce, drain pineapple juice from pineapple pieces and reserve.
2. Mix together tomato ketchup, soy sauce, vinegar, sugar, cornflour and seasoning. Stir in to pineapple juice.
3. Heat half the oil in large frying pan or wok, add onions and stir fry for 2 – 3 mins. Add celery and carrots and stir fry for 2 mins. Set aside.
4. Heat remaining oil, add prawns and fry for 1 min. Pour in sauce and bring to boil, stirring until thickened.

5. Add chestnuts and pineapple and cook for 2 mins. Stir in onions, celery and carrot and cook for 1 min. Serve on a bed of boiled rice.

Nutritional Information		
Calories	Fat	Fibre
1250 total (serves 4) 312 per serving	Low	Low
Low in fat, low in calories		

Plaice Rolls (England)

For 4 servings
- 4 large plaice fillets
- salt and pepper
- grated rind and juice of 1 lemon
- 1 teaspoon chopped parsley
- 4 rashers streaky bacon
- 1 oz. butter
- 1 tablespoon milk
- 1 small onion
- 1 small tin tomatoes
- dash Worcester sauce

Preparation time
20 minutes

Cooking time
30 minutes

Preparation
1. Skin the fillets. Season well with salt and pepper. Lay each fillet skinned side up. Sprinkle with lemon rind, juice and parsley. Roll up head to tail. Remove the bacon rinds and wrap a rasher around each fillet. Dot each with butter using not more than ½ oz. altogether, place on plate and add milk.
2. Steam over a pan of hot water for 20 minutes.
3. Melt remaining butter in small pan. Peel and grate onion, add to butter and fry until transparent. Add tomatoes, Worcester sauce and seasoning of choice, e.g. basil, mixed herbs or dash garlic salt. Cook rapidly for 5 minutes.

4. Carefully remove fish rolls, turn on to side and grill for 2-3 minutes to brown bacon. Arrange the tomato mixture in a serving dish and place fish rolls in centre.

Nutritional Information		
Calories	Fat	Fibre
940 total (serves 4) 232 per serving	Low	Low
Good source of protein.		

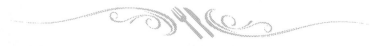

Potted Shrimps

Origin: England

You will need
- 2 pints shrimps
- 4 oz. butter
- juice of ½ lemon
- pinch ground mace
- 3 oz. butter, clarified
- 1 bunch watercress

Preparation time
20 minutes

Preparation:
1. Pick the shrimps, chop and mix with the butter. Beat well. Add the lemon juice and mace, beat well.
2. Divide the mixture into small pots, press firmly and cover with clarified butter. Allow to cool.
3. Cover pots and keep in cold place. To serve, place moulded shrimps into bed of lettuce leaves or shredded lettuce or arrange pots on a small tray. Garnish with watercress.

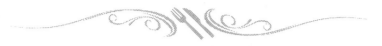

Russian Fish Pie

Origin: Russia

For 4 servings
- 375g (12oz) haddock OR cod, skinned
- 50ml (2fl oz) water
- 150ml (¼ pt) dry white wine
- 25g (1oz) butter
- 1 onion, sliced
- 4 tbsp plain flour
- 150ml (¼ pt) milk
- Salt and pepper
- 2 tbsp chopped parsley
- 2 tbsp chopped dill
- 2 hard boiled eggs chopped
- 450g (1lb) puff pastry
- Beaten egg, to glaze.

Preparation:
1. Put fish in shallow pan, add water and wine. Bring to boil, cover and poach gently for 6-8 minutes until tender. Strain and reserve juices.
2. Flake fish, discarding any bones. Melt butter in saucepan and sauté onion until lightly browned. Stir in flour and cook for 30 seconds.
3. Remove from heat and gradually stir in juices and milk. Return to heat and bring to boil, stirring until thickened. Stir in fish, parsley, dill, eggs. Season and cool.
4. Preheat oven. Roll out pastry into 35cm (14in) square. Cut into 2 strips, one 2.5cm (1in) wider than the other. Put filling on smaller piece of pastry. Brush edge with beaten egg and top with larger piece, sealing edges. Cut slits on top.

5. Place on dampened baking tray, brush with beaten egg and bake for 30 mins.

Nutritional Information		
Calories	Fat	Fibre
Total serves 4 584 per serving	Low	Low
Good source of Protein.		

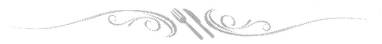

Salmon Chaudfroid (France)

You will need…
- 4 salmon steaks
- 1 oz. breadcrumbs
- Lemon juice
- ¼ pint mayonnaise
- ¼ pint aspic jelly (made from packet crystals)
- ½ fresh red pepper, blanched
- Few capers
- 1 lettuce
- Bunch watercress

Preparation time
40 minutes

Cooking time
10 minutes

Preparation:
1. Steam fish on greased plate over pan of hot water for 10 minutes. Drain, remove skin and centre bone, keeping the fish whole. Leave to cool. Mix breadcrumbs with enough lemon juice to bind, use to fill cavity in each steak.
2. Mix mayonnaise with half the aspic. Leave until cold and beginning to set. Stand fish on wire rack with plate underneath and pour sauce over, coating evenly. When set, gently pour remaining aspic over, catching the surplus for later use. Leave until set.
3. Cut pepper into strips and arrange over Chaudfroid, place capers between pepper strips. Place salmon steaks on lettuce and garnish with watercress in centre. Serve very cold.

Seafood Gratin

For 4 servings:
- 1 tbsp vegetable oil
- 2 shallots, chopped
- 150ml (¼ pt) dry white wine
- 8 queen scallops, trimmed and washed
- 8 large prawns, peeled
- 175g (6oz) mussels
- 150ml (¼ pt) milk
- 1 tbsp lemon juice
- salt and black pepper
- 25g (1oz) unsalted butter
- 1 tbsp plain flour
- 50g (2oz) Gruyere cheese, grated

Preparation
1. Heat oil in a sauce- pan and sauté the shallots for 10 mins, until softened. Add wine and bring to boil.
2. Add scallops, prawns and mussels and simmer for 4 mins. Using a slotted spoon, transfer the seafood to a plate and keep warm.
3. Boil juices rapidly until reduced to about 4 tbsp. Stir in milk, lemon juice and seasoning.
4. Blend together butter and flour. Bring sauce to boil. Gradually add butter mixture, stirring until blended.
5. Reduce heat and stir sauce until thickened. Arrange seafood in four scallop shells, or flameproof serving dishes. Pour over sauce and sprinkle with cheese.
6. Cook under a pre- heated grill for 5 mins until golden. Serve immediately.

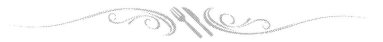

Seafood Supreme

Origin: France

For 4 servings
- 4 plaice fillets, skinned and halved
- 100g (4oz) garlic and herb cream cheese,
- Salt and pepper
- 225g (8oz) peeled prawns, thawed if frozen
- 25g (1oz) butter
- 25g (1oz) plain flour
- 150ml (¼ pt) fish stock
- 150ml (¼ pt) white wine
- 50g (2oz) Emmanthal cheese, grated
- 450g (1lb) potatoes, mashed

Preparation
1. Preheat oven. Spread garlic and herb cream cheese over skinned side of fillets and roll up carefully. Put in an ovenproof dish, season and scatter over prawns.
2. Heat butter in a saucepan, add flour and cook, stirring, for 2 mins. Remove from heat and gradually stir in stock and wine until well blend-ed. Return to heat and bring to boil, stirring, until thickened. Remove from heat and stir in cheese.
3. Pour sauce over fish, covering well. Using a piping bag fitted with a large star-shaped nozzle, pipe mashed potato around edge.
4. Bake for 30 mins, until golden brown. Serve with a light salad or green vegetable.

Nutritional Information		
Calories	Fat	Fibre
1685 total (serves 4) 421 per serving	Low	Low
Good source of protein.		

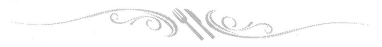

Sole Veronique

Origin: France

For 4 servings
- 8 medium fillets
- salt and pepper to taste
- 1 wine glass dry wine
- 1 ½ oz. butter
- 1oz. flour
- ¼ pint milk
- 4oz. white grapes

Preparation time
10 minutes

Cooking time
10 minutes

Oven setting
375oF; Gas Mark 5

Preparation:
1. Roll each filet. Well butter a baking dish and arrange fillets in this. Sprinkle with salt and pepper and pour over the wine. Cook uncovered for about 10 minutes in a moderately hot oven. Lift the fish carefully on to a warm serving dish.
2. Meanwhile heat the butter, stir in the flour and a measured half pint of liquid made up of juices from the fish and milk.
3. Bring to the boil and cook, stirring until smooth and thick.
4. Taste and correct seasoning.

5. Pour over the fish and decorate with the grapes, seeded and halved

Nutritional Information		
Calories	Fat	Fibre
1100 total (serves 4) 275 per serving	Low	Low
Good source of protein.		

Stuffed Easter Sole

Origin: England

For 4 servings:
- 175g (6oz) cooked peeled prawns
- 2 hard boiled eggs, chopped
- 2 spring onions, sliced
- 1 tsp chopped fresh dill
- 4 large sole fillets, approximately 225g (8oz) each
- 25g (1oz) butter
- 150mls (¼ pint) dry vermouth
- 2 egg yolks
- 1 tsp tomato puree
- 125ml (4 fl oz) double cream
- salt and pepper
- dill sprigs.

Preparation:
1. Mix together prawns, eggs, spring onions and dill. Put fillets in a large frying pan. Spread half the fillet with prawn mixture and fold over. Dot with butter and sprinkle with vermouth.
2. Cover tightly and simmer gently for 10-15 minutes until fish is warmed through. Using a slotted spoon, transfer to serving plates and keep warm.
3. Blend together egg yolks, tomato puree and cream. Stir into pan juices and heat until thickened. Season. Pour around lid and serve, garnished with dill sprigs.

Nutritional Information.		
Calories	Fat	Fibre
2008 total (serves 4) 502 per serving	Med	Low

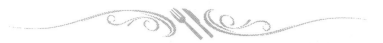

Tagliatelle with Haddock and Avocado

Origin: Italy

For 4 servings
- 350g (12oz) fresh haddock fillets, skinned
- 2.5ml (½ cup) each ground cumin, ground coriander and turmeric
- 150ml (1/4 pt) ½ cup fromage frais
- 150ml/ ¼ pt/ ½ cup double cream
- 15ml (1 tbsp) lemon juice
- 25g/1oz/2tbsp butter
- 1 onion, chopped
- 15ml (1tbsp) plain flour
- 150ml/ ¼ pt/ ⅔ cup fish stock
- 350g (12oz) tagliatelle
- 1 avocado, peeled, stoned and sliced
- 2 tomatoes, seeded and chopped
- Salt and ground black pepper
- Fresh rosemary sprigs, to garnish

Preparation
1. Carefully cut the haddock into bite size pieces
2. Mix together all the spices, seasoning, fromage frais, cream and lemon juice.
3. Stir in the haddock to coat. Cover the dish and leave to marinate overnight.
4. Heat the butter in a frying pan and fry the onion for about 10 minutes until softened. Stir in the flour then blend in the stock until smooth.
5. Carefully stir in the haddock mixture until well blended. Bring to the boil, stirring, cover and simmer for about 30 seconds. Remove from the heat.

6. Meanwhile, cook the pasta in plenty of boiling salted water according to the instructions on the packet.
7. Stir the avocado and tomatoes into the haddock mixture.
8. Drain the pasta thoroughly and divide among four serving plates. Spoon over the sauce and serve immediately, garnished with fresh rosemary.

Trout with Almonds

(Origin: France)

You will need...
- 4 trout
- 1 tablespoon seasoned flour
- 3oz. butter
- 3 oz/ flaked almonds
- 1 tablespoon cooking oil
- 2 tablespoon lemon juice
- few sprigs parsley

Preparation time
10 minutes

Cooking time
10 minutes

Preparation:
1. Toss the cleaned fish in seasoned flour. Melt 1 oz. butter in frying pan. Add the almonds, fry until lightly browned, then remove from pan and keep on one side.
2. Add remaining butter to pan with the oil. Fry the trout gently for about 10 minutes or until nicely browned, turning once during the cooking.
3. To serve, sprinkle with the browned almonds and lemon juice. Decorate with parsley.

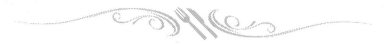

Tuna Vermicelli

Origin: Italy

For 4 servings
- 3 tbsp olive oil
- 2 cloves garlic, crushed
- 400g (14oz) plum tomatoes or canned tomatoes
- Salt and pepper
- 350g (12 oz) Vermicelli or capellini
- 2x200g (7oz) cans tuna in brine
- 6 anchovy fillets, chopped
- Chopped parsley, to serve.

Preparation
1. Heat 1tbsp oil in a saucepan, add garlic and cook for 1-2 minutes until soft.
2. Add tomatoes and seasoning and slowly bring to boil. Simmer for10-15 minutes, stirring occasionally.
3. Meanwhile, cook pasta in a large pan of boiling salted water for 6-17 minutes until tender.
4. Heat remaining oil in a frying pan, break tuna into chunks and add to pan. Heat gently for 3-4 minutes.
5. Add anchovies and cook for 2 minutes. Stir tuna mix into tomato sauce.
6. Drain pasta and serve, topped with tuna sauce. Garnish with parsley.

Nutritional Information		
Calories	Fat	Fibre
2112 total (serves 4) 528 per serving	Low	Med
Good source of Omega 3.		

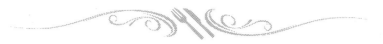

Whiting Meuniere

(France)

For 4 servings
- 2 whiting, filleted
- plain flour
- salt and pepper
- 4oz butter
- few lemon slices
- few beetroot slices
- juice of ½ lemon
- 2 teaspoons chopped parsley

Preparation time:
15 minutes

Cooking time:
10 minutes

Preparation:
1. Wipe the fish and dust well with flour, salt and pepper. Melt the butter and fry the fillets on both sides for about 10 minutes. Remove to a dish and keep hot.
2. Arrange the lemon slices around the edge of a large platter. Place the fish in the centre. Cut the beetroot into diamonds and arrange between the lemon slices.
3. Lightly brown remaining butter in the pan, add lemon juice and parsley, mix well and pour over the fish. Serve immediately.

Nutritional Information		
Calories	Fat	Fibre
912 total (serves 4) 223 per serving	High	Low
Good source of protein.		

VEGETARIAN

Aubergine Tagliatelle

For 4 servings:
- 350g (12oz) fresh tagliatelle
- 50g (2oz) ricotta cheese
- fresh basil, to garnish

Sauce:
- 1 tbsp vegetable oil
- 1 onion, chopped
- 1 clove garlic, crushed
- 2 tbsp tomato puree
- 1 tbsp paprika
- 450ml (3/4 pt) passata or sieved tomatoes
- 100g (4oz) stuffed olives, sliced
- 1 tbsp dried oregano
- salt and pepper
- 1 aubergine
- 1 tbsp fresh chopped basil

Preparation
1. To make the sauce, heat oil in a pan and cook the onion and garlic for 10 mins, until softened.
2. Add tomato purée and paprika and cook for 2 mins. Stir in passata, olives, oregano, salt and pepper.
3. Bring to boil, cover and simmer for 10 mins.
4. Slice aubergine. Put in a colander and sprinkle with plenty of salt. Leave to stand for 10 mins. Rinse thoroughly and pat dry with kitchen paper.
5. Cook pasta in a pan of boiling salted water for 10 mins.

6. Meanwhile, heat oil in a frying pan and fry aubergine for 4 mins on each side, until brown.
7. Stir aubergine and basil into sauce. Drain pasta and transfer to warmed serving plates. Spoon over sauce, top with ricotta and garnish with basil.

Blue Cheese Risotto

For 4 servings:
- 65g (2½ oz) butter
- 1 onion, chopped
- 350g (12oz) risotto
- 900ml (1½ pt) vegetable stock
- 150ml (¼ pt) dry white wine
- 100g (4oz) blue cheese
- 50g (2oz) walnuts
- salt and pepper

Preparation
1. Melt 50g (2oz) butter in a large pan and cook onion for 5 mins.
   Add rice and cook, stir- ring occasionally, for 2 mins. Add stock, 150ml (1/4pt) at a time, waiting until liquid is absorbed each time before adding any more.
2. Dice blue cheese and chop walnuts.
3. Add wine to rice and cook gently, stirring, until liquid is absorbed and risotto looks thick and creamy.
4. In a large frying pan, dry fry walnuts for 2 mins, until browned. Add blue cheese, rice and seasoning and heat gently, stirring, for 2 mins. Stir in remaining butter and serve.

Chilli fiesta

For 4 servings
- 450g (1lb) tomatoes
- 1 small green pepper
- 1 small red pepper
- 1 small yellow pepper
- 100g (4oz) baby corn
- 50g (2oz) button mushrooms
- 225g (80z) courgettes
- 1 green chilli, chopped
- 1 tbsp olive oil
- 1 onion, sliced
- 2 gloves garlic, crushed
- ½ tbsp chilli powder
- ½ tbsp ground puree
- 25g (1oz) plain flour
- 600ml (1pt) vegetable stock
- 432g (15oz) can red kidney beans
- salt and pepper
- 1 ½ tbsp chopped fresh coriander

Preparation
1. Cut a cross in top of each tomato and put in a bowl of boiling water for 2-3 mins, until skins began to peel off. Remove skins, and seed and chop tomatoes.
2. Seed and chop peppers. Halve corn and mushrooms. Slice courgettes.
3. Heat oil in a flame- proof casserole and sauté onion and garlic for 5 mins.
4. Add chilli powder, cumin, tomato puree and flour Cook, stirring for 1 minute. Add stock and bring to boil.

5. Add chilli, peppers, corn, mushrooms and courgettes. Stir in drained kidney beans and season to taste.
6. Stir in coriander, cover and simmer gently for 1 hr or until vegetables are tender.
7. Adjust seasoning, garnish and serve with soured cream and tortilla chips or brown rice.

Flaky Spinach Pie

For 8 servings:
- 900g (2lb) fresh spinach, roughly chopped
- 2 tbsp vegetable oil
- 1 glove garlic, crushed
- 2 onions, finely sliced
- 50g (2oz) butter, melted
- 200g (8oz) feta cheese
- 4 eggs
- ½ tbsp grated nutmeg
- black pepper
- 450g (1lb) filo pastry

Preparation:
1. Wash spinach and drain well. Heat oil in a large frying pan and add garlic and onions. Fry gently for 5 mins. Add spinach cover with a lid and leave to cook gently for 8 mins.
2. Uncover, increase heat and stir spinach until all liquid has evaporated.
   Add parsley and allow to cool.
3. Mash feta cheese with fork and whisk in eggs. Stir in spinach and season with nutmeg and black pepper.
4. Preheat oven. Brush a Swiss roll tin with melted butter. Layer half of the filo sheets into the tin, brushing each sheet with melted butter.
5. Spread filling on top and cover with remaining filo pastry, brushing each sheet with butter. Brush top generously with remaining butter and bake for 1 hr until pie is crisp. Serve warm or cold with a Greek salad.

Greek Pasta with Avocado Sauce

Origin: Greece
Healthy Option

For 4 servings
- 3 ripe tomatoes
- 2 large ripe avocados
- 25g/1oz/2tbsp butter, plus extra for tossing the pasta
- 1 garlic clove, crushed
- 330ml/12fl or 1½ cups double cream
- Dash of Tabasco sauce
- 450g/1lb green Tagliatelle
- Salt and ground black pepper
- Freshly grated Parmesan Cheese, to garnish
- 60ml (4tbsp) soured cream, to garnish

Preparation
1. Halve the tomatoes and remove the cores. Squeeze out the seeds and dice the flesh. Set aside until required
2. Halve the avocados, remove the stones and peel. Roughly chop the flesh. If hard-skinned, scoop out the flesh with a spoon.
3. Melt the butter in a saucepan and add the garlic. Cook for 1 minute, then add the cream and chopped avocados. Increase the heat, stirring constantly to break up the avocados.
4. Add the diced tomatoes and season to taste with salt, pepper and a little Tabasco sauce. Keep the mixture warm.
5. Cook the pasta in plenty of boiling salted water according to the instructions on the packet. Drain well through a colander and toss with a knob of butter.
6. Divide the pasta among four warmed bowls and spoon over the sauce. Sprinkle with grated Parmesan cheese and top with a spoonful of soured cream.

Italian Style Asparagus

Origin: Italy

For 4 servings:
- 450g (1lb) asparagus
- 1 small leek
- 25g (1oz) butter
- 1 onion, finely chopped
- 25g (1oz) plain flour
- 125ml (4fl oz) dry white wine
- 300ml (1/2pt) vegetable stock
- 3 egg yolks
- salt and pepper
- 1 tsp dried thyme
- 50g (2oz) cream cheese
- flat leaf parsley, to garnish (optional)

Timing
Preparation:
5mins

Cooking:
20mins

Preparation
1. Prepare the asparagus by cutting off the woody base and peeling the lower half of each spear
2. Line a steamer with foil, put asparagus and leek in steamer and cover with lid. Put over a pan of boiling water and steam for about 10 mins, or until tender.
3. Meanwhile, melt butter in a small saucepan and gently sauté onion until soft.

4. Stir in flour. Remove from heat and add white wine and stock, stirring until blended. Return to heat and cook, stirring until sauce thickens and boils.

5. Remove from heat and allow to cool slightly. Whisk in egg yolks, seasoning and thyme.

6. Return to heat. Cut cream cheese into 3 pieces and whisk into sauce one at a time. Reheat gently, stirring, until almost boiling.

7. Cut leek into long strips and use to tie asparagus into bundles. Arrange on top of sauce and garnish with parsley, if using. Serve warm.

Nutritional Information		
Calories	Fat	Fibre
819 total (serves 4) 204 per serving	Med	High

Mediterranean Pasta Twists

For 4 servings:
- 225g (8oz) courgettes
- 1 aubergine
- 1 green pepper
- 2 tbsp olive oil
- 1 onion, chopped
- 1 clove garlic, crushed
- 450g (1lb) ripe tomatoes, skinned and chopped
- 2 tbsp tomato puree
- 1 tbsp chopped oregano OR 1 tbsp dried oregano
- salt and pepper
- 350g (12oz) pasta twists
- grated Parmesan cheese
- basil sprigs (optional)

Preparation
1. Slice courgettes, dice aubergine and seed and chop green pepper.
2. Heat oil in a heavy- based pan, add onion and garlic and cook for 4-5 mins until soft.
3. Add courgettes, aubergine, pepper, tomatoes, tomato puree, oregano and seasoning. Bring to the boil, stirring, then cover and simmer gently for 20-30 mins, stirring occasionally, until vegetables are tender.
4. Towards the end of cooking time, put pasta in a large pan of boiling, salted water and cook for 10-12 mins.
5. Drain pasta. Top with vegetables, sprinkle with cheese and garnish with basil.

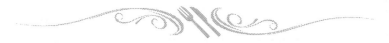

Onion Tart

Origin: England

For 4-6 servings:

Pastry:
- 175g (6oz) plain flour
- ½ tbsp salt
- 100g (4oz) butter or margarine
- 1 egg yolk

Filling
- 50g (2oz) butter
- 3-4 onions, halved and thinly sliced
- 1 tbsp plain flour
- 3 eggs, beaten
- 50g (2oz) grated Parmesan cheese
- salt and pepper
- 200ml (7fl oz) single cream

Preparation
1. Sift flour and salt together, add butter or margarine and rub in until mixture resembles fine breadcrumbs. Mix to a firm dough with egg yolk and 4-5 tbsp cold water. Wrap and chill for 30 mins.
2. Melt butter in a large pan and fry onions for 10-12 mins until soft. Leave to cool.
3. Preheat oven. Roll out pastry on a lightly floured surface and use to line a 23cm (9in) fluted flan tin.
4. Line pastry with greaseproof paper, add baking beans and bake blind for 15 mins.

5. Lower oven temp to 180C/ 35OF/gas 4. Remove beans and paper and return pastry case to oven for 5 mins.
6. Raise oven temp to 200C/ 400F/gas 6. Mix together onions, flour, eggs, cheese, seasoning and cream.
7. Add to pastry case and cook for 25-30 mins.

Spaghetti with Feta Cheese

Origin: Italy
Healthy Option

For 2-3 servings:
- 115g (4oz) spaghetti
- 1 garlic clove
- 30ml (2tbsp) extra virgin olive oil.
- 8 cherry tomatoes, halved
- A little freshly ground nutmeg
- Salt and ground black pepper
- 75g (3oz) feta cheese, crumbled
- 15ml (1tbsp) chopped fresh basil
- A few black olives, to serve (optional)

Preparation
1. Cook the spaghetti in plenty of boiling salted water according to the instructions on the packet, then drain well.
2. In the same pan gently heat the garlic clove in the olive oil for 1-2 minutes, then add the halved cherry tomatoes.
3. Increase the heat to fry the tomatoes lightly for 1 minute, then remove the garlic and discard.
4. Toss in the spaghetti, season with the nutmeg and salt and pepper to taste, then stir in the crumbled feta cheese and basil.
5. Check the seasoning, remembering that feta can be quite salty, and serve hot topped with black olives if desired.

Spanish Omelette

(Origin: Spain)

Serves 2.

Ingredients
- 2 small tomatoes
- 1 small onion
- 1 tablespoon French Beans (cooked)
- 1 medium potato (cooked)
- 1oz (25g) smoked garlic sausage
- 4 eggs (free range eggs recommended)
- 1 tablespoon peas (cooked)
- Salt and pepper to taste
- 1 teaspoon olive oil

Preparation:
1. Peel and chop tomatoes removing seeds. Chop the onion and French beans, dice the potato and sausage. Beat the eggs lightly, add the vegetables, sausage, salt and pepper.
2. Melt the oil in a frying pan, pour in the egg mixture and cook for 3 minutes. Place for a further minute under a hot grill to brown.
3. Slide out without folding onto a hot plate.

Stir Fried Vegetables with Pasta

Origin: Italy
Suitable for vegans

Serves 4
- 1 carrot
- 175g/6oz small courgettes
- 175g/6oz runner or other green beans
- 175g/6oz baby sweetcorn
- 450g/1lb ribbon pasta, such as tagliatelle
- salt, to taste
- 30ml/2tbsp corn oil, plus extra for tossing the pasta
- 1cm/ ½ in piece fresh root ginger, peeled and finely chopped
- 2 garlic cloves, finely chopped
- 90ml/6tbsp yellow bean sauce
- 6 spring onions, sliced into 2.5cm/1in lengths
- 30ml/2tbsp dry sherry
- 5ml/1 tsp sesame seeds, to garnish

Preparation
1. Slice the carrot and the courgettes diagonally into chunks. Slice the beans diagonally. Cut the baby sweetcorn diagonally in half.
2. Cook the pasta in plenty of boiling salted water according to the instructions on the packet. Drain, then rinse under hot water. Toss in a little corn oil.
3. Heat 30ml/2tbsp oil until smoking in a wok or frying pan and add the ginger and garlic. Stir fry for 30 seconds, then add the carrots, beans and courgettes.
4. Stir-fry for 3-4 minutes, then stir in the yellow bean sauce. Stir-fry for 2 minutes, add the spring onions, sherry and pasta and stir-fry for 1 minute or until piping hot. Sprinkle with sesame seeds and serve immediately.

Shepherd's Pie (Vegetarian)

Serves 4

- 6oz (175g) brown/green lentils
- 4oz (100g) split peas green or yellow
- 1 pint (500mls) hot water
- 1 medium onion, peeled and chopped
- ½ green pepper, chopped
- 2 carrots, chopped
- 2 sticks celery, chopped
- 1 clove garlic, crushed
- ½ teaspoon dried mixed herbs
- 2 pinches ground mace
- ¼ teaspoon cayenne pepper
- 25g low fat margarine
- Sprinkle of flaxseed

For the topping

- ½ 1lb tomatoes (200g) peeled and sliced
- 1 ½ lbs cooked potatoes (700g)
- 3oz (75g) cheddar cheese, grated
- 1 small onion, chopped
- 2oz low fat margarine (50g)
- 2 tablespoons milk
- Salt and freshly milled black pepper.

Wash the lentils and split peas then put them in a saucepan with hot water and simmer gently covered for approximately 45 – 60 minutes, or until the peas and lentils have absorbed the water and are soft. Pre heat the oven to gas mark 5, 375°F (190°C).

Meantime melt some low fat margarine in a frying pan, add the celery, onion, carrots and chopped pepper, and cook gently until softened. Then mash lentil mixture and add to the vegetables. Add seasoning and a pinch of salt. Then spoon the mixture into a large pie dish (3 pint or 1.75 litre) and arrange the sliced tomatoes on top.

Next prepare the topping by softening the onion in low fat margarine in a small pan, then mash the potatoes, add the cooked onion, margarine, milk and grated cheese and mix thoroughly. Season well then spread on top of the ingredients in the pie dish. Bake for about 20 minutes or until the top is lightly browned. Sprinkle with a tsp flaxseed.

As an alternative to a low fat margarine instead of butter, you can compromise and use half butter, half margarine available in most supermarkets.

For a meat shepherd's pie just replace lentils and split peas with 1lb minced steak.

Winter Vegetable Gratin

For 4 servings
- 225g (8oz) red lentils
- 2 leeks, sliced
- 2 carrots, chopped
- 1 parsnip, grated
- 1 small turnip, grated
- 400g (14oz) Passatta
- 1 tbsp chopped fresh parsley
- 1 tsp chopped fresh sage
- 1 tsp chopped fresh thyme
- ½ French mustard
- Salt and pepper
- 100g (4oz) Cheddar cheese, grated.

Preparation
1. Preheat oven. Put lentils, leeks and carrots in a saucepan. Cover with water and bring to boil. Simmer for about 10 mins, until vegetables are tender.
2. Add parsnip and turnip and cook for a further 2-3 mins. Drain.
3. Stir in passatta, herbs, mustard and seasoning. Mix well.
4. Put in an ovenproof dish and top with cheese. Bake for 15-20mins or until cheese is golden and bubbling. Serve immediately.

Nutritional Information		
Calories	Fat	Fibre
1500 total (serves 4) 375 per serving	Low	High
Good source of Vitamin A, D, B6 and calcium		

VEGETABLE ACCOMPANIMENTS

VEGETABLE ACCOMPANIMENTS

Broccoli Gratin

For 4 servings
- 900 (2lb) broccoli florets
- 50g (2oz) butter
- 2 onions, chopped
- 50g (2oz) plain flour
- 600mls (1 pint) milk
- 200g (8oz) mozzarella cheese, cubed
- 100g (4oz) blue cheese, crumbled
- 2 red peppers, halved, seeded, and sliced
- Salt and pepper
- 100g (4oz) cheddar cheese, grated

Timing
Preparation:
25mins

Cooking:
20 – 25 minutes

Cooking temperature
200C/400F/gas 6

Preparation
1. Preheat oven. Put broccoli in pan of lightly salted boiling water and cook until just tender, about 10 minutes.
2. Meanwhile, melt butter in a saucepan, add onion and cook for 3-4 minutes until softened.
3. Stir in flour, remove from heat and gradually add the milk, stirring until blended

4. Bring to the boil, stirring continuously until thickened. Stir in the mozzarella, blue cheese, red peppers and seasoning. Add broccoli and stir well to coat.
5. Divide between four individual dishes, top with grated cheese and place in a preheated oven for 10 – 15 minutes.

Nutritional Information		
Calories	Fat	Fibre
3160 total (serves 4) 790 per serving	High	High

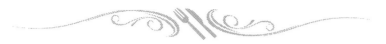

Carrots in Parsley Sauce

For 4 servings
- 575g (1¼ lbs) young carrots
- 25g (1oz) plain flour
- 25g (1oz) butter
- 125ml (4fl oz) single cream.
- 150ml (5fl oz) vegetable stock or milk
- 1 egg yolk
- ½ tsp oregano
- 2 tbsp hand chopped fresh parsley
- Salt and pepper.

Timing
Preparation:
10mins

Cooking:
15mins

Preparation
1. Cook carrots in a pan of lightly salted boiling water until just tender.
2. Meanwhile melt butter in a saucepan. Stir in flour, and then gradually add cream and stock or milk. Bring to boil stirring until thickened.
3. Add a little sauce to the egg yolk, whisk together, and then add to pan. Stir to combine

4. Add oregano, half the parsley and seasoning. Drain carrots and serve topped with sauce. Sprinkle remaining parsley over top of dish.

Nutritional Information		
Calories	Fat	Fibre
896 total (serves 4) 224 per serving	Low	Med
Good source of Vitamin A.		

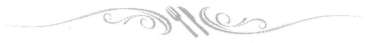

Cauliflower Cheese

- 1 medium cauliflower
- 1 tbsp plain flour
- 25g low fat margarine
- 500mls skimmed milk
- 25g cheddar cheese
- 1 tsp mustard (optional)

1. Break cauliflower into small pieces. Boil cauliflower in boiling water for 20 minutes.
2. Melt margarine and stir in plain flour until it becomes like a small ball of dough.
3. Slowly add milk stirring constantly until it reaches a smooth consistency.
4. Add grated cheddar cheese and stir into the mixture. A teaspoon of mustard is optional.
5. Stir mixture over cauliflower and serve.

Cauliflower Cheese Deluxe

For 4 servings
- 1 large cauliflower, cut into florets
- 50g (2oz) butter
- 1 small onion cut into wedges
- 1 small red pepper, seeded and sliced
- 50g (2oz) plain flour
- ½ tsp dry mustard
- 600mls (1 pint) milk
- 225g (8oz) cheddar cheese
- Salt and pepper
- 1 tbsp chopped fresh parsley
- parsley to garnish.

Timing
Preparation:
5 minutes

Cooking:
25 – 30 minutes

Preparation
1. Cook cauliflower in a large saucepan of boiling salted water for 10 minutes until tender.
2. Meanwhile, heat butter in a saucepan and cook onions and peppers for 5 minutes until softened
3. Stir in flour and mustard and cook for 2 minutes. Remove from heat and gradually milk, stirring until well blended. Return to heat and bring slowly to boil, stirring until thickened.
4. Stir in ¾ of cheese, season and cook for 2 mins, stirring gradually until cheese has melted. Stir in parsley.

5. Preheat grill. Put cauliflower in an oven proof serving dish and spoon over sauce. Sprinkle with remaining cheese. Grill for 2 minutes until golden.

6. Garnish with fresh parsley and serve.

Nutritional Information		
Calories	Fat	Fibre
1560 total (serves 4) 390 per serving	High	Low

Champ

1lb sliced potatoes
¼ pint skimmed milk
1 tsp low fat spread
6 spring onions (scallions)

Boiled potatoes or cook in a steamer. When cooked mash them.

Mix chopped spring onion, milk and low fat spread together with potato until creamed. Serve with a knob of butter or low fat spread.

Cheese and Herb Potatoes

For 4 servings
- • 4 Spring onions
- • 100g(4oz) smoked bacon
- • 750g (2lb) cooked potatoes, cut into chunks
- • salt and pepper
- • 100g (4oz) garlic and herb cream cheese
- • (or 2tbsp chopped chives and 1 clove crushed
- • garlic to plain cream cheese)
- • 150ml (¼ pint) milk
- • 50g (2oz) grated cheddar cheese

Timing
Preparation:
15 minutes

Cooking:
45 minutes

Cooking temperature
180C/350F/gas 4

Preparation
1. Preheat oven. Cut spring onions into 5cm (2in) lengths. Cut bacon into thin strips.
2. Melt butter in a frying pan and fry bacon until crisp.
3. Mash cream cheese with a fork. Add the milk and blend together.

4. Butter an ovenproof dish and add potatoes, spring onions, bacon, and seasoning.

5. Pour milk over the potatoes and top with grated cheese. Bake for 30 minutes until golden. Serve hot.

Nutritional Information		
Calories	Fat	Fibre
2270 total (serves 4) 567 per serving	High	Med

Homemade Chunky Oven Chips

(Serves 2)

Ingredients:

- 3 large potatoes such as Roosters, Maris Piper, King Edward, Desirée
- 1 tbsp olive oil
- 1 tsp celery salt (optional)
- Low salt to serve

Method:

1. Heat oven to 180°C. Peel potatoes and chop into chip chunks.
2. Blanch in boiling water for 5-10 minutes.
3. Lay onto baking tray, toss with oil and celery salt and pop in oven for 40-45 minutes, tossing about a few times so as the chips don't stick to tray.
4. When cooked they should be golden brown and crisp with a light fluffy centre. Scatter on sea salt to serve.

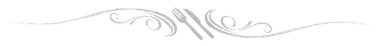

Creamy Potato Gratin

For 4 servings
- 900g (2lb) potatoes, thinly sliced
- Salt and pepper
- 1 tsp grated nutmeg
- 1 clove garlic, crushed
- 150ml (¼ pint) single cream
- 100ml (4 fl oz) milk
- 75g (3oz) Gruyere or cheddar cheese grated.

Timing
Preparation:
15 mins

Cooking:
45 mins

Cooking temperature
220C/425F/gas 7

Preparation
1. Preheat oven. Cook potatoes in boiling salted water for 5 minutes, then drain well.
2. Arrange potatoes in layers in a greased, shallow, ovenproof dish, sprinkling each layer with salt, pepper, nutmeg and garlic.
3. Mix cream and milk together and pour over potatoes. Sprinkle with cheese. Cover with aluminium foil and cook for 30 minutes.

4. Remove foil and cook for a further 15 minutes until the potatoes are tender and the cheese topping has browned.

Nutritional Information.		
Calories	Fat	Fibre
1640 total (serves 4) 410 per serving	Med	Low
Good source of Vitamin C		

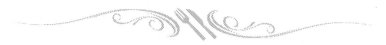

Glazed Spring Vegetables

For 4 servings
- 450g (1lb) small carrots
- 450lg (1lb) small turnips
- 2 tbsp butter
- 2 tbsp brown sugar
- 1 tsp salt
- Chopped parsley to garnish

Timing
Preparation:
5 mins

Cooking:
12 mins

Preparation
1. Scrape carrots and peel turnips. Cover with water and boil for 10 minutes until tender.
2. Melt butter in a frying pan and add brown sugar and salt
3. Add vegetables and stir until coated with golden glaze. Sprinkle with chopped parsley and serve.

Nutritional Information		
Calories	Fat	Fibre
480 total (serves 4) 120 per serving	Med	High.

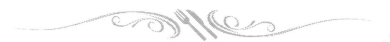

Green Beans with Hazelnuts

For 4 servings
- 550g (1½ lbs) French green beans
- 50g (2oz) butter
- 50g (2oz) chopped or flaked hazelnuts
- 2 tbsp lemon juice
- 2 tbsp flat leaf parsley, chopped
- Salt and pepper

Timing
Preparation:
15 minutes

Cooking:
12 minutes

Preparation
1. Trim the beans and rinse. Bring saucepan of water to the boil.
2. Add beans, cover and simmer for 10-12 minutes until just tender but still slightly crisp.
3. Meanwhile, melt butter, add hazelnuts and sauté for 3-4 minutes to brown slightly. Stir in lemon juice.
4. Drain beans, toss with parsley and seasoning. Put in serving dish, pour over hazelnut butter and serve.

Nutritional Information		
Calories	Fat	Fibre
831 total (serves 4) 208 per serving	Low	Med
Good source of Vitamin C + E		

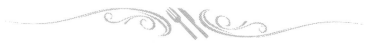

Italian Baked Mushrooms

Origin: Italy

For 4 servings:
- 575g (1¼ lb) button mushrooms
- 50g (2oz) butter
- 440g (1lb) jar pasta sauce with onions and garlic
- 2 tbsp chopped fresh parsley
- 6 tbsp parmesan cheese
- 8 spring onions, finely chopped

Cooking temperature
190C/375F/gas 5

Timing
Preparation:
10mins

Cooking:
30mins

Preparation:
1. Preheat oven. Wipe the mushrooms with kitchen paper. Melt butter in a large frying pan, add mushrooms and sauté for 5 minutes.
2. Add tomato sauce and parsley and stir well to combine. Heat for 2-3 minutes.
3. Transfer to shallow oven proof dish. Sprinkle over the cheese and bake for 15-20 minutes.
4. Remove from oven, sprinkle with spring onions and serve.
5. Serve on a bed of rocket.

Nutritional Information		
Calories	Fat	Fibre
336 total (serves 4) 84 per serving	Low	Med

Leek and Potato Pasties

For 4-6 servings:
- 1 onion
- 2 leeks
- 225g (8oz) potatoes
- 1 tbsp olive oil
- 1 tbsp plain flour
- 125ml (4fl oz) vegetable stock
- 4tsp single cream
- 3 tbsp fresh dill, chopped, optional
- 325g (12oz) puff pastry
- beaten egg, to glaze

Preparation
1. Preheat oven. Chop onion and leek. Scrub potatoes and cook until just tender. Leave to cool and dice.
2. Meanwhile, heat oil in saucepan; add onion and leek and sauté for 4-5 mins. Stir in flour, then gradually add stock, cream and dill, if using. Bring to boil, stirring continuously, until thickened.
3. Add the potatoes, and stir well. Leave to cool.
4. Roll out pastry into a rectangle 30x 45cm (12x18in). Cut into six 15cm (6in) squares. Divide filling between squares. Brush pastry edge with beaten egg, fold over to form triangles and press with a fork to seal. Brush with egg and bake for 20-25 mins.

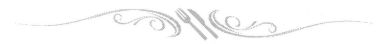

Leeks with Lemon

For 4 servings
- 4 leeks
- Salt and pepper
- 1 tbsp olive oil
- 1 tbsp grated lemon rind

Timing
Preparation:
10mins

Cooking:
10 mins

Preparation
1. Trim and wash leeks
2. Cut into 7cm (3in) lengths
3. Put in a saucepan of lightly salted boiling water and cook for 10 minutes, or until just tender. Drain and arrange in a serving dish.
4. Mix olive oil and lemon juice together. Season with salt and pepper. Pour over leeks, sprinkle with lemon rind.

Nutritional Information		
Calories	Fat	Fibre
220 total (serves 4) 55 per serving	Low	Low
Good source of Vitamin B, iron.		

Mediterranean Pasta Twists

For 4 servings:
- 225g (8oz) courgettes
- 1 aubergine
- 1 green pepper
- 2 tbsp olive oil
- 1 onion, chopped
- 1 clove garlic, crushed
- 450g (1lb) ripe tomatoes, skinned and chopped
- 2 tbsp tomato puree
- 1 tbsp chopped oregano OR 1 tbsp dried oregano
- salt and pepper
- 350g (12oz) pasta twists
- grated Parmesan cheese
- basil sprigs (optional)

Preparation
1. Slice courgettes, dice aubergine and seed and chop green pepper.
2. Heat oil in a heavy- based pan, add onion and garlic and cook for 4-5 mins until soft.
3. Add courgettes, aubergine, pepper, tomatoes, tomato puree, oregano and seasoning. Bring to the boil, stirring, then cover and simmer gently for 20-30 mins, stirring occasionally, until vegetables are tender.
4. Towards the end of cooking time, put pasta in a large pan of boiling, salted water and cook for 10-12 mins.
5. Drain pasta. Top with vegetables, sprinkle with cheese and garnish with basil.

Mediterranean Vegetables

(Serves 3-4)

Ingredients:

- 2 medium sized red onions chopped
- 1 red pepper & 1 orange pepper chopped
- 1 courgette chopped into chunks
- 1 packet cherry tomatoes washed
- 1 tbsp olive oil
- 2 tsp Cajun spice (Schwartz)

Method:

1. Preheat oven to 180°C
2. Lay vegetables on a baking tray or in a shallow casserole dish
3. Drizzle on oil and sprinkle with Cajun spice
4. Bake in the oven for about 20-30 minutes or until vegetables are softened.

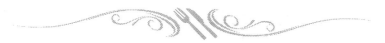

Spicy Potatoes

For 4 servings
- 750g (11½) potatoes
- 25g (1oz) butter
- 2 tbsp vegetable oil
- 2 tsp curry paste
- salt and pepper
- parsley to garnish

Timing
Preparation time:
10mins

Cooking time:
45mins

Cooking temperature
220°C/425f/gas 7

Preparation
1. Preheat oven. Scrub the potatoes and cut into large chunks. Cook in lightly salted boiling water for about 15 minutes, or until just tender. Arrange in a shallow baking tray.
2. Heat and oil in a small pan. Add curry paste and cook, stirring constantly, for 1 minute until well blended.
3. Pour curry mix over potatoes making sure they are well coated. Season and bake for 25-30 minutes, until crispy, turning over after 15 minutes.
4. Serve garnished with parsley.

Nutritional Information		
Calories	Fat	Fibre
1060 total (serves 4) 265 per serving	Low	Low
Good source of Vitamin C.		

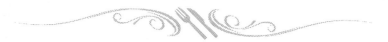

Sweetcorn with Lemon Butter

Origin: England

For 4 servings:
- 75g (3oz) butter
- 2 tbsp chopped fresh parsley
- grated rind of 1 lemon
- salt and freshly ground black pepper
- 4 fresh corn cobs
- Lemon wedges to serve.

Timing
Preparation:
10mins

Cooking:
20mins

Preparation:
1. Soften the butter in a mixing bowl. Blend in the parsley and grated lemon rind. Season well.
2. Put the butter on a sheet of grease proof paper and roll up to form a cylinder. Seal the ends and chill in the fridge for 20 minutes.
3. Meanwhile, remove the outer leaves
4. Remove butter from the fridge and unwrap. Cut into thick slices and quarter each slice.
5. Drain the corn and transfer to a serving plate. Top with butter shapes and serve with lemon wedges.

Nutritional Information		
Calories	Fat	Fibre
1118 (serves 4) 280 per serving	Med	Med
Good source of Vitamin E		

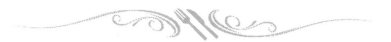

Winter Vegetable Gratin

For 4 servings
- 225g (8oz) red lentils
- 2 leeks, sliced
- 2 carrots, chopped
- 1 parsnip, grated
- 1 small turnip, grated
- 400g (14oz) Passatta
- 1 tbsp chopped fresh parsley
- 1 tsp chopped fresh sage
- 1 tsp chopped fresh thyme
- ½ French mustard
- Salt and pepper
- 100g (4oz) Cheddar cheese, grated.

Preparation
1. Preheat oven. Put lentils, leeks and carrots in a saucepan. Cover with water and bring to boil. Simmer for about 10 mins, until vegetables are tender.
2. Add parsnip and turnip and cook for a further 2-3 mins. Drain.
3. Stir in passatta, herbs, mustard and seasoning. Mix well.
4. Put in an ovenproof dish and top with cheese. Bake for 15-20mins or until cheese is golden and bubbling. Serve immediately.

Nutritional Information		
Calories	Fat	Fibre
1500 total (serves 4) 375 per serving	Low	High
Good source of Vitamin A, D, B6 and calcium		

SALADS

SALADS

Apple and Celery Salad

1 Eating Apple
2 sticks of celery
1 tbsp low fat (light) mayonnaise

Cut apple into small cubes, slice celery into small chunks

Mix apple and celery with mayonnaise and serve.

Cod with Orange Salad

(England)

For 4 servings
- 4 cod cutlets
- Salt and pepper
- 1oz butter
- 1oz white breadcrumbs
- 1oz cheese, grated
- 3 small oranges
- 1 tablespoon oil
- 1 teaspoon lemon juice
- 1 bunch watercress

Preparation time
15 minutes

Cooking time
10 minutes

Preparation
1. Wipe the fish and season well. Dot with half the butter and grill for 5 minutes. Mix breadcrumbs and cheese together. Turn cutlets and cover with cheese mixture, dot with remaining butter and grill for another 5 minutes.
2. Meanwhile, peel oranges, removing all pith. Cut into thin slices and mix with oil and lemon juice.
3. Arrange cutlets on long serving platter. Drain oranges and arrange around the fish. Garnish with watercress.

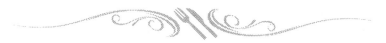

Egg and Prawn Salad

Origin: England

For 4 servings:
- 4 hard-boiled eggs
- 100g (4oz) peeled prawns
- 1 avocado, peeled, stoned and sliced
- ¼ curly endive, washed
- Snipped chives, to garnish (optional)

Dressing:
- 6 tbsp mayonnaise
- 2 tbsp lemon juice
- 1 tsp paprika
- 2 tbsp Greek yoghurt
- Salt and pepper
- 1 tsp tomato ketchup
- 1 clove garlic, crushed (optional)

Preparation:
1. Mix together mayonnaise, lemon juice, paprika and yoghurt, salt and pepper, tomato ketchup and garlic if using.
2. Shell hard-boiled eggs and cut into quarters. Put in a large bowl with the prawns. Add avocado and toss gently.
3. Tear endive into small pieces and arrange on serving plates.
4. Divide prawn mixture between plates and spoon over dressing. Garnish with snipped chives and serve.

Nutritional Information		
Calories	Fat	Fibre
1830 total (serves 4) 457 per serving	Med	Low
Good source of protein		

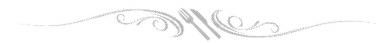

Greek Salad

For 4 servings
- ½ cucumber
- 4 tomatoes
- 1 green pepper
- 1 onion
- 225g (6oz) feta cheese
- 12 black olives

Dressing
- 3 tbsps olive oil
- Salt and pepper to taste
- 1 tbsp white wine vinegar

Timing
Preparation: 15 minutes

Preparation
1. Cut cucumber in 5cm (2in) slicks. Quarter tomatoes, seed and slice green pepper, slice onion. Arrange vegetables in a salad bowl.
2. To make the dressing whisk the oil and seasoning together. Gradually whisk in the vinegar. Pour over the salad and toss gently to cook.
3. Slice or crumble the feta cheese and sprinkle over salad. Garnish with black olives and serve.
4. For a real Greek flavour serve with warm pitta bread. This dish can be served as a side salad with kebabs or a barbeque.

Nutritional Information		
Calories	Fat	Fibre
1188 total (serves 4) 297 per serving	Medium	Low
Good Source of Vitamin C		

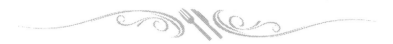

Pasta Salad with Olives

Origin: Italy
Healthy Option
Suitable for vegans

For 6 servings:
- 450g (1lb) short pasta, such as medium shells, farfalle or penne
- 60ml (4tbsp) extra virgin olive oil
- 10 sun-dried tomatoes, thinly sliced
- 30ml (2tbsp) capers, in brine or salted
- 115g/4oz/1cup stoned black olives
- 2 garlic cloves, finely chopped
- 45ml (3tbsp) balsamic vinegar
- 45ml (3tbsp) chopped fresh parsley.
- Salt and ground black pepper.

Preparation
1. Cook the pasta in plenty of boiling salted water until *al dente*. Drain and rinse under cold water to stop the cooking. Drain well and turn into a large bowl. Toss with the olive oil and set aside until required.
2. Soak the tomatoes in a bowl of hot water for 10 minutes. Do not discard the water. Rinse the capers well. If they have been preserved in salt, soak them in a little hot water for 10 minutes. Rinse again.
3. Combine the olives, tomatoes, capers, garlic and vinegar in a small bowl. Season with salt and ground black pepper.
4. Stir the olive mixture into the cooked pasta and toss well. Add 30-45ml/2-3tbsp of the tomato soaking water if the salad seems too dry. Toss with the parsley and allow to stand for 15 minutes before serving.

DESSERTS

DESSERTS

American Apple Cake

For 4 servings:
- 450g (1lb) cooking apples
- 50g (2oz) sultanas
- 125g (5oz) caster sugar
- 1 tbsp lemon juice
- 75g (3oz) butter
- 25g (1oz) dark muscavado sugar
- 1 egg, lightly beaten
- 150g (5oz) self-raising flour
- ½ tsp ground cinnamon.
- 1-2tbsp milk
- whipped double cream, or ice cream to serve (optional).

Timing:
Preparation:
10 mins

Cooking:
50 mins.

Preparation:
1. Preheat oven. Grease a 5cm (2in) deep ovenproof dish. Peel and core apples. Slice and arrange in base. Sprinkle over sultanas, 50g (2oz) caster sugar and lemon juice.
2. Cream together the butter, remaining caster sugar and muscavado sugar until fluffy. Gradually beat in egg.
3. Sift flour and cinnamon together and fold into creamed mixture with sufficient milk to give a dropping consistency. Spread over the apples.
4. Bake for 45-50 mins until sponge is cooked. Test sponge with a skewer and if it comes out clean the cake is ready. Serve warm with cream or ice cream.

Apple Strudel

For 10 servings
- 225g (8oz) strong plain flour
- ½ tsp salt
- 2 tbsp vegetable oil
- 1 egg, lightly beaten
- 5 tbsp lukewarm water
- 700g (1½ lb) cooking apples, peeled, cored and diced.
- 100g (4oz) sultanas
- 50g (2oz) walnuts, chopped
- 40g (1oz) caster sugar
- 2 tsp mixed spice
- 2 tsp grated lemon rind
- 2 tsp cornflour
- 2 tbsp fresh white breadcrumbs
- 40g (1½ oz) butter
- 3 tbsp icing sugar

Timing
Preparation:
40mins plus resting

Cooking:
40 mins

Cooking temperature:
200C/400F/gas 6.

Preparation:
1. Mix flour, salt, oil, egg and sufficient water to make a soft, slightly sticky dough.

2. Work dough until it forms a ball. Knead for 10 mins. Wrap and leave in a warm place for 30 mins.
3. Mix together the apples, sultanas, walnuts, sugar, spice, lemon rind, cornflour and breadcrumbs
4. Preheat oven. On a floured tea towel, roll out pastry into a rectangle 0.3mm (½ in) thick. Melt butter and use to brush over dough.
5. Stretch dough by gently lifting it on backs of hands. Stretch from centre to the edges, keeping a good rectangular shape. Continue until paper thin. Trim edges.
6. Spread apple mix at one end of dough, leaving a 2.5cm (1in) border. Fold side edges over filling. With fruit nearest to you, carefully lift tea towel and roll strudel forwards to form a sausage shape.
7. Put onto baking sheet, seam down and form into a horseshoe. Brush with remaining butter and bake for 35-40 mins. Sprinkle with icing sugar to serve.

Nutritional Information		
Calories	Fat	Fibre
2682 total (serves 10) 268 per serving	Low	Med

Baked Raspberry Roll

For 6 servings
- 225g (8oz) self raising flour
- 1 tsp baking powder
- ½ tsp salt
- 100g (4oz) shredded suet
- 3 tbsp sugar
- 175g (6oz) raspberry jam
- 50g (2oz) chopped walnuts
- ½ tsp ground cinnamon.

Timing:
Preparation:
20mins

Cooking:
30 – 35 mins

Cooking temperature:
200C/400F/gas 6.

Preparation:
1. Preheat oven. Sift together the flour, baking powder and salt. Stir in suet and 1 tbsp sugar. Using a knife, mix in 150ml (¼ pt) of water, to form a dough. Knead until smooth.
2. Roll out into a rectangle 20x30cm (8x12in). Spread with jam to within 2.5cm (1in) of edges. Sprinkle with nuts.
3. Dampen edges with water and roll loosely lengthways. Fold the ends under. Brush top of roll with water.
4. Mix cinnamon with remaining sugar and sprinkle over the roll. Put on a greased baking sheet and bake for 30-35mins.
5. Serve immediately with whipped cream or custard.

Banana Split

For 4 servings:
- 4 bananas
- 250ml (8fl oz) double cream
- 8 scoops vanilla ice cream
- 4 tbsp hazelnuts, roughly chopped

Chocolate sauce:
- 175g (6oz) plain chocolate, broken into pieces
- 40g (1½ oz) butter
- 2 tbsp water

Preparation:
1. To make chocolate sauce, put chocolate and butter in a bowl over a saucepan of hot water and stir until melted. Stir in water.
2. Peel bananas and cut them in half lengthways. Whip cream until it forms soft peaks.
3. Put bananas in four dishes. Add ice cream, pour over sauce and top with whipped cream and hazelnuts. Serve immediately.

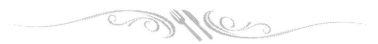

Banoffee Pie

For 6 servings
- 175g (6oz) shortcrust pastry
- 3 bananas
- 1 tbsp lemon juice
- 200g (7oz) sweetened full cream condensed milk
- 50g (2oz) caster sugar
- 50g (2oz) unsalted butter
- 1 tbsp golden syrup

To decorate:
- 150ml (5fl oz) double cream
- 2 bananas

Preparation
1. Preheat oven. Roll out pastry on a floured surface and use to line a 20cm (8in) fluted flan tin.
2. Chill for 30 mins. Prick base, line with grease-proof paper, fill with baking beans and bake blind for 15 mins. Remove paper and beans and cook for a further 5 mins until base is firm and set.
3. Leave to cool.
4. Put condensed milk, sugar, butter and golden syrup in a heavy based saucepan and heat gently until sugar has dissolved.
5. Bring to boil and simmer for 5 mins, stirring all the time, until light brown in colour.
6. Remove from heat and cool slightly. Pour over bananas and allow to cool thoroughly.
7. Slice the remaining bananas and use to decorate the top. Whip cream until it forms soft peaks and pipe around the edge of pie.

Barbecued Fruit Cups

For 4 servings:
- 4 pink grapefruit
- 1 large orange, segmented
- 1 large banana, sliced
- 2 red dessert apples
- 1 tbsp rum (optional)
- 25g (1oz) desiccated coconut
- lemon balm, to decorate.

Timing:
Preparation:
30mins

Marinating:
2hrs

Cooking:
15mins.

Preparation:
1. Cut a thin slice from the base of each grapefruit to allow it to stand upright. Using a sharp knife, cut halfway down each side of the fruits, leaving a 6mm (¼ inch) wide "handle" in the centre.
2. Cut a wedge shaped piece either side of the handle and remove. Peel and segment each of the wedges and reserve.
3. Segment the remaining "bowls" of the grapefruit and reserve. Put segments in a bowl with the orange and banana.
4. Core the apples and cut into chunks. Add to the bowl of fruit, stir in the rum, cover and marinate for 2 hours.
5. Spoon the fruit into the baskets and top with coconut. Wrap in foil and cook over a hot barbeque for 15 mins. Decorate with lemon balm and serve with pouring cream.

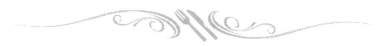

Blackcurrant Meringue Soufflé

For 4-6 servings:
- 350g (12oz) fresh blackcurrants, stalks removed
- 225g (8oz) caster sugar
- 1 tbsp powdered gelatine, dissolved in 3tbsp water.
- 6 eggs, separated
- 300ml (½ pt) double cream, whipped
- 25g (1oz) flaked almonds.

Timing
Preparation:
30mins

Chilling:
2hrs

Cooking:
13mins

Cooking temperature:
230C/450F/gas 8.

Preparation:
1. Put blackcurrants and 50g (2oz) sugar in a saucepan and heat gently until sugar has dissolved and blackcurrants are soft. Puree in a food processor.
2. Whisk together 3 egg yolks and 75g (3oz) sugar until pale and thick. Fold in blackcurrant puree and gelatine. Fold in cream.
3. Whisk 3 egg whites until stiff. Fold into puree mixture. Pour into 1 litre (2pt) soufflé dish, cover and chill until set.
4. Preheat oven. Whisk remaining egg whites until stiff. Whisk in half remaining sugar. Fold in remaining sugar. Spread over blackcurrant mixture.
5. Sprinkle with flaked almonds and bake on top shelf for 3-5 mins, until golden.

Cappuccino Sundae

For 4 servings:
- 350ml (12fl oz) sweetened strong black coffee
- 150ml (5fl oz) double cream
- 1 tbsp caster sugar
- 1 litre (2pt) dairy vanilla ice cream
- 2 tsp cocoa powder
- 1 tbsp whole unbalanced almonds, chopped

Timing:
Preparation:
20 minutes

Preparation:
1. Divide half of coffee between four chilled sundae glasses. Reserve the remaining liquid.
2. Whip cream with sugar until it forms soft peaks. Put in a piping bag fitted with a large star nozzle.
3. Place 2 scoops of ice cream in each sundae glass. Pour over remaining coffee. Pipe cream on top.
4. Sprinkle with cocoa powder. Top with almonds and serve immediately.

Cheesecake

For 10 Servings:
Base
- 175g (6oz) digestive biscuits
- ½ tsp ground cinnamon
- 75g (3oz) unsalted butter.

Filling:
- 450g (1lb) full fat soft cheese
- 75g (3oz) caster sugar
- 2 eggs, separated
- 2 tbsp plain flour
- 1 tsp vanilla essence
- grated rind and juice ½ lemon
- 225g (8oz) red cherry conserve
- 100g (4oz) crème fraiche

Timing
Preparation:
25mins

Cooking:
45-50 mins

Oven temperature
180C/350F/gas 4

Preparation
1. Crush biscuits into fine crumbs. Add cinnamon. Melt butter and add to crumbs, stirring well.
2. Grease a 24cm (9½ in) spring form cake tin. Press biscuit mixture over the base.

3. Mix together soft cheese, sugar, egg yolks, flour, vanilla essence and lemon rind and juice.
4. Whisk the egg whites until stiff then fold into the cheese mixture. Spread over biscuit base.
5. Bake for 45-50 mins until set. Leave to cool and refrigerate.
6. Mix cherry conserve with 3 tbsp water and heat gently to combine. Leave to cool.
7. Spread crème fraiche over cheesecake. Remove from tin. Serve with cherry sauce.

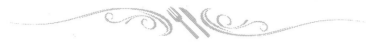

Chilled Chocolate Brûlée

For 4 servings:
- 600ml (1pt) double cream
- 50g (2oz) plain chocolate
- 50g (2oz) white chocolate
- 4 egg yolks
- 5 tbsp muscavado sugar
- grated white chocolate and chocolate curls, to decorate.

Timing:

Preparation:
15mins

Chilling:
2-3 hours

Cooking:
40mins.

Preparation:
1. Pour the cream into a bowl and place over pan of hot water, ensuring the water does not touch base of bowl. Heat gently until the cream reaches scalding point (52C/125F)
2. Melt the plain and white chocolate in separate bowls. Pour half the cream into each, mixing well.
3. Cream the egg yolks with 1 tbsp of the sugar and whisk half into each chocolate mixture.
4. Put bowls over pans of hot water and heat gently until mixture is thick enough to coat back of a wooden spoon. Do not boil.
5. Spoon white mixture into 4 ramekins. Spoon plain mixture on top. Leave to cool. Cover and chill for 2-3 hours.
6. Sprinkle remaining sugar on top of each ramekin and place under a hot grill for 10 mins, until sugar melts. Decorate and serve immediately.

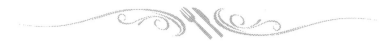

Chocolate Pancakes

For 4 servings
- 90g (3 ½ oz) plain flour
- 15g (½ oz) cocoa powder
- 1 egg, beaten
- 300ml (½ pt) skimmed milk
- 2 tbsp vegetable oil
- 450g (1lb) strawberries
- 8 scoops vanilla ice cream
- 8 tbsp ready made chocolate sauce
- Lemon balm, to decorate (optional).

Preparation
1. Sieve flour and cocoa powder into a bowl. Make a well in centre and gradually whisk in egg and milk, drawing flour in from sides to form a smooth batter. Cover and leave to stand for 30 mins.
2. Heat oil in a 15cm (6in) pan until hot. Tilt pan to coat and pour off excess oil.
3. Pour about a tablespoon of batter into pan, tilting it to cover base. Cook for 2 mins or until underside is cooked. Flip pancake and cook for another 2 mins. Remove and stack between sheets of greaseproof paper. Repeat to make 7 more pancakes.
4. Wash and hull strawberries. Slice thinly. Put strawberries on quarter of each pancake. Fold pancakes over strawberries.
5. Put a couple of scoops of ice cream on top of the pancakes. Spoon chocolate sauce over ice cream. Decorate with lemon balm, if using and serve immediately.

Nutritional Information		
Calories	Fat	Fibre

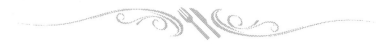

Crème Brûlée

For 4 servings:
- 600ml (1pt) double cream
- 6 egg yolks
- 2 tbsp caster sugar
- 1 tbsp cornflour
- few drops vanilla essence
- 100g (4oz) demerara sugar

Preparation
1. Put cream in a saucepan and bring to boil. Beat together egg yolks, sugar, cornflour and vanilla essence.
2. Gradually pour cream into egg mixture and stir until well blended. Return to pan and bring almost to the boil, stirring constantly, until thickened.
3. Pour into 4 ramekins
4. Sprinkle sugar over top of each custard and put under a pre-heated grill for 5 mins, or until the sugar has melted and caramelised.
5. Leave to cool. Chill for 1 hour before serving.

Crepes Suzettes

For 4 servings:
- 100g (4oz) plain flour
- pinch salt
- 1 egg
- 300ml (½ pt) milk
- vegetable oil, for frying

Sauce
- 50g (2oz) butter
- 25g (1oz) caster sugar
- grated rind and juice of 1 orange
- 3 tbsp orange- flavoured liqueur
- 4 tbsp brandy
- 50g (2oz) almonds, cut into thin slivers

Preparation
1. Sift flour and salt into a bowl. Gradually beat in the egg and milk to form a smooth batter.
2. Heat a little oil in an 18cm (7in) frying pan and pour off excess.
3. Add sufficient batter to thinly coat the base of the pan.
4. Cook for 1-2 mins until underside is golden, turn over and cook second side. Transfer to a plate and keep warm. Repeat with remaining batter to make 8 pancakes.
5. Melt butter for the sauce in a large, heavy frying pan. Add the sugar, orange rind and juice and liqueur and heat until sugar dissolves. Fold each pancake in half then in half again and arrange in sauce in frying pan.
6. Warm brandy, pour over the pancakes and set alight. Serve immediately, garnished with almond slivers.

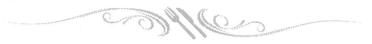

Dutch Pancake Dessert

For 4 servings:
- 225g (8oz) plain flour
- pinch of salt
- 2 eggs
- 600ml (1pt) milk
- vegetable oil
- 225g (8oz) cream cheese
- 150ml (¼ pt) double cream
- 8 tbsp strawberry jam

Preparation
1. Mix together flour and salt in a large bowl. Make a well in the centre and break in eggs. Add half the milk and gradually stir eggs and milk into flour. Beat until smooth.
2. Add remaining milk and beat well.
3. Stand for 30 mins.
4. Coat small frying pan with oil and heat. Pour in just enough batter to cover base and cook over a moderate heat for 1 min. Turn over and cook for a further 30 seconds. Slide onto a plate.
5. Repeat with remaining batter to make 14 pancakes, stacking them as they are made.
6. Mix together cream cheese and cream. Put a pancake on serving plate and spread with a little cream and then jam. Repeat layers, finishing with jam. Serve.

Easter Ice Cream Cake

For 8 servings:
- 225g (8oz) chocolate digestive biscuits, crushed
- 50g (2oz) butter, melted
- 1 litre (2pt) chocolate and nut ice cream
- 500ml (1pt) orange sorbet
- 350g (12oz) chocolate flakes

Timing:
Preparation:
10 mins

Freezing:
3 hrs

Preparation:
1. Add melted butter to crushed biscuits and mix well. Press into the base of a greased 20cm (8in) loose-bottomed cake tin.
2. Allow ice cream and sorbet to soften slightly. Spread half chocolate and nut ice cream over biscuits. Top with half orange sorbet. Repeat layers.
3. Crumble flakes and sprinkle over ice cream cake. Cover and freeze for 3 hours. Remove from cake tin and serve.

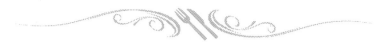

Flambéed Bananas

For 4 servings:
- 150ml (¼ pt) whipping cream
- ¼ tsp vanilla essence
- 1 tbsp caster sugar
- 2 tbsp flaked almonds, toasted
- 100g (4oz) 'no need to soak' dried apricots
- 1 tbsp lemon juice
- 25g (1oz) butter
- 4 bananas
- 4 tbsp rum or brandy

Preparation
1. Whip together the cream, vanilla essence and sugar until it forms soft peaks. Put in a small serving dish, sprinkle with almonds and chill.
2. Put apricots, lemon juice and 150ml (¼ pt) water in a saucepan and cook gently for 10-15 mins, until tender. Puree in a food processor or push through a sieve. Gently heat butter in a frying pan. Peel bananas and cut into half lengthways.
3. Add to pan and brown on both sides.
4. Pour over rum or brandy. Ignite, if wished, then let flames die down. Add apricot puree, stirring well to combine.
5. Serve bananas with sauce poured over and topped with vanilla cream.

Nutritional Information		
Calories	Fat	Fibre
1265 total (serves 4) 314 per serving	Med	High
Good source of Vitamin A, B6		

Fudgy Apple Pudding

For 4 servings:
- 675g (1½ lb) Bramley cooking apples, peeled, cored and chopped.
- 150ml (¼ pt) single cream
- 50g (2oz) cream cheese
- 1 egg
- 50g (2oz) sugar
- 2-3 drops vanilla essence
- rind and juice of 1 lemon
- 2 tbsp cornflour.

Topping:
- 50g (2oz) soft brown sugar
- 50g (2oz) rolled oats
- 1 tsp cinnamon
- 50g (2oz) plain flour
- 50g (2oz) butter.

Timing:
Preparation:
10mins

Cooking:
35-40mins

Cooking temperature:
200C/400F/gas 6

Preparation:
1. Preheat oven. Whisk together cream, cream cheese and egg. Add sugar, vanilla essence, lemon rind and juice and

cornflour. Whisk again until smooth. Add apples and put into a shallow ovenproof dish.

2. Mix together the brown sugar, oats, cinnamon and flour. Rub in the butter until it resembles coarse breadcrumbs. Sprinkle evenly over the apple mixture.

3. Bake for 35-40 mins until apples are soft and the topping crisp. Serve warm with whipped cream.

Hot Chocolate Soufflés

For 4 servings:
- 100g (4oz) cooking chocolate
- 50g (2oz) caster sugar
- 4 eggs, separated
- 2 tbsp coffee liqueur
- icing sugar, to dust
- raspberry sauce, to serve (optional)

To prepare soufflé dishes:
- 25g (1oz) butter
- caster sugar.

Timing:
Preparation:
15mins

Cooking:
15mins

Cooking temperature:
200C/400F/gas 6

Preparation:
1. Gently melt chocolate in a bowl over a pan of simmering water. Meanwhile, prepare soufflé dishes by greasing the sides and bottom with butter and dusting with caster sugar.
2. In a large bowl, beat egg yolks with the sugar until light and fluffy. Add coffee liqueur and melted chocolate and gently stir.
3. Preheat the oven. Whisk egg whites until they form soft peaks. Fold half of the egg white into the chocolate mixture. Fold in remaining egg white.
4. Divide the mixture between the 4 soufflé dishes. Cook for 15mins until just firm. Dust with icing sugar and serve immediately with raspberry sauce, if wished.

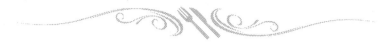

Ice Cream Cake

For 8 servings:
- 225g (8oz) hazelnut cookies, crushed
- 50g (2oz) hazelnuts, chopped
- 100g (4oz) unsalted butter, melted
- 700ml (1 pt) chocolate soft scoop ice cream
- 700ml (1pt) vanilla soft scoop ice cream

Topping
- 100g (4oz) plain chocolate
- 4 tbsp double cream
- flaky chocolate bar, to serve

Preparation
1. Line the base of a 22cm (8in) spring- form cake tin with silicone paper. Mix together biscuits, hazelnuts and butter.
2. Press biscuit mixture over cake tin base.
3. Freeze for 30 mins.
4. Remove ice cream from freezer for 5 mins to soften. Put spoonfuls of each ice cream in a bowl and gently mix together until rippled. Spread over biscuit base and freeze for 2 hours.
5. To make topping, break chocolate into pieces and put into a bowl over a pan of hot water. Heat until melted.
6. Remove from heat and stir in cream.
7. Spread topping over ice cream.
8. Freeze for 2 hours.
9. Crumble chocolate bar and use flakes to decorate cake. Serve.

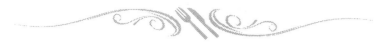

Ice Cream with Orange Sauce

(Origin: England)

For 4 servings
- 200ml (7fl oz) orange juice
- 1 tbsp sugar
- 2 tbsp orange liquer
- 1 egg
- 2 tbsp cornflour
- 150ml (5 fl oz) double cream
- ½ litre (18 fl oz) chocolate ice cream
- Toasted flaked almonds
- 12 strawberries
- Lemon mint leaves to decorate (optional)

Preparation
1. In a non stick pan mix together orange juice, orange liquor, egg, cornflour and double cream. Whisk together over a very gentle heat until thick. Remove from heat and leave to cool.
2. Divide sauce between 4 small serving plates. Put 2 scoops of chocolate ice cream on each plate and sprinkle with toasted almonds.
3. Arrange 3 strawberries on each plate and decorate with lemon mint if using. Serve immediately.

Nutritional Information		
Calories	Fat	Fibre
1015 total (serves 4) 293 per serving	High	Low

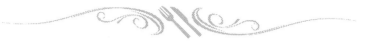

Kiwi Chocolate Cups

For 4 servings
- • 100g (4oz) plain chocolate, broken into pieces
- • 1 ½ kiwi fruit, peeled
- • 1 egg white
- • 25g (1oz) caster sugar
- • 1 tbsp fromage frais
- • 15g (½ oz) toasted almonds, cut into slivers.
- • Mint leaves to decorate (optional)

Timing

Preparation 30mins
Chilling   2hrs.

Preparation
1. Put chocolate in a bowl over a saucepan of simmering water. Stir until melted. Remove from heat and allow to cool slightly.
2. Using a fine brush, paint chocolate onto 4 paper cake cases. Leave to set. Repeat process until chocolate case is quite thick. Leave to set for 2 hours.
3. Finely chop 1 kiwi fruit. Thinly slice remaining half.
4. Whisk egg white until stiff. Add half sugar and whisk until stiff and glossy. Gently fold in remaining sugar. Stir in fromage frais.
5. Add egg white and half the almonds to chopped kiwi fruit.
6. Carefully peel paper cases away from chocolate. Divide kiwi mixture between cases. Sprinkle with remaining almonds and serve, decorated with kiwi slices and mint leaves if using.

Nutritional Information		
Calories	Fat	Fibre
827 total (serves 4) 206 per serving	Med	Low

Knickerbocker Glory

For 4 servings.
- 225g (8oz) frozen raspberries, defrosted
- 2 tbsp icing sugar
- 150ml (¼ pt) double cream
- 1 small can fruit cocktail
- 1 small can stoned red cherries
- 4 scoops vanilla ice cream
- 4 scoops strawberry ice cream
- 4 scoops pineapple ice cream
- 50g (2oz) chopped walnuts
- 4 maraschino cherries

Preparation
1. Put the raspberries and icing sugar in a food processor or blender and puree. Pass through a sieve to remove pips.
2. Whip cream until it forms soft peaks.
3. Place a spoonful of fruit cocktail in the bottom of each glass.
4. Top with vanilla ice cream, cherries, then the raspberry puree.
5. Continue the layers with fruit and remaining ice creams and purée.
6. Top each sundae with whipped cream, chopped nuts and a maraschino cherry.

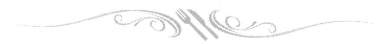

Layered Fruit Salad

For 6-8 servings
- 225 (8oz) black grapes
- 2 bananas
- 5 peaches
- 225g (8oz) raspberries
- 3 oranges
- 3 kiwi fruit
- 200ml (7fl oz) orange juice
- 2 tbsp orange liquor

Preparation
1. Slice bananas and peaches. Peel and slice kiwi fruit. Halve grapes and remove seeds.
2. Arrange grapes in a large glass serving dish. Add bananas, peaches, and raspberries in separate layers.
3. Peel oranges, cut into segments in half and arrange in the serving dish. Arrange kiwi fruit on top.
4. Mix together the orange juice and liquor. Spoon over fruit and serve.

Timing

Preparation   35 minutes.

Children will love this fresh fruit salad without the orange liquor.

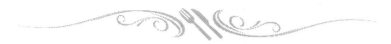

Lemon and Lime Syllabub

(Origin: England)

For 4 servings
- 150ml (½ pt) dry white wine.
- 75g (3oz) caster sugar
- Grated rind and juice of 1 lime
- Grated rind and juice of 1 lemon
- 300ml (½ pt) double cream
- Rind of ½ lemon, to decorate

Preparation
1. Mix together wine, sugar and lime and lemon rind and juice. Cover and leave to infuse for 3 hours.
2. Add cream to wine infusion and whisk until mixture holds its shape.
3. Spoon mixture into individual serving glasses or dishes. Chill for at least 2 hours.
4. Decorate syllabub with lemon rind and serve with sweet dessert biscuits.

Timing

Preparation   20mins
Chilling   5 hours

Nutritional Information		
Calories	Fat	Fibre
1711 total (serves 4) 428 per serving	Med	Low

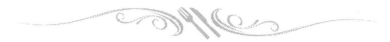

Lemon Clouds

For 4 servings:
- 5 egg yolks
- 450ml (¾ pt) milk
- 50g (2oz) caster sugar
- 1 tbsp cornflour
- ½ tsp vanilla essence
- 2 tbsp lemon juice
- grated rind of 1 lemon
- 4 tbsp fromaige frais
- pared rind of 1 lemon, to decorate (optional)

Meringues:
- 1 egg white
- 2 tbsp caster sugar

Preparation
1. Put egg yolks, milk, caster sugar and cornflour in a saucepan and heat gently, stirring constantly until custard has thickened. Remove from heat.
2. Stir in the vanilla essence and lemon juice and rind. Leave to cool. Stir in fromage frais until well blended. Spoon into four serving dishes and chill.
3. To make meringues, whisk egg white until stiff. Whisk in caster sugar until stiff.
4. Put some cold water in a large frying pan and heat until gently simmering. Using a tablespoon, shape meringue into four oval shapes and spoon into water. Poach for about 5 mins, turning once, until set.
5. Remove meringues with a slotted spoon, drain on absorbent paper and carefully put on top of lemon mixture.

Nutritional Information		
Calories	Fat	Fibre
1041 total (serves 4) 260 per serving	Med	Low

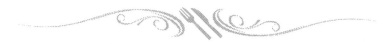

Lemon Cream Dessert

For 4 servings:
- 2 eggs, separated
- 75g (3oz) caster sugar
- 200ml (7fl oz) milk
- 1 tbsp gelatine
- juice 3 lemons
- finely grated rind 1 lemon
- 200ml (7fl oz) double cream
- sugared lemon slices, to decorate

Preparation
1. Beat together egg yolks and sugar until thick and creamy. Heat milk in a pan until almost boiling then pour onto egg mixture, stirring well.
2. Return to pan and heat gently, stirring, until slightly thickened.
3. Do not boil. Strain into a bowl and cool.
4. In a small bowl, sprinkle gelatine into lemon juice. Put over a pan of hot water and heat until dissolved. Stir into custard mixture.
5. Add lemon rind and chill until it begins to thicken.
6. Whip cream until it forms soft peaks and fold in. Whisk egg whites until stiff and fold in. Divide between four individual bowls and chill for 2-3 hours until set.
7. Decorate with lemon slices and serve.

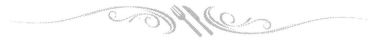

Lemon Ice Cream with Chocolate

For 8 servings
- 2 eggs, separated
- 75g (3oz) caster sugar
- ½ tsp vanilla essence
- Grated rind and juice of 1 lemon
- 200ml (7fl oz) Greek yoghurt
- 200ml (7fl oz) whipping cream
- 150g (5oz) dark cooking chocolate
- Crystallized flowers and silver balls, to decorate (optional)

Timing

Preparation   25 mins
Freezing   4 hours

Preparation
1. Whisk egg yolks with caster sugar and vanilla essence until pale and thick. Beat in lemon rind and juice and yoghurt.
2. Whip cream until it forms soft peaks. Whisk egg whites until stiff. Fold egg whites and cream into lemon mixture.
3. Spoon mixture into a container suitable for freezing and freeze for at least 4 hours.
4. Break chocolate into chunks. Put in a bowl over a pan of simmering water and heat until melted. Allow to cool slightly.
5. Remove ice cream from freezer and turn out onto a serving plate. Pour over chocolate, decorate as wished and serve.

Nutritional Information		
Calories	Fat	Fibre
2400 total (serves 4) 300 per serving	High	Low

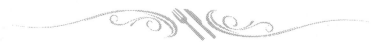

Parisian Apple Flan

For 6-8 servings:
- 225g (8oz) plain flour
- pinch of salt
- 2 tbsp caster sugar
- 100g (4oz) butter
- 1 egg yolk
- 3-4 tbsp water
- 450g (1lb) dessert apples, peeled, cored and sliced
- 3 tbsp apricot jam, sieved
- 1 tbsp Calvados OR water
- 2 tbsp granulated sugar

Timing:
Preparation:
20mins

Chilling:
30mins

Cooking:
20-25mins

Cooking temperature:
200C/400F/gas 6.

Preparation
1. Sift flour and salt into a bowl. Stir in caster sugar. Rub in butter until mixture resembles fine breadcrumbs. Stir in egg yolk and water until mixture forms a soft dough. Knead lightly, cover in cling film and chill for 30 mins.

2. Preheat oven. Line a baking tray with greaseproof paper. Roll out pastry on a lightly floured surface and trim to a circle 30cm (12in) in diameter. Put on baking tray and prick with a fork.
3. Arrange apple slices on pastry, leaving a 2.5cm (1in) border.
4. Put apricot jam and Calvados or water in a pan and heat until melted. Remove from heat and brush onto apples. Sprinkle with granulated sugar.
5. Bake for 20-25 mins until apples are golden and tender. Serve warm, topped with whipped cream.

Peach Melba

For 4 servings:
- 4 ripe peaches
- 50g (2oz) granulated sugar
- 300ml (½ pt) water
- 225g (8oz) raspberries
- 2-3 tbsp icing sugar
- 25g (1oz) butter
- 50g (2oz) split almonds
- 4 scoops vanilla ice cream

Preparation
1. Halve and stone peaches. Put sugar and water in a saucepan. Bring to boil and simmer for 5 mins.
2. Add peaches and poach for 10 mins or until tender. Remove from syrup and leave to cool.
3. Put raspberries and icing sugar in a food processor and purée until smooth. Sieve to remove raspberry seeds. Chill.
4. Melt butter in a frying pan, add almonds and fry gently until lightly browned.
5. Peel peaches.
6. Arrange in four serving dishes and add a scoop of vanilla ice cream to each.
7. Pour over raspberry sauce, sprinkle with almonds and serve.

Profiteroles

For 6 servings:
- 75g (3oz) margarine or butter
- 200ml (7fl oz) cold water
- 100g (4oz) plain flour
- 3 eggs, lightly beaten
- 300ml (10fl oz) double cream

Sauce:
- 50g (2oz) caster sugar
- 175g (6oz) plain chocolate
- 300ml (½ pint) cold water
- 1 tsp butter

Preparation
1. Preheat oven. Put butter or margarine in saucepan with water and bring to boil.
2. Remove from heat and immediately tip in all of flour. Beat thoroughly with wooden spoon until smooth.
3. Gradually beat in eggs. Cover 3 baking trays with baking parchment. With medium nozzle, pipe walnut sized balls on to trays.
4. Bake for 25-30 mins until crisp.
5. Make slit in side of each profiterole to release steam. Leave to cool on wire rack.
6. To make sauce, put sugar, chocolate and water in a saucepan. Heat gently, stirring occasion- ally, until dissolved.
7. Bring to boil and simmer for 10-15 mins, stirring occasionally, until a thick pouring consistency.
8. Stir in butter, remove from heat and leave to cool.
9. Whip cream until stiff and fill profiteroles.
10. Arrange on serving dish, pour over a little sauce and serve remaining sauce separately.

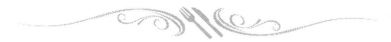

Raspberry Fool

(Origin England)

For 4 servings:
- 200g (7oz) raspberries
- 40g (1oz) icing sugar
- 2 tbsp cherry brandy
- 3 tsp powdered gelatine
- 125ml (4fl oz) double cream
- 2 egg whites.

Preparation
1. Reserve 4 raspberries for decoration and put remainder in a food processor. Add icing sugar and blend to a puree. Sieve to remove seeds.
2. Mix cherry brandy with 1tbsp cold water. Sprinkle gelatine on top. Put bowl over pan of hot water and stir until gelatine dissolves. Stir into puree.
3. Whisk cream until it forms soft peaks. Fold into puree. Chill for 5-10 minutes until mixture thickens.
4. Whisk egg whites until stiff and fold into puree.
5. Spoon mixture into individual dishes. Chill for about 1 hr until set. Decorate and serve.

Timing

Preparation   15mins
Chilling   65-70mins

Nutritional Information		
Calories	Fat	Fibre
788 total (serves 4) 197 per serving	Med	Med
Good source of Vitamin C		

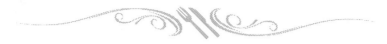

Strawberries Romanoff

For 4 servings:
- 450g (1lb) strawberries
- grated rind of 1 orange
- juice of 2 oranges
- 75-100ml (3-4fl oz) curacao
- 200ml (7fl oz) double cream
- 1 tbsp vanilla sugar
- orange rind and lemon balm, to decorate (optional).

Timing:
Preparation:
15mins

Chilling:
1-2 hours.

Preparation:
1. Hull the strawberries and put into a bowl. Mix together orange rind and juice.
2. Pour orange rind and juice and curacao over the strawberries. Toss lightly and chill for 1-2 hours.
3. Whip cream and sugar until thick. Decorate strawberries with strips of orange rind and lemon balm, if wished, and serve with vanilla cream.

Strawberry And Banana Smoothie

Ingredients
- 2 punnets of fresh strawberries
- 2 large bananas
- 1 medium glass of pure orange juice
- 1 tub of Low fat Onken yoghurt
- Other fruits can be used including:
- Raspberries
- Mango
- Blueberries
- Melon
- Passion Fruit
- Kiwi Fruit
- Nectarines
- Pears
- Blackberries
- Or frozen fruit can be used.

Method.
Chop fruit into small pieces, add orange juice and yoghurt, and blend in a liquidiser until smooth. Serve in a tall glass and drink through a straw.

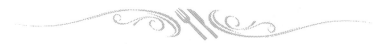

Strawberry Shortcake

For 8 servings:
- 225g (8oz) plain flour
- 3 tbsp baking powder
- ½ tbsp salt
- 50g (2oz) caster sugar
- 50g (2oz) butter or margarine
- 1 egg
- 75ml (3fl oz) milk

Filling
- 350g (12oz) strawberries, hulled and sliced
- 2 tbsp caster sugar
- 150ml (¼ pt) whipping cream

Preparation
1. Preheat oven. Sift flour, baking powder and salt into a bowl. Stir in sugar and rub in fat until mixture resembles fine breadcrumbs.
2. Make a well in centre. Add egg and sufficient milk to form soft dough. Knead lightly, then form into 8 balls. Flatten to make small shortcakes.
3. Put on a baking tray and brake for 10-15 mins until risen and brown. Transfer to a wire rack to cool.
4. Whip together cream and sugar until mixture forms soft peaks. Halve shortcakes. Sandwich together with cream and strawberries. Serve

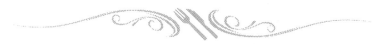

Summer Fruit Flan

For 8 servings
- 3 eggs
- 75g (3oz) caster sugar
- 50g (2oz) plain flour
- 40g (1½ oz) butter, melted
- 25g (1oz) ground almonds
- 3 tbsp almond liqueur, optional
- 12 strawberries, halved
- 75g (3oz) blueberries
- 100g (4oz) seedless green grapes, halved
- 200g (7oz) can mandarin oranges
- 3 tbsp apricot jam.

Timing:

Preparation: 45mins
Cooking   40mins

Cooking temperature
180C/350F/gas 4

Preparation
1. Preheat oven. Grease a 23cm (9in) round cake tin and line the base.
2. Put eggs and sugar in a bowl over a pan of hot water and whisk until creamy. Remove from heat and beat until cool.
3. Using a metal spoon, gently fold the flour into the egg mixture. Fold in the melted butter and ground almonds. Pour into the prepared tin and bake for 30-35 mins until risen and beginning to shrink from the sides of the tin.

4. Turn out and leave to cool. Sprinkle with almond liqueur, if using.

5. Arrange fruit on top of the sponge, placing the strawberries and the blueberries in the centre and the grapes and mandarins around the edge.

6. Put the jam and 2 tbsp cold water in a saucepan. Heat gently, stirring, until it boils. Simmer for 1 minute. Sieve and brush over fruit. Allow jam to cool and set before serving.

Nutritional Information		
Calories	Fat	Fibre
1700 total (serves 6) 213 per serving	Low	Low

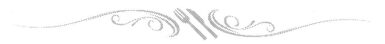

Tipsy Orange Soufflé

For 4 servings
- 50g (2oz) caster sugar
- 4 eggs, separated
- 4 tbsp plain flour
- 2 tsp arrowroot
- 300ml (½ pt) milk
- 25g (1oz) butter
- 2 tsp grated orange rind
- 4 tbsp orange liqueur
- icing sugar, to serve.

Timing
Preparation:
15mins

Cooking:
45mins

Cooking temperature
180C/350F/gas 4

Preparation:
1. Preheat oven. Grease a 1.4litre (2½ pt) soufflé dish
2. In a saucepan, mix together sugar, 1 egg yolk, flour, arrowroot and 3 tbsp milk.
3. Pour on remaining milk and mix until smooth. Bring to boil, stirring continuously. Simmer for 2 mins.
4. Remove from heat and beat in butter, remaining egg yolks orange rind and orange liqueur.
5. Whisk egg whites until stiff and gently fold into sauce. Pour into soufflé dish and bake for 40 mins until well risen, firm to touch and pale golden.
6. Quickly dust with icing sugar and serve.

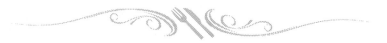

Winter Fruit Salad

For 4 servings:
- 100g (4oz) dried apricots
- 50g (2oz) dried pears
- 50g (2oz) prunes
- 200ml (7fl oz) orange juice
- 2 tbsp dark rum
- 2 green apples
- 50g (2oz) toasted flaked almonds
- Greek yoghurt, to serve

Preparation
1. Cut dried fruits in half and put in a large bowl.
2. Add orange juice and rum. Cover and leave to soak for 2 days.
3. Just before serving, roughly chop apples and mix with dried fruits.
4. Transfer to serving dish, sprinkle with toasted almonds and serve with Greek yoghurt.

Nutritional Information		
Calories	Fat	Fibre
643 total (serves 4) 160 per serving	Low	High

Apple and Celery Salad

1 Eating Apple
2 sticks of celery
1 tbsp low fat (light) mayonnaise

Cut apple into small cubes, slice celery into small chunks

Mix apple and celery with mayonnaise and serve.

REFERENCES

Sources of Information:

Department of Human Nutrition and Dietetics, Glasgow Caledonian University, Glasgow, Scotland

Department of Health and Social Care, Southern Regional College, Armagh, Northern Ireland

Department of Health and Social Care, The Open University, Milton Keynes

1983 "The Composition of Foods" McCance & Williamson

2000 "The Optimum Nutrition Bible", Patrick Holford Ch13,18,27,31,33 and 42

1987 "Nutritional Medicine" Dr Stephen Davies and Dr Alan Stewart

Part 1 p10-21 and Part 3 p227-230

1999 "Journal of American College of Nutrition"

2000 "A Case for Vitamin C" © Welder Publications. Townsend et al 1998

White paper: Saving Lives: Our Healthier Nation (DOH 1999)

White paper: Faculty of Health Promotion (DOH 1992. WHO 1978)

Dennis et al 1982, Downie et al 1990, Henesey 1998, McKee 1994, Townsend et al 1998, Blaxter 1990, Carragher and MacNab 1996, Dreyer and White, Health 1997

"Ministry of Agriculture, Fisheries and Food: The Manual of Nutrition 10th Edition" London HMSO 1995

Bender E. and Bender D.A. "Food Tables" Oxford University Press 1986

Department of Health "Dietary Reference Values – A Guide" London HMSO 1991

Gregory S., Foster K., Tyler H., Wiseman M. "The Dietary and Nutritional Survey of British Adults" HMSO 1990

1998 "Health Promotion: Foundations for Practice" Jennie Naidoo and Jane Willis Ch4 P63-77

2000 "Promoting Health, Knowledge and Practice" Edited by Jeanne Katz, Alyson Perberdy and Jenny Douglas.
Second Edition Ch1 P3-5, Ch4 P69, Ch7 P109, Ch10 P171

2002 "Working for Health," edited by Tom Heller, Rosemary Muston, Moyra Siddell and Cathy Lloyd

2004 "Debates and Dilemmas in Promoting Health a Reader," edited by Moyra Siddell, Linda Jones, Jeanne Katz and Alyson Perberdy

2002 "The Challenge of Promoting Health Exploration and Action" edited by Jones, Moyra Siddell and Jenny Douglas, Second Edition
Second Edition Ch8 P161, Ch11 P229

2004 "Promoting Health Knowledge and Practice", edited by Jeanne Katz, Alyson Deberdy and Jenny Douglas

------ "Holy Bible" – English Standard Version

1999 "Health Promotion Models and Values Second Edition", R.S. Downie, Carol Tannahill, Andrew Tannahill

1984 "Health and Disease – A Reader", edited by Nick Black, David Boswell, Alastair Gray, Seán Murphy & Jennie Popay

1994 "Health Promotion Foundations for Practice", Jennie Naidoo and Jane Wills Ch6 P109, Ch10 P188

1982 "Professor McArdle – City University of New York - Fundamentals of General, Organic and Biological Chemistry", John R. Holum.

Sources of Information:

1991   "Simply Delicious Readers Digest Recipe File"
1983   "Hamlyn All Colour Cook Book"
1992   "Pasta Flip Books for Cooks", edited by Gabrielle Rossi
1981   "Family Meals", Elizabeth Seldon

1996   "Pasta & Pizza Presto", Maxine Clarke and Shirley Gill

1983   "Human Nutrition and Dietetics (Seventh Edition)", Sir Stanley Davidson, R. Passmore, J.F. Brock, A.S. Truswell

1985   "Family Medical Encyclopaedia – An Illustrated Guide"
        "Men and Women of Science – The World Book Encyclopaedia of Science"

Printed in the United States
By Bookmasters